Emotionally Disturbed

Emotionally Disturbed

A History of Caring for America's Troubled Children

DEBORAH BLYTHE DOROSHOW

The University of Chicago Press
Chicago and London

The University of Chicago Press, Chicago 60637
The University of Chicago Press, Ltd., London

Published 2019
Printed in the United States of America

28 27 26 25 24 23 22 21 20 19   1 2 3 4 5

ISBN-13: 978-0-226-62143-2 (cloth)
ISBN-13: 978-0-226-62157-9 (e-book)
DOI: https://doi.org/10.7208/chicago/9780226621579.001.0001

Library of Congress Cataloging-in-Publication Data

Names: Doroshow, Deborah Blythe, author.
Title: Emotionally disturbed : a history of caring for America's troubled children / Deborah Blythe Doroshow.
Description: Chicago ; London : The University of Chicago Press, 2019. | Includes bibliographical references and index.
Identifiers: LCCN 2018042377 | ISBN 9780226621432 (cloth : alk. paper) | ISBN 9780226621579 (ebook)
Subjects: LCSH: Child psychopathology—United States. | Children—Institutional care—United States
Classification: LCC RJ501.A2 D676 2019 | DDC 362.20830973—dc23
LC record available at https://lccn.loc.gov/2018042377

♾ This paper meets the requirements of ANSI/NISO Z39.48-1992 (Permanence of Paper).

In memory of Louise Lorden, who taught me to play with feeling and never worried about a few wrong notes

CONTENTS

ILLUSTRATIONS

Introduction

In 1934, Marty arrived at the Children's Ward of Bellevue Hospital's psychiatric division. The six-year-old had been referred there because of his increasingly strange behavior, which had started two years earlier. As his doctor, child psychiatrist Lauretta Bender, later described, Marty "seemed to live in his own fantasy world."[1] He refused to keep his clothes on and wouldn't eat unless he was spoon-fed. He didn't talk much, and when he did, it was nonsensical. As he explained, "The blood is coming from the red eyes of a fish."[2] Most concerning of all was his disinterest in other children. He preferred to keep to himself.[3]

Marty stayed at Bellevue for six months of observation and treatment. Every day was predictable: breakfast at eight, school at nine, lunch with the psychiatric residents and nurses' aides at noon, and so on. At 9 PM came bedtime with toothbrushing, washing up, and some time to watch television or listen to a story read out loud.[4] What Marty and the other children might not have realized was that this routine was part of their treatment.[5] Daily activities—school, music therapy, art therapy, and even puppet therapy—were meant to allow the staff to observe and diagnose the children and to give the children opportunities to express themselves and learn to play cooperatively with other children.[6] Marty also received individual psychotherapy every week.[7] And because staff members felt he needed to develop what Dr. Bender called "the normal aggressive tendency of the 6 year old," he was given a cowboy outfit and toy gun.[8]

Before the 1940s, most children like Marty would have had few options. They might have been placed in a state mental hospital or asylum, an institution for the so-called feebleminded, a training school for delinquent children, or perhaps kept at home quietly.[9] Bellevue's unit, one of the first of its kind, was founded in 1920 and had few counterparts during its first decade of operation.[10] But starting in the 1930s and 1940s, more specialized institutions began to open all over the country with the goal of treating these children. The centers were not affiliated with any one academic or charitable organization, and on a superficial level, they had little in common. Some, like the Langley Porter Clinic at the University of California, San Francisco, were part of university teaching hospitals. Others, like the Hawthorne Cedar Knolls School in Westchester, New York, were run by charitable agencies. Several were part of state mental hospital systems, like the Arthur Brisbane Treatment Center in Allaire, New Jersey. Residential treatment centers (RTCs), as staff members and child mental hygiene professionals called them, ranged from large urban institutions like Bellevue to the tiny Child Guidance Center of Cincinnati, which could only care for a maximum of twelve children at any one time.[11]

What they shared, though, was a commitment to helping children like Marty who couldn't be managed anywhere else. The staff who worked at RTCs adopted a similar integrated approach to treatment, employing talk therapy, schooling, and other activities in the context of a therapeutic environment. That environment, which they called the therapeutic milieu (or the milieu, for short), would be their legacy long after residential treatment had gone out of vogue. RTC professionals shared the goal of helping these children become productive members of society. They positioned their institutions as active sites of observation, diagnosis, and treatment, taking great pains to emphasize that their institutions were an enlightened alternative to asylums, state institutions for the feebleminded, or training schools for delinquent youth, which they (sometimes simplistically) characterized as custodial warehouses for society's castoffs. This particular narrative took on added significance as RTCs rose to prominence just as deinsitutionalization was taking hold in adult psychiatry.

Emotionally Disturbed considers the history of troubled children in twentieth-century America by examining a set of spaces and the people who inhabited them. These young boys and girls did not quite fit in the existing landscape of children's care. In the late nineteenth and early twentieth centuries, so-called juvenile delinquents were adjudicated in newly established juvenile courts, where they might be sent to reform schools or counseled by the judge.[12] Starting in the 1910s, children who were perceived as predelinquents or even just deemed troublesome were taken by their mothers to child guidance clinics, where they received psychological testing and individual counseling.[13] Meanwhile, intellectually disabled children were sequestered in large custodial institutions for the feebleminded, which were overflowing with children as fewer and fewer were returned to the community.[14] The children at RTCs lay somewhere in between.

In the early twentieth century, the mental hygiene movement represented the preventive core of American psychiatry. Mental hygiene efforts, though aimed at improving the mental health of all Americans, were especially directed toward children, who were simultaneously the most vulnerable and most promising. Young truants and thieves were labeled juvenile delinquents and taken to new juvenile courts or disciplined on the street by policemen. Delinquency was considered a primordial form of mental illness, and the law a form of preventive treatment.[15] By the 1920s, child guidance clinics became the primary loci for child mental hygiene. There, teams of child psychiatrists, psychologists, and social workers sought to diagnose and treat "predelinquent" or troublesome children.[16] But some children were too troubled to be treated in this outpatient setting. As child mental hygiene professionals realized the limitations of child guidance clinics, they began to transform existing institutions for neglected children into RTCs specifically engineered to help children whose behavior was so perplexing that outpatient treatment was no longer a possibility. While child guidance provided an important professional and intellectual model for residential treatment, RTC professionals—a term I use to describe the psychiatrists, psychologists, nurses, and social workers who worked at and ran RTCs—were forced to seek out novel therapeutic approaches and professional structures to treat this newly identified, seriously troubled group of children.

Emotionally Disturbed explores children's experiences of residential treatment by analyzing mediated evidence like transcribed comments, analyzed artwork, and reports of children's actions. In the process, I explore how it felt to leave home for an RTC, to undergo individual therapy for troubles that one might acknowledge or deny experiencing, and to live among other troubled children in a structured, planned environment. For some children, being separated from their parents was a godsend, a respite from a painful home environment. For others, it was just another place that adults put them when they misbehaved. Some children embraced the therapeutic milieu, forming tight bonds with staff members and other children, while others were physically and emotionally aggressive to everyone around them and rejected the entire premise of residential treatment. At RTCs, children and adults negotiated for power in an environment where traditional authority structures operated with a great deal of leeway. This environment, RTC professionals believed, gave children the opportunity to develop their own voices while learning how to submit their own preferences to those of a group's in order to function successfully in social environments.

This is the story of how a certain kind of person came to be. As RTCs emerged as new spaces with a fresh therapeutic perspective, RTC professionals identified a new kind of person: the emotionally disturbed child. In this sense, the creation of spaces and the creation of new types of people were codependent; the identification of a population of emotionally disturbed children was necessary for the creation of RTCs, and the development of RTCs was critical to the understanding of who the disturbed child was and how he or she might best be helped. Of course, these children didn't emerge out of thin air. But as philosopher of science Ian Hacking has suggested, the confluence of a variety of social and cultural factors at discrete moments in time gives rise to fertile environments for certain "kinds" of people.[17] Children like Marty existed before the Bellevue ward was built. But RTCs and the people who worked there built physical and conceptual structures that identified a population of children who were alike in distinctive ways.

This new type of child and the novel institutions needed to treat her attracted public attention far beyond the walls of RTCs, which were small and few in number. In fact, RTCs were featured on television, in the popular media, and on the radio. Many were funded by community chests and local philanthropies, demonstrating a remarkable public investment in the disturbed child. This engagement was a reflection of larger American concerns about mental hygiene, normalcy, and about juvenile delinquency in particular. Emotional disturbance became a diagnosis, a policy problem, and a statement about the troubled state of postwar American society, all at the same time.

Emotionally Disturbed is a story about Americans trying to achieve normality after World War II. For them, normality was an almost unattainable ideal fueled by experts who told them in movies, magazines, and books that they should strive in every way to be "perfectly average."[18] At RTCs, treating emotional troubles and building normal children were inextricably intertwined. Although scholars have demonstrated that the reality of family life and its members' ability to enact traditional gender roles were far from perfect and that our vision of "the good old days" is mostly nostalgic, they have also demonstrated the immense cultural pressure individuals felt to strive for normality, even though the personal cost of these efforts was often great.[19]

As staff members attempted to understand and treat these decidedly abnormal children, they simultaneously wrestled with the question of what made a child normal. "Normal" was to be both the yardstick against which emotional disturbance was measured and the goal of successful treatment, and RTC professionals worked to categorize the ways in which a child might deviate from this ideal. In their eyes, normal meant moderate. The normal child was neither too quiet nor too overbearing, neither too obedient nor too unruly; he or she represented a delicate balance between conformity and individuality. The normal child also came from a normal family. This family was not broken, as were many of those from which RTC patients came, but was led by two parents occupying traditionally imagined gender roles.

Although normality remained a distant, even unreachable, goal for most children in residential treatment, RTC professionals grounded their therapeutic approach within this ideal. Centers were to resemble white, middle-class homes and organize children in family-like groups with adults playing the roles of parents. Individual talk therapy and art and music therapies fostered a child's creativity and self-expression, while group activities and community interactions demanded conformity to basic social expectations. After discharge, a successfully treated child would ideally return to his or her family, school, and community to become a productive citizen. In this way, the story of emotional disturbance and residential treatment is also a story about the pressure to belong in mid-twentieth-century America and efforts to restore broken children to full citizenship.

The process of treating emotionally disturbed children was an experimental one, subject to great successes, abysmal failures, and negotiation about how best to approach a difficult patient population. The individuals who took on the challenge of residential treatment in the 1940s, 1950s, and 1960s perceived themselves as pioneers in the untamed wilderness of child mental health. With little historical tradition to build on, they worked together to provide a multifaceted treatment program for a group of children formerly considered by their families and communities to be intractably damaged.

Structurally, *Emotionally Disturbed* consists of several chapters of thick description, bookended by chapters that focus more on change over time. I first explain how RTCs came to exist amid a broad landscape of institutional and community-based therapeutic options for children considered abnormal. The bulk of the book then explores the elements of a child's stay, in which he or she was admitted, became familiar with the physical environment, met the staff members and the other children who worked and lived there, and experienced the different modes of treatment. Finally, the book concludes with the child's discharge from the RTC, an evaluation of efficacy, and the gradual dissolution of RTCs as a sustainable answer to a perceived crisis in child mental health. In addition to representing a "golden age" of residential treatment, the central chapters are purposefully bookended by chapters that explore the creation and disintegration of emotional disturbance as a meaningful organizational category. These chapters focus on change over time during the 1930s–40s and the 1970s onward, while the bulk of the book (chaps. 2–6) is chronologically fixed, covering approximately 1945–65. This twenty-year period represents a time of relative therapeutic constancy in which little substantial change occurred in how residential treatment was conceptualized and delivered in the United States. Elsewhere, I have argued for increased attention to the often-slow pace of clinical change; in *Emotionally Disturbed*, I argue that in the 1940s, 1950s, and early 1960s continuity largely characterized the history of residential treatment.[20] Ultimately, the structure of *Emotionally Disturbed* shows the reader why the emergence and closure of RTCs and the creation and fragmentation of emotional disturbance were concurrent developments.

Chapter 1 traces the emergence of RTCs in the 1930s and 1940s. Overlapping developments in child welfare—the codification of mothers' pensions as Aid to Families with Dependent Children in the 1935 Social Security Act, the development of child psychoanalysis, and the emergence of mental hygiene and the related juvenile justice and child guidance movements—led to the recognition of a population of children too troubled to be treated by any existing agencies or institutions. A confluence of local factors led to the transformation of existing individual institutions into RTCs, inspiring origin stories that emphasized RTCs' dissimilarity from existing custodial institutions for children and their pioneering approach to emotional disturbance. These two elements were central to the professional identities of the people who worked there. Chapter 2 shows how this pioneering attitude made staff members more willing to experiment in what was essentially a brand-new venture and abandon the strict division of professional roles they had learned in graduate school. Chapter 3 explores how RTC professionals described, categorized, and made visible a new population of emotionally disturbed children, whom they identified primarily by the presence of strange or disruptive behavior that the adults around them had given up trying to live with or fix. In their view, emotional disturbance—whether manifested by aggressive and acting-out behavior or by withdrawn and anxious behavior—was rooted in pathological family relationships.

This definition of emotional disturbance guided the therapeutic rationales of most RTCs, which called for the temporary separation of a child from her pathological home environment accompanied by simultaneous outpatient work with her parents with the aim of healing the entire family. Consistent with this reasoning, residential treatment consisted of three main components: individual therapy, casework with parents, and the therapeutic milieu. Chapter 4 focuses on the first two. Individual therapy was a protected space where children and adults could interact in nontraditional ways to express themselves, learn about one other, and gain self-knowledge. Casework with parents, a modified form of individual therapy, was intended to provide an opportunity to repair so-called "broken" parenting styles and address parents' own emotional troubles.

Chapters 5 and 6 examine the therapeutic milieu, arguably the most original therapeutic aspect of residential treatment. At RTCs, staff strove to create an environment that was in itself therapeutic. It was to be warm, welcoming, and permissive, a noninstitutional institution differentiating RTCs from punitive, custodial institutions for children, such as training schools. Most importantly, the milieu would foster normality. RTC professionals engineered the physical environments of their facilities to resemble typical, white, middle-class American homes so that the children living there would have corrective experiences to erase the effects of their pathological ones at home. In this milieu, every activity and interaction was theoretically imbued with therapeutic potential, aimed at shaping normal children who represented moderation: a balance between creativity and conformity, between self-expression and subjugation to the will of the group, and between energetic participation and quiet time alone. There, RTC staff members enacted and promulgated their complex vision of normal childhood in mid-twentieth-century America.

By the late 1960s and early 1970s, the stability of emotional disturbance as an organizing concept was in jeopardy. In chapter 7, I discuss how RTCs found themselves on shaky ground in the face of increased costs, reduced funding, growing anti-institutional sentiment, and the community mental health movement. Faced with these realities, RTCs were forced to become multiservice organizations offering a spectrum of services from residential treatment to more community-oriented options like day hospitals and group homes in order to stay afloat. In the context of a perceived crisis in child mental health, even these efforts were not enough to make residential treatment a viable solution for the hundreds of thousands of children newly identified as needing treatment. Meanwhile, special education legislation, increased attention to autism, and a broken juvenile justice system contributed to the breakdown of emotional disturbance as a category by fragmenting disturbed children symbolically and physically. By the late 1970s, residential treatment as an optimistic, progressive treatment option for the emotionally disturbed child was relegated to the margins of mental health care. In its place were thousands of children in need of treatment and a maze of disjointed agencies and professionals with no organized way of helping them.

By the 1980s and 1990s, a child like Marty might not have made it to an RTC. Instead, he probably would have been admitted to a psychiatric ward for a one- or two-week stay, followed by weekly outpatient therapy with medication, as long as his parents had ample insurance. Other children with fewer means would not have been as lucky. They might have been incarcerated or transferred among mental health and child welfare specialists who likely did not communicate with one another. Chapter 8 concludes our story by examining the increasingly fractured nature of the child mental health infrastructure since 1980. Faced with financial stressors and a cultural narrative that prized "family-centered" care, RTCs found themselves on the defensive, forced to justify their very existence. But for at least thirty years, many children like Marty had a place to go, a label that got them there, and a treatment plan that attempted to treat them holistically and attempted to return them to their families and communities. The simultaneous development of RTCs and emotional disturbance as a category provided children and families with one last option for treatment and child mental health with a professional model for its future.

ONE

O Pioneers!

When medical journalist Albert Deutsch visited the Illinois State Training School for Boys in the late 1940s, he was told that corporal punishment was not used as a tool of discipline for the delinquent children who lived there. Yet he later learned that boys who misbehaved received so-called hydrotherapy, for which they were forced to strip, face a wall, and have a fire hose sprayed against them. As one boy explained, "It's like needles and electricity running all through you. . . . You yell bloody murder and try to climb the wall. Your blood freezes. It lasts a few minutes, but it seems like years."[1] The Illinois State Training School for Boys was just one of fourteen highly reputable training schools, or reformatories, that Deutsch visited for his 1950 exposé of institutions for delinquent youth, *Our Rejected Children*. In it, he explicitly detailed for the American public the horrendous conditions persisting in many training schools.

Despite continuing assurances from administrators that the institutions had undertaken major reforms, Deutsch found quite the opposite. Instead, he found a new euphemistic vocabulary wherein "whips, paddles, blackjacks and straps were 'tools of control.' Isolation cells were 'meditation rooms.'"[2] Psychiatric care was nonexistent at most of the schools he visited. At the Indiana State School for Delinquent Boys, Deutsch was introduced to a fifteen-year-old boy who had a history of physical abuse, child labor, and multiple orphanage and foster home stays who had killed his foster mother. When Deutsch asked a staff member if the boy should be seen by a psychiatrist, the staff member replied, "Psychiatry for what? He doesn't misbehave and that's all we ask."[3] At the Indiana State School, delinquency was a criminal problem with a disciplinary solution; psychological treatment played no role.

Amid the despair of the children he interviewed, Deutsch found reason for hope. In a chapter on private training schools, he noted that some institutions specifically sought out the most troubled children and attempted to better understand the roots of their delinquency and administer meaningful treatment.[4] A specific subset of private institutions was notable: "One of the most interesting and significant developments . . . has been the establishment . . . of small 'study homes' and 'treatment centers' where delinquents with especially marked behavior disorders can be subjected to intensive study and/or treatment by highly qualified experts."[5] Even to Deutsch, a critic of psychiatric institutions, something about these "treatment centers" was very different from the other places he had visited.

These residential treatment centers, as founders and staff members called them, were unlike any existing institution for children. They were small, sometimes serving fewer than twenty children at a time, and equipped with a staff that outnumbered the children staying there. They housed children from across the socioeconomic spectrum, with some centers focusing on middle- or upper-middle-class children who likely never would have been sent to a training school or orphanage. Most importantly, RTCs were therapeutically oriented. They employed a psychiatric model to understand and actively treat a new population of children they targeted and labeled as emotionally disturbed. This goal, they believed, differentiated them from many of the more custodial institutions to which children might be sent. While children might remain at an RTC for several months or even one or two years, these were short stays compared to the multiyear stays at many institutions like orphanages or training schools.

The emergence of residential treatment centers occurred in the context of several related developments in child welfare and psychiatry. Growing attention to child mental health and welfare, coupled with increasing public and private funds to care for dependent and mildly troublesome youth in the community, left many existing institutions for children aimless. At the same time, these processes also led to a recognition of a new population of children whose needs were not met at home, in school, in juvenile courts, or even in child guidance clinics. These children, grouped under the vague label "emotionally disturbed," were often defined by their rejection in every other arena of care. Guided in part by the perception of a leftover group of children who fit poorly into the existing landscape of social welfare and influenced by the work of psychoanalysts who had established therapeutic environments for troubled children, many administrators reimagined their struggling institutions as therapeutic, short-term centers for these disturbed children. The processes of institutional transformation and recognition of the emotionally disturbed child as a new kind of person went hand in hand; emotional disturbance and residential treatment developed as codependent ways of organizing people and their care.

On the local level, a series of circumstances often worked to gradually transform orphanages, schools for intellectually disabled children deemed "feebleminded," and training schools into RTCs. Though these processes often occurred by happenstance, staff members developed institutional origin stories that characterized their centers as progressive, treatment-oriented institutions, providing care for children otherwise doomed to life in a custodial training school or state mental hospital. Of course, these portrayals were often oversimplistic, ignoring advances being made in other institutions. However, these origin stories allowed administrators to fashion themselves as pioneers with little precedent to follow, granting themselves freedom to experiment with novel therapeutic techniques. By the mid-1950s, residential treatment as a concept and profession had coalesced, with growing numbers of RTCs, a representative organization and publications, and a large professional network of individuals exchanging ideas and experiences.

The Web of Child Welfare

Residential treatment centers emerged in the context of several generations of child welfare work that initially sought to place children in large institutions away from home in the mid- to late-nineteenth century before struggling against this model in the 1920s and 1930s. The result was a continued push to help a wide variety of children without a clear place for them to go.

Starting in the mid-nineteenth century, an enthusiastic generation of mostly women reformers had become concerned with ensuring the physical and emotional wellbeing of neglected and dependent children.[6] They founded organizations opposing cruelty to children, built lodging houses for working boys and girls, and sent poor children to live with families in rural areas in the Orphan Train Movement.[7] Before then, many unwanted or dependent children had lingered in houses of refuge, punitive institutions where they were often subject to abuse and horrid physical conditions. In the mid-nineteenth century, reformers constructed orphanages to provide a more kindly place for dependent children to stay.[8] These children, considered unfortunate and blameless, ranged from true orphans to children of impoverished single parents.

By the late nineteenth century, reform efforts swelled into a full-fledged child-saving movement, which focused on improving the welfare of dependent and neglected children by ending child labor, promoting compulsory progressive education, and creating a multitude of agencies designed to help dependent children.[9] In 1912, the federal government announced its involvement in child saving with the creation of the U.S. Children's Bureau, which quickly became an authoritative voice on child welfare.[10] In the 1910s and 1920s, state governments also began to provide a modicum of financial support to "deserving" single mothers (typically widows) and their children, a program that was expanded by the 1935 Social Security Act under the new title of Aid to Dependent Children.[11] As Linda Gordon has argued, these federal and state reform programs promoted the dominant family ideal, with a breadwinning father (even if he was absent) and a dependent mother and child.

While federal aid policies promoted the preservation of the family, early twentieth-century reformers were growing wary of the very institutions their predecessors had erected to "save" neglected children. Many believed that institutions were often impersonal and devoid of the love that made family life so important for children, more than a hundred thousand of whom were living in orphanages by 1910.[12] At the inaugural White House Conference on the Care of Dependent Children in 1909, several hundred child welfare workers expressed their strong belief that children should remain at home if at all possible. Many declared their strong opposition to placing children in institutions. In many cases, explained the secretary of the Indiana State Board of Charities, institutions "simply boarded" children without truly caring for them.[13] Rabbi Emil Hirsch of the National Conference of Jewish Charities of Chicago went further, declaring that children in institutions "are of necessity trimmed and turned into automatons. . . . Spontaneity of the emotional and volitional sides of child nature certainly is dwarfed, if not destroyed."[14] Reformers almost universally proclaimed that options like foster care and direct financial aid to families were superior solutions, which would help keep children situated in families, even if they were not their own.[15]

Institutions like orphanages attempted to counter this growing criticism by promoting a family-like atmosphere in small cottages led by staff members called housemothers.[16] However, change came slowly, and in many cases, these reformed institutions were no better than their original incarnations.[17] Governmental aid and foster care served as alternate means of keeping families together. In particular, placing children into foster or adoptive families became an increasingly common practice for social workers in the 1920s and 1930s.[18] If they could not be part of their biological families, children would at least belong to *some* kind of family. In 1921, the Child Welfare League of America (CWLA) was founded for the express purpose of establishing standards for foster family care to keep children out of institutions. Ultimately, CWLA officials hoped to reunite each child with his birth parents, but frequently endorsed foster care as the optimal stopgap measure.[19] Still, the number of institutionalized children continued to rise, with over 132,000 living in institutions by 1923.[20]

Anti-institutional sentiment increased in the 1920s and 1930s as physicians became concerned about the implications of institutional care for a child's development. Pediatrician and child welfare reformer Henry Chapin found that children raised in institutions were more likely to become intellectually disabled or die young.[21] In 1941, child psychiatrists Lauretta Bender and Helen Yarnell of Bellevue Hospital described 250 dependent young children who had been raised in institutions, many of whom had few opportunities to play or interact with others.[22] When these children were moved to foster homes, they were hostile toward other children, "hyperkinetic and distractible," and "unable to accept love, because of their deprivation in the first three years."[23] In summary, they argued, children "cannot be raised in an institution without risking [their] normal personality development."[24] Research such as this contributed to a growing backlash against children's institutions.

In the setting of increased governmental aid, more adoption and foster care placements, and growing anti-institutional sentiment, the number of institutionalized children finally began to fall by the mid-1930s.[25] As a result, a leftover population of children began to emerge who were too troubled or odd to be kept at home and did not qualify for placement in a foster or adoptive family.[26] As the staff of the Chicago-based Illinois Children's Home and Aid Society observed in 1946, they had been left to care for the most troubled children because "the needs of the normal dependent child are being progressively better met by such public resources as aid to dependent children . . . [and] by the public child-placing services of the Children's Division of the Chicago Welfare Administration."[27] The normal children, they believed, had been accounted for; those who remained needed more than they were equipped to offer.[28]

The Preventive Model

This leftover group of very troubled children also became more visible because adults were looking harder for them. In the first half of the twentieth century, leaders of the mental hygiene movement were bringing psychiatry out of the asylum and into the larger community, shifting their attention from treatment to prevention. Because of its preventive focus, mental hygiene was especially directed toward children, who were simultaneously deemed the most vulnerable and the most promising sector of American society.[29] The primary target of mental hygiene experts was the problem known as "juvenile delinquency," fundamentally defined as illegal activity committed by a minor.

Prior to the rise of mental hygiene, children deemed delinquent had been sent to reform schools or houses of refuge, punitive institutions which hoped to instill in their inmates middle-class moral values by demanding hard physical labor. Despite reforms like the introduction of cottages and housemothers, these institutions retained a prisonlike atmosphere.[30] This approach changed in the early twentieth century with the introduction of juvenile courts. These unusual institutions were conceived as rehabilitative agencies, with judges who redefined delinquency as a representation of psychological and socioeconomic stressors.[31] Working-class children were sent to juvenile courts for both petty and serious crimes and for status offenses, or age-inappropriate behaviors like drinking, gambling, or running away from home. In the court, which had no jury or lawyers, the judge would offer individualized guidance and a probation officer would serve as the child's mentor.[32] Sadly, some juvenile courts became mere detention or distribution centers for unwanted children.[33] Still, they signified an important shift in the way delinquency was understood. By the time the White House Conference on Child Health and Protection was held in 1930, the Committee on Delinquency declared that "delinquent acts are but symptoms of deeper stresses and difficulties," a "natural and expected sequel of some deeper trouble."[34] No longer were delinquent children merely lawbreakers; their behavior had become an expression of psychological stress.

Mental health experts hoped to use their institutional clout to create programs that would not only treat but also prevent delinquency. In 1922, the National Committee for Mental Hygiene, the flagship organization of the mental hygiene movement, collaborated with the Commonwealth Fund, a philanthropic organization interested in child welfare, to found the Program for the Prevention of Delinquency.[35] The program placed social workers in schools to identify children in need of help, created the Bureau of Children's Guidance in New York City to train psychiatric social workers, offered psychiatric consultation to juvenile courts, and used public outreach to raise awareness of the importance of good mental hygiene. As part of the program, the fund and the National Committee for Mental Hygiene set up demonstration clinics to treat delinquent children.[36]

Between 1922 and 1942, the number of child guidance clinics had grown from two to sixty.[37]

Child guidance clinics were initially intended to treat delinquent children referred there from juvenile courts. But almost immediately, clinic professionals also began to identify a new population of patients: "predelinquent" children. These typically middle-class, troublesome, or problem children had minor emotional and behavioral problems ranging from bedwetting to temper tantrums and truancy. Most importantly, experts believed these children had a better prognosis than delinquent children, many of whom came from poverty and tended to be repeat offenders.[38] At child guidance clinics, teams of psychiatrists, psychologists, and social workers worked with children and their parents to understand the origin of the problematic emotions or behavior, often tracing it to a child's relationships with his parents, especially his mother.[39]

The efforts of mental hygiene experts, including child guidance professionals, to identify and treat a vast, previously unidentified population of troublesome children had important consequences for the burgeoning field of child mental health. With increased efforts to identify and work with problem children, experts identified a large number of children requiring help. One psychiatrist observed in 1935 that, "with the excellent work accomplished by [child guidance], or rather in spite of it, there is a steadily increasing number of children under 15 years of age requiring . . . treatment."[40] This phenomenon, he explained, might also be due to a rising number of children with problems.[41] However, the active work of the National Committee for Mental Hygiene and other mental hygiene organizations to promote mental health and identify at-risk children in schools certainly contributed to the perception of this increase. Moreover, the "delinquent" children who were no longer the primary target of child guidance clinics were still in need of treatment.

Child guidance clinics, despite their growing number, had limitations. Children with mild, easily treated troubles could be managed at the clinics, while seriously ill or disabled children with conditions like epilepsy, intellectual disability, or schizophrenia were referred elsewhere.[42] As the Committee on Delinquency of the 1930 White House Conference found, "more and more there is left for commitment to the correctional institution only the most difficult cases."[43] This included a large group of children still referred to as delinquent, identified by their behavior but increasingly grouped with other troubled children who had never broken the law. While child guidance clinics were successfully identifying and helping to treat troublesome children in the community, they were simultaneously uncovering a population of severely troubled children who had nowhere to go for the treatment they required.

This population would never have been identified as in need of care if it were not for the interaction of a broad spectrum of child welfare and public health efforts, several of which collaborated to create a new population of leftover children. Progressive child-saving interventions like financial assistance to poor families and professionalized foster care, combined with increasing anti-institutional sentiment, kept many poor children out of institutions like orphanages and identified a new group of children who were too troubled to be kept at home or taken in by a foster family. Mental hygiene interventions for troublesome children like child guidance clinics provided community care for many children with behavioral and emotional problems. Yet by excluding severely troubled children, some of whom would previously have been merely labeled delinquent, they further helped to identify a group of children who could not even be treated by these new forms of psychiatric and psychological intervention.

A Different Kind of Institution

Throughout the 1930s, 1940s, and 1950s, child welfare professionals struggled to find a place for these children, who did not fit the mold of any existing community resources. They had often been rejected by their families, their schools, and their communities for being unruly, unmanageable, or incomprehensible. Many of them were sent to custodial institutions after failed attempts to help them at home, at school, and in the community.[44] The landscape of children's institutions in the early twentieth century consisted of state mental hospitals, which rarely accepted children for treatment; orphanages, which focused on impoverished children; reform or training schools, which were primarily aimed at delinquent children; and institutions for so-called feebleminded, or intellectually disabled children. Residential treatment centers, their founders imagined, would be the antidote to these institutions, against which they specifically positioned themselves. They would serve as havens for these rejected children, whom social workers Joseph Reid and Helen Hagan characterized as "incorrigible, untreatable . . . ousted from public schools, and rejected by the neighborhood and community."[45]

While residential treatment as a movement developed in the context of larger reform efforts and professional developments, individual RTCs typically began as other types of institutions and transformed their focus to the care of this new population, which they labeled emotionally disturbed. In this way, the development of residential treatment and the creation of the emotionally disturbed children were inextricable, each dependent on the other. As local forces interacted with larger trends like anti-institutional sentiment and the psychologization of delinqency, child welfare professionals declared they would be the ones to respond to the needs of this newly identified population. In the process, they developed origin stories that emphasized their difference from the custodial institutions from which they had arisen. These origin stories did important work for RTCs and their staff members, giving rise to institutional identities and practices that reflected staff members' perceptions of their own work as progressive and experimental.

Perhaps the most odious type of institution from which RTC professionals distanced themselves was the state mental hospital. It was rare, but not unheard of, for a child to be sent to a state mental hospital; in 1934, 130 children under the age of fifteen were admitted to one in the state of New York.[46] Only two years later, *Life* magazine published a photographic exposé of the horrid conditions in state mental hospitals in Ohio and Pennsylvania; institutions like these were perceived as a last resort.[47] Hoping to avoid this stigma, the New Jersey State Hospital purchased a large semirural estate and turned it into the Arthur Brisbane Child Treatment Center, complete with an outdoor pool and tennis court.[48] Brisbane's first annual report described a comfortable, explicitly noninstitutional atmosphere where "friendliness and informality pervade the whole house. The child quickly feels at home, this constituting the best medium for therapy."[49] From the beginning, Brisbane administrators were crafting a narrative that placed themselves in opposition to state mental hospital care. Instead, it was noninstitutional and even homelike.

The Former Orphanage

More frequently, RTCs emerged from orphanages. Although child welfare experts had expressed their clear preference that such children remain at home since the 1909 White House Conference, the number of children living in such institutions rose until the mid-1930s.[50] At that point, this statistic decreased as more children were placed into fee-for-service foster homes and Aid to Dependent Children helped more children remain with their families. Hurting for money and often finding that the leftover children they served were emotionally troubled, many orphanages reframed themselves as therapeutic institutions for this demanding population.[51]

Bellefaire, founded in 1868 as the Cleveland Jewish Orphan Home, initially catered to poor and otherwise dependent children from sixteen states.[52] By the late 1930s, Bellefaire was increasingly seeing children from two-parent homes with emotional and behavioral problems as opposed to the poor children from single-parent homes who had previously made up the bulk of its population.[53] In 1939, the institution commissioned the CWLA and Council of Jewish Federations and Welfare Funds to conduct a thorough study of their practices, which identified emotionally disturbed children as an underserved population.[54] As a result, Bellefaire administrators decided it was time to change course and focus their efforts entirely on treating this group of children.

On the weekend of March 15, 1942, Bellefaire held a conference for local child welfare professionals that "helped dispel the impression that we are an old-line institution."[55] From that point on, Bellefaire administrative and professional staff identified themselves in opposition to the culturally dominant perception of institutions, hoping their institution would become characterized by its individualized, psychologically minded treatment. In 1940, several caseworkers joined the Bellefaire staff. Although their function was still evolving, the superintendent explained that they were there "to neutralize if not to dissipate wherever possible the tendency of the campus to move as a mass," decreasing the congregate feel of what remained a large institution.[56] Individual casework services would ideally help to offer "for every child, the kind of care he needs," a statement that emphasized the personalized approach staff members hoped to take.[57]

As Bellefaire's population grew dramatically in the 1940s and early 1950s, so, too, did its staff. In 1952 and 1953 alone, the center hired a new caseworker, increased the hours of its psychiatrists, mandated psychiatric interviews for all new children, and hired a new clinical psychologist to perform psychometric testing and conduct research. Administrators had to think creatively about how to integrate these new staff members into the daily texture of the children's lives.[58] A pilot program assigned a unit social worker to groups of three cottages, or residential living units. Instead of sitting at a desk in another building, the unit social worker's office was inside one of the cottages, allowing him or her to observe and supervise cottage life and work directly with children who had difficulty adapting to group life.[59] Not only did this impart a psychiatric, therapeutic character to daily life, it also created a smaller scale on which Bellefaire could operate. As Bellefaire's newsletter described, the unit social worker "makes it possible . . . to have all the advantages of small, relatively independent living units while at the same time being able to utilize the central treatment facilities that only a large institution can provide."[60] Bellefaire administrators prided themselves on embarking on a brand new kind of service. As executive director and social worker Leon Richman explained, "The treatment of emotionally disturbed children is still in the experimental stage, and is now appreciated only by the most progressive leaders."[61] Bellefaire, formerly a congregate institution for dependent children, now offered an advanced, novel approach to caring for a newly identified population.

The Former Training School

In Westchester County, New York, the Hawthorne Cedar Knolls School had emerged from a different kind of large custodial institution—a training school for delinquent youth. These institutions were descendants of the large, primarily punitive reformatories and houses of refuge of the mid-nineteenth century.[62] In the early twentieth century, many reformatories undertook self-examination and reform. They adopted a philosophy that theoretically emphasized education, individualized treatment, and a psychological approach to understanding delinquent behavior and rebranded themselves as "training schools" and "industrial schools."[63] A Children's Bureau study of these institutions between 1929 and 1932 described how many had shifted in tone and purpose from punitive to therapeutic.[64] At the State Agricultural and Industrial School in New York, for example, boys moved about freely, lived in "colonies" of twenty-five or fewer where they spent rainy days playing checkers and dominoes in "homelike" living rooms, and were treated by psychologists and psychiatrists from an on-site clinic who helped to plan and manage the boys' care on a daily basis.[65]

These changes were not uniform, however. A 1929 study of fifty-seven training schools for delinquent girls found that although many institutions were adopting constructive methods of discipline like point systems and student governments, corrective or punitive forms of discipline were still common.[66] Most of the schools still used solitary confinement, and nine "had prison-like steel cells or strong wooden cages" to confine misbehaving girls. More than half used whipping as a form of discipline.[67] A progressive approach to delinquency, reimagining illegal behavior as a symptom of psychological dysfunction, was slow to take hold. While most administrators interviewed favored the integration of psychologists and psychiatrists into their work, more than half the schools surveyed had neither on site.[68]

Plenty of training schools remained prisonlike. At the Boys' Industrial School in Lancaster, Ohio, the boys wore military-style uniforms and marched two by two in "long, silent, shuffling lines."[69] They ate meals in silence, lived in cottages of forty to ninety boys, and spent their evenings reading silently in "bare" living rooms while two larger boys "walked back and forth around the tables, apparently watching for any relaxation in attitude or any movement."[70] The boys at Lancaster were subject to corporal punishment by paddling and received almost no psychiatric or psychological attention.[71] It was institutions like this to which RTC professionals compared themselves, especially those at RTCs that had previously existed as training schools. The origin story of Hawthorne Cedar Knolls, told in large part by the social worker and administrator who presided over its transformation to an RTC in the 1940s, spoke to RTC professionals all over the country who disparaged what they saw as training schools' overwhelming failure to meet the complex psychological needs of the children in their care.

In 1902, Hawthorne Cedar Knolls' predecessor, the Jewish Protectory and Aid Society, had been founded in Hawthorne, New York, for the care of "unruly and wayward youth."[72] The boys referred there (Hawthorne became coed in 1917) were typically from poor, immigrant families, and staff members attributed their delinquent behavior to deficient upbringing in the slums.[73] Life at Hawthorne was difficult and punitive. Treatment involved learning good habits, attending school, learning and performing vocational skills, and attending frequent religious services, all of which occurred in a military atmosphere.[74] Explained the superintendent in the institution's 1908 annual report: "The discipline of strict daily routine is invaluable. He must arise with others at the first bugle call. He must march with others to the synagogue for united worship."[75] Corporal punishment was common, and an isolation area was used for children who had misbehaved particularly badly.[76] "'Abandon Hope All Ye Who Enter Here,' that was the reputation of the place," remembered Herschel Alt, executive director of Hawthorne's parent agency, several decades later.[77]

Change came slowly to Hawthorne. In the 1920s, staff members started to identify more deeply troubled boys who were very difficult to help. They founded a small "study and treatment cottage" on the grounds, reflecting their "growing belief that many problems of the maladjusted boy might be solved through a psychotherapeutic approach."[78] Several new professionals arrived to help, including psychiatrists, psychologists, and social workers, who spoke to the staff about the psychological basis of delinquency. However, they spent only limited time with a few of the most troubled children, and the tenor of the place remained custodial and punitive.[79] Meaningful change only took place after a 1933 study of the institution by the prestigious Columbia Teachers' College suggested that Hawthorne focus less on punishment and more on treatment. In 1941, social worker Herschel Alt was hired as Hawthorne's new director, complementing a professional staff of five caseworkers, a part-time psychologist and two part-time psychiatrists. No longer were the children identified as delinquents, defined solely by their criminal past. Now, Alt explained, they were children whose troubled pasts had caused them to commit crimes. Their needs would be met at the on-campus child guidance clinic and in individual cottages, where staff members known as cottage parents would become agents of therapy and familial comfort. Soon, mass drills and isolation rooms gave way to more individualized treatment in an environment more akin to a home than a prison.[80]

Although Hawthorne did undergo a major transformation after the 1933 report, it was neither easy nor sudden. Alt and his new psychologically oriented colleagues, hoping to escape the institution's past, gave the children more latitude, reducing scheduled activities and introducing more coed mixing. The unhappy result was that, in the cottages, "the beds were unmade, filth accumulated, and the place became infested with vermin."[81] With unlocked doors and little threat of physical punishment, many children rebelled by rioting and running away.[82] The cottage parents, holdovers from the reformatory years, continued to espouse the institution's prior philosophy and a few continued to employ corporal punishment.[83] Although Hawthorne ultimately became a leader in residential treatment, it was never able to completely shake off its training school past. Later in his career, Herschel Alt admitted that Hawthorne continued to struggle with how to achieve the right balance "between the degree of restriction some children require for stable living and the degree of freedom and flexibility which fosters healthful growth."[84] But the need for residential treatment centers was so great, Alt argued, that it was critical that existing institutions—especially other training schools—adapt themselves for this purpose.[85]

Of course, RTC professionals like Alt were comparing themselves to the dominant cultural perception of training or industrial schools. In fact, training schools themselves were continuing to undergo changes just as RTCs were becoming a real alternative. In the 1950s, the American Psychiatric Association and the Children's Bureau independently published standards for training schools, which argued that delinquency was both a legal and a psychological problem and that training schools should focus on the social rehabilitation of youngsters who had strayed from community norms. Both organizations strongly recommended the integration of psychiatrists, psychologists, and social workers into training school life and disparaged the use of old-line disciplinary tactics like corporal punishment and humiliation.[86] While much of this rhetoric may have been a response to Albert Deutsch's inflammatory 1948 exposé of the horrid conditions in many American training schools, it reflected reform efforts that had been ongoing since the early twentieth century.

Studies of training school practices suggested that while some changes were being made, many training schools had difficulty adopting more psychologically grounded philosophies and remained punitive in nature. In Rhode Island, neither the boys' nor the girls' training school had a full-time psychologist or psychiatrist.[87] A study of three New York state training schools found that all had "limited or token clinical services," were overcrowded, and meted out disciplinary measures unevenly and sometimes arbitrarily. At the Otisville State Training School, boys had generally "very good relationships" with staff members, while at the New York State Training School for Boys in Warwick, the report authors noted that "in one cottage the boys may not talk while eating and may be 'chopped' (i.e., the next home visit deferred by a half day) for dropping a spoon" while another cottage might have "a casual atmosphere."[88] As the authors concluded, the training schools they visited were "former custodial institutions that are struggling, under serious difficulties, to become treatment-oriented institutions which aim at rehabilitation and not just custody."[89] Still, the cultural perception that training schools were uniformly dark, custodial, and often punitive persisted and were seized on by RTC professionals who sought to differentiate their small, progressive programs in the larger mental hygiene landscape. Notably, most training schools accepted only teenagers while RTCs often admitted school-age children. Yet RTC administrators rarely mentioned this critical difference, instead focusing on what they were not.

Whether RTCs had emerged from state mental hospitals like Brisbane, orphanages like Bellefaire, or training schools like Hawthorne Cedar Knolls, RTC professionals took care to describe their center's radical transformation from an old-fashioned institution to an enlightened, progressive one. Promoting this image would become an essential component of their efforts to attract patients, staff members, and funding amid widespread public and professional suspicion of all institutions for children.

The Analytic Answer

A few early RTCs were founded to care for troubled children according to the psychoanalytic model of August Aichhorn, an Austrian psychoanalyst and educator. Ultimately, the work done at these RTCs influenced the development of others throughout the United States. In 1918, Aichhorn had founded a residential school for delinquent adolescent children, based on the belief that their behavior was rooted in neglect in their early years. These children, he argued, "come into conflict with society because of an unsatisfied need for tenderness and love in their childhood."[90] The answer, he believed, was to construct a therapeutic milieu, an environment that was itself accepting and supportive of these love-starved children.

The milieu Aichhorn built and spoke about was based on psychoanalytic concepts circulating widely in Europe at the time. For example, he believed a child's improper impulses might be sublimated, or transformed, into productive activities, a concept that drew on the Freudian concepts of the id, with its strong and inappropriate urges, and sublimation, which made these urges into acceptable behaviors. Aichhorn described one sixteen-year-old boy who struggled with aggression and was able to get this out through physical labor in the vegetable garden. A seventeen-year-old boy who had expressed homosexual interests "was put to work in the tailor shop because we assumed that the making of men's clothes could serve as a sublimation for his homosexual strivings."[91] Not only did the boy become an excellent tailor and obtain employment as one after discharge from the institution, but as Aichhorn noted, he only approached one other boy sexually during the rest of his stay.[92] Like many American RTC professionals would soon do, Aichhorn emphasized the differences between his kindly, warm institution and the military atmosphere of older-style reform schools where "a cautious, distrustful, antagonistic attitude" reigned.[93]

In the 1940s, Austrian psychoanalysts Bruno Bettelheim and Fritz Redl explicitly established RTCs in the United States on Aichhorn's model. Bettelheim, an Austrian psychoanalyst and concentration camp survivor, did so at an existing institution, though his academic contributions and questionable claims about his background would later make him one of the most contentious figures in the history of child mental health.[94] The Orthogenic School in Chicago had been founded in 1915 as a day program for intellectually disabled children. It became formally associated with the University of Chicago in 1934, by which point the school was primarily residential and shifting its focus to emotionally troubled children.[95] In August 1944, Bettelheim was appointed director of the Orthogenic School. There, he implemented a therapeutic milieu, which he defined as "the application of psychoanalytical concepts to the specific task of creating a setting for emotionally disturbed children."[96] Simply put, Bettelheim hoped to engineer an environment in which the children felt in control and where their needs would be met consistently, an idea he had in part borrowed from Aichhorn.[97]

Viennese psychoanalyst Fritz Redl had trained with Aichhorn himself. In 1946, he founded Pioneer House, a residential center for ten aggressive, low-income boys in Detroit. Like the Orthogenic School, Pioneer House sought to give children a secure, accepting, and therapeutic environment with a psychoanalytic bent. Although the institution operated for only two years due to financial difficulties, Redl went on to found the Children's Psychiatric Service at the National Institutes of Health, where he trained a number of influential child psychiatrists and obtained extensive publicity.[98] In their writings, Redl and his trainees consistently acknowledged their debt to the "classic contribution" of Aichhorn.[99]

For anyone writing about residential treatment in the mid-twentieth century, it was pro forma to mention Aichhorn.[100] "Aichhorn" could even become a label for authentic residential treatment. In an oral history interview, social worker Herschel Alt described the transformation of the Hawthorne Cedar Knolls School from a custodial reformatory to "an Aichhorn type of facility."[101] The line of succession continued as younger RTC professionals paid homage to Bettelheim and Redl as pioneers whose zeal and hard work were "contagious" and spurred on the development of new RTCs across the United States.[102] When psychiatrist Earle Silber heard that Fritz Redl would be coming to the National Institutes of Health in 1953 to start a new children's psychiatric unit, he "jumped" at the opportunity to work with him, having read his and Aichhorn's books.[103]

To many RTC professionals, the work of pioneers like Aichhorn, Bettelheim, and Redl suggested that residential treatment provided in a psychoanalytically oriented environment was an optimal way of treating delinquent and other emotionally disturbed children. This made sense in an America becoming accustomed to the psychoanalytic worldview, particularly as it pertained to children. In the late 1920s, Anna Freud in Vienna and Melanie Klein in London, among others, had begun to write about and practice psychoanalysis with young children.[104] During World War II in Britain, the evacuation of children to the countryside without their parents provided fertile ground for this new generation of European child psychoanalysts, who published and spoke widely about their findings.[105] By the time RTCs were being founded in America, most child mental hygiene experts were operating within a psychodynamic, or modified psychoanalytic, context.[106] In many ways, residential treatment embodied the practical application of psychoanalysis to daily life beyond the traditional therapy hour.

The Pioneers of Residential Treatment

As RTC administrators sought attention for their new institutions, they embraced the role of intrepid explorers. This enabled them to move beyond pointing out what they were not and embrace what they wanted to be: a novel, progressive place to treat a new kind of child. Pioneer narratives gave their work meaning and proved central to their efforts to fundraise for their small, expensive institutions.

Southard School was another name for the children's division of the foremost psychiatric institution in the country: the Menninger Clinic in Topeka, Kansas. From the time of its founding, Southard embraced its identity as a leading institution. Founded in 1926 by two sisters to deal with the large number of children who were referred to Menninger, Southard School was initially intended for children with intellectual disabilities.[107] In the 1930s, it was extremely common for intellectually disabled children, at that time lumped together under the term "feebleminded," to be institutionalized. The institutions to which they were sent, often called schools (even though many children never graduated), were typically custodial and emphasized vocational training.[108] But to many mental hygiene professionals, such schools were not promising sites for research or advancement. In fact, most RTC professionals would go on to specify that intellectually disabled children were not appropriate for admission, suggesting that this population was seen as fundamentally different, and perhaps less interesting, than emotionally disturbed children.[109]

This was certainly the case at Southard School. By the 1930s, Southard staff were considering changing their emphasis from intellectually disabled children to emotionally disturbed ones. As director Dr. Earl Saxe explained, the switch would pay many dividends: "Interesting and deserving cases might be admitted, and thereby we would obtain material to report on and write about, and as a result accomplish worth-while publicity."[110] Saxe did not feel the existing population of children at Southard was going to inspire any notable research. Unlike administrators at Hawthorne and Bellefaire, Southard staff had not noticed an increasing number of disturbed children referred, nor did they want to change course solely to meet a large community need. Instead, they hoped treating emotionally disturbed children would reap rewards beyond mere service, providing interesting cases for research that might raise Southard's public profile.

In 1939, Southard administrators decided to make the switch formally. Their focus would move from caring for children with mental disabilities to treating disturbed children without intellectual deficits.[111] The staff sent letters to physicians all over the country to inform them of the new policy, stating that "only boys and girls of average or superior intelligence with behavior problems or personality disorders will be accepted."[112] From the beginning, Southard staff members identified this new mission as uncharted territory. The institution's 1940 annual report proclaimed that "our effort . . . is in a very real sense a pioneering effort."[113] Yet the unfamiliarity of this venture also made it a risky one. "There are no guideposts for us and we must grope our way," the report continued.[114] Comments like these were common among RTC administrators, who adopted overly humble descriptions of their efforts while positioning themselves as leaders in a new field.

In the 1940s and 1950s, the Menninger Clinic was the premier center for psychoanalytic treatment and training in the United States.[115] Given Southard's affiliation with the Menninger, it is not surprising that administrators there sought to establish a leadership role in the field of child psychiatry. In 1946, Southard School officially joined the Menninger Foundation, and in 1955, an ad hoc committee suggested it be rechristened the Children's Division to emphasize the connection, as "the name Southard in connection with the school does not have nearly the drawing power that a more prominent use of the name Menninger would have."[116] By that time, Southard administrators conceived of their institution as a national leader in child psychiatry.[117] Not only had their work uncovered new insights into both normal and abnormal children, they argued, Southard served as a model for other fledgling residential treatment centers and trained new child psychiatrists and psychologists who would run these new programs.[118] Ultimately, they hoped to "act as a consultant on a national level . . . in developing the concept of residential treatment as an effective tool for helping many disturbed and delinquent children."[119] Just as the Menninger Clinic was a model for psychoanalytically oriented treatment of adult patients, Southard administrators hoped their center would become a model for the emerging field of residential treatment.

Despite ambitious dreams and a new name, the Menninger Children's Division was still housed in two dilapidated mansions separated by a busy interstate highway. A 1951 progress report on the division described the "ancient and uninviting appearance of the building," noting that "the battered front door, through which guilty, defensive parents enter for the first time, is inscribed with a four-letter word."[120] Administrators worried that their physical setup, which came with a hefty price tag, was off-putting to the parents of potential patients, many of whom "found it hard to believe that a first-rate clinical program could be housed in such a third-rate plant."[121] For Southard administrators, it was critical that the physical plant reflect the organization's prestige.

Throughout the long fundraising process for a new campus in the 1950s, administrators repeatedly turned to one aspect of the division's origin narrative that emphasized its identity as a leader in the field. Southard School had been named for Harvard psychiatrist Elmer Ernest Southard, Karl Menninger's professor at Harvard Medical School, who had (according to subsequent lore) encouraged him to include children in his plans to build a psychiatric mecca in the Midwest. This story became central to fundraising campaigns for the new building. A 1954 fundraising brochure for the division began with a large, cartoonish drawing of Southard and the following words: "One of the great leaders of American psychiatry was Dr. Ernest Southard, professor at Harvard Medical School until 1920. *'Go back to Kansas,'* he said to Dr. Karl Menninger, *'and establish a psychiatric clinic; but don't forget the children! It is from them that we are going to learn most about the human mind and therefore about mental health.'*"[122] Ernest Southard was a nationally known psychiatrist and the director of Boston's Psychopathic Hospital, where he had played an instrumental role in directing psychiatry's attention away from the asylum and toward the troubles of everyday life.[123] This fable assigned him the role of a revered leader ordering his disciple to found a children's unit for the benefit of mankind. The Children's Division would not just treat disturbed children; it would use them to learn more about mental illness and ultimately, the human mind. If the Children's Division was to be a national leader, it needed a first-rate campus.

Once the new buildings were completed in 1961, the story gained new currency. Children's Division Director Robert Switzer described the saga of building the new facilities at the annual meeting of the American Association for Children's Residential Centers in Chicago. Predictably, he began by invoking Southard's advice to Menninger: "Before returning to Topeka . . . Dr. Karl Menninger went to see his great teacher and dear friend, Dr. Elmer Ernest Southard. Doctor Southard advised Doctor Karl to come back to Kansas and start a psychiatric hospital. He also told him not to forget the children."[124] In this case, the Southard myth helped Switzer justify the division's substantial financial commitment to the new campus and proclaim its continued leadership in residential treatment to an audience of peers. The myth lived on in various forms; a 1964 update of the 1954 fundraising pamphlet repeated the Southard tale almost verbatim, and a 1986 history of the institution by children in a journalism class there was entitled *Don't Forget the Children: A History of Southard School, 1926–1986*.[125] It is certainly possible that Southard told Karl Menninger to include children in his Topeka clinic. But by invoking this hyperbolic origin myth, division staff and children ensured that no one (including themselves) would forget that their work had broken new ground.

Administrators at many other RTCs identified themselves as innovators, adopting a falsely humble tone to boast of their accomplishments. Arthur Ruggles, who had helped to found the Emma Pendleton Bradley Home (later Hospital) in 1931, later reflected, "We had absolutely no precedent to go by."[126] While Bradley was one of the earliest RTCs, this proclaimed narrative of uncertainty persisted for some time. Psychiatrist Wrenshall Oliver of the Napa State Hospital Children's Unit (which identified itself as an RTC despite being located in a hospital) explained in 1949 that, "from the purely psychiatric standpoint, we are babes in the woods of the youngest branch of a young science."[127] Administrators equated newness to bravado; the most literal example was Fritz Redl's Pioneer House in Detroit, where children were referred to by staff as "pioneers."[128]

Being "the first" took on great importance. Administrators of at least three RTCs credited themselves with inventing residential treatment altogether.[129] Others argued that their institution had been "the first"—in one way or another. The Cincinnati Child Guidance Home was "the first inpatient home in a medical setting for the study and treatment of problem children to be established in the United States."[130] The Arthur Brisbane Child Treatment Center in New Jersey was "the first state-operated treatment center for children presenting emotional problems which is not on the grounds of a state hospital."[131] And in perhaps the biggest stretch, staff of the Children's Ward of the Illinois Neuropsychiatric Institute declared it was "the only public, non-profit, treatment and study center for disturbed children in a therapeutically controlled, psychiatrically-oriented environment, which is an integral part of both a research hospital . . . and a public child guidance clinic."[132] Even though these statements seem somewhat ridiculous today, they were a common way of asserting that an RTC, which might otherwise seem like yet another child welfare institution to an outsider, was in fact a novel experiment.

Why the intense desire to be a pioneer or the first? In a brand-new field, being "the first" gave an RTC increased legitimacy. Brisbane's 1952 annual report boasted that, because it was the first publicly funded residential treatment center, "visitors from twenty-two foreign countries and from eighteen States" had come to observe its activities.[133] Visitors helped build a network of referring mental health professionals, some of whom provided opportunities like providing consulting services for states developing their first RTCs.[134] Regardless of whether a center was actually the first, being part of a pioneering venture could help attract philanthropic funds for a worthy cause, as Southard School learned. But most importantly, being a pioneer meant adopting an attitude of openness to experimentation. As one social work student explained about the Illinois Neuropsychiatric Institute, everything they did on the unit counted as research, because the entire field was experimental.[135] This attitude was essential to RTC professionals' development of novel staffing and treatment approaches. Because the whole undertaking was brand-new and the children so troubled, there was little to lose.

The Interracial Pioneers of Wiltwyck

The Wiltwyck School in Esopus, New York, was novel in a different way. Wiltwyck was founded in 1937 when liberal Children's Court justice Justine Wise Polier recognized that she had nowhere to send young African American boys referred to her court for delinquent behaviors. Most local foster organizations and institutions for delinquent children excluded African Americans, and the nearby training school, Warwick, only accepted teenagers. After she expressed this need to her friend and New York City mayor Fiorello La Guardia, the New York Protestant Episcopal Mission Society founded Wiltwyck, which initially served as a custodial summer camp for this population. When money troubles surfaced in 1942, the school was reorganized under the leadership of Polier, First Lady Eleanor Roosevelt, and philanthropist Marshall Field, with a board of directors comprising a variety of liberals from the National Association for the Advancement of Colored People and the American Jewish Congress.[136]

Over the next fifteen years, the board worked hard to transform the now year-round institution into a residential treatment center for emotionally disturbed boys, a broader and more psychologically oriented category that included boys who previously would have been labeled delinquent. In 1955, Wiltwyck's mission statement was updated to reflect this change, while still reflecting its emphasis on treating racial minorities. While an earlier statement had stated that Wiltwyck was intended to treat "neglected, abandoned, destitute, delinquent and pre-delinquent children, without discrimination as to race or color," the revised draft described the target population as "**dependent**, neglected, abandoned, destitute, delinquent and **emotionally disturbed** ~~pre-delinquent~~ children, without discrimination as to race or color [bolded and struck through words as per original]."[137] As the school grew under its board of prominent liberals, African American celebrities like Harry Belafonte and Floyd Patterson became prominent supporters.[138]

By the 1960s, the school was drawing on its interracial legacy to attract donors. A 1966 pamphlet called *The Wiltwyck Story*, intended to help raise funds for the school's new campus, described the school's dramatic origin story as a haven for troubled young African American boys: "A shaking little 10-year-old stood before the Court, charged with habitual delinquency. His probation officer told the judge, 'There is nothing to do, Your Honor, until he is 12 or commits a felony. Then he can be sent to the State Training School.' The reason given was that the 10-year-old was Negro. After twenty such cases were presented to the Mayor in the single year of 1936, the New York Episcopal City Mission Society was prevailed upon to start an experimental summer camp for delinquent and homeless Negro boys."[139] Now, the pamphlet proclaimed, "The Wiltwyck School program today is an interracial, non-sectarian, residential treatment center which serves . . . about 200 disturbed boys aged 8 to 12."[140] Similar language filled the pages of glossy programs produced for benefit concerts at Lincoln Center. In the program for "Ed Sullivan Presents at Philharmonic Hall," a 1966 Wiltwyck benefit, Justine Wise Polier reflected that, "when segregation and exclusion of Negro children were prohibited by law, Wiltwyck was first to welcome the change and open its doors to all children."[141] By 1970, Wiltwyck leaders were envisioning themselves as treaters not only of troubled African American boys but also of the most vulnerable sector of society. A fact sheet about the institution boasted that "Wiltwyck is the *only* agency which undertakes treatment of every member of poverty-stricken, minority-group families in addition to the boy in residence."[142] The 1966 fundraising pamphlet *The Wiltwyck Story* featured photograph after photograph of African American and white boys playing on swings together, standing with their arms around one another, huddled around Eleanor Roosevelt to hear her read a book, and playing the drums together (fig. 1.1). For Wiltwyck's founders and supporters, the institution's origin story was continually shaping and reshaping its legacy and identity, even twenty years after its transformation into an RTC.

A Common Goal

In its early years, residential treatment as a movement started small and grew quickly. In 1952, the Children's Bureau counted thirty-six RTCs in existence.[143] At the end of the decade, residential treatment had expanded

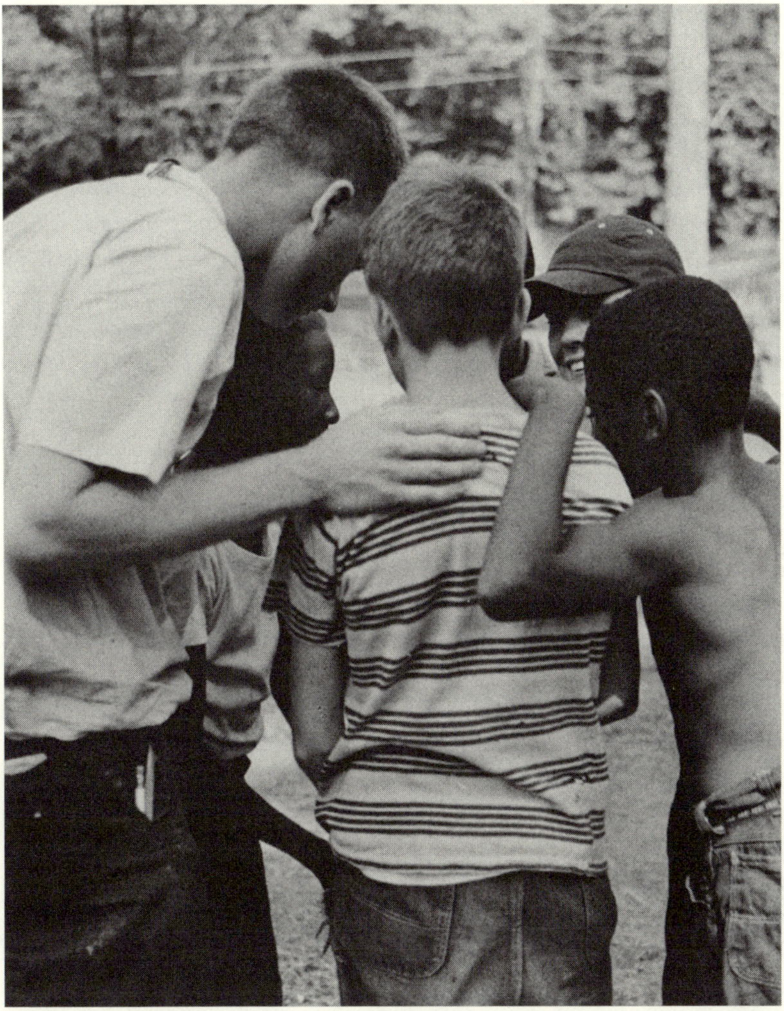

1.1. Boys at Wiltwyck School, 1960s. ("The Wiltwyck Story," Box 48, Folder 20, WR.)

geographically with centers in Mississippi, New Mexico, and Puerto Rico.[144] RTC professionals acknowledged that, although their centers were superficially very different, they were engaged in a common project. Joseph Reid, who was by then the executive director of the CWLA, reflected in 1958 that "'residential treatment center' was soon applied to a small, varied group of inpatient or resident facilities which concentrated exclusively on trying to help children who could not be treated in any other way."[145] Self-identification as an RTC became a critical step to the recognition of residential treatment as a national movement.

In the 1950s, "residential treatment center" and "residential treatment" became standard terms used to describe these heterogeneous treatment locales and the support they provided. Two RTC social workers explained that "residential treatment institutions exist today in a variety of forms and settings. They may be called schools, centers, study homes, hospital wards, etc."[146] The work done in these centers by definition went beyond taking a child out of his home environment and doing intensive psychotherapy, these experts explained. Residential treatment involved interdisciplinary therapy from social workers, psychotherapists, teachers, and residential workers that was individualized in nature.[147] Treatment was administered in a therapeutic environment or milieu, "the complement of adult-child relationships and experiences which can be clinically manipulated and controlled in the interests of therapy."[148] Most importantly, as we will see, RTCs identified one another as taking part in the treatment of emotionally disturbed children, a population they would define and in essence, create.

Although these concepts might seem vague today, in the 1950s, RTC professionals strongly identified with this definition of residential treatment and its related terminology. Conferences and symposia on residential treatment brought together mental health professionals from disparate regions and types of institutions to discuss common principles. In 1953, a symposium titled "The Education of Emotionally Disturbed Children" at the annual meeting of the American Orthopsychiatric Association (the professional association for child mental hygiene professionals) became a broader discussion about residential treatment, with speakers addressing education in the residential setting, professional roles in RTCs, and the purpose of residential treatment.[149] The next year, the annual meeting offered a symposium titled "The Role of Residential Treatment for Children" and featured Edward Greenwood of the Menninger Children's Division, Bruno Bettelheim of Chicago's Orthogenic School, and Morris Mayer of Bellefaire, among others.[150] During the same meeting, a group of participants began planning a new organization specifically devoted to residential treatment. In 1956, they founded the American Association of Children's Residential Centers, which brought together a small, selective group of practitioners to discuss their new profession.[151]

The largest gathering on residential treatment was held in October 1956 under the auspices of the American Psychiatric Association and the recently founded American Academy of Child Psychiatry, with funding from the National Institute of Mental Health. The five-day conference was intended largely for psychiatrists, although it was also attended by social workers and psychologists. It was preceded by one year of data gathering from a number of RTCs and preparatory work by subcommittees on topics like therapy, professional roles, and education.[152] The conference represented a national movement to recognize residential treatment as a new venture and resulted in the publication of a book on the topic in 1957.[153] Other publications by national groups like the CWLA and Children's Bureau further solidified the concept of residential treatment, providing academic bibliographies, listings of existing centers with brief summaries of their activities, and in-depth descriptions of their work.[154]

Communication between staff members at different institutions was instrumental to establishing a network of RTC professionals. During Brisbane's first three years of operation in New Jersey, the center's many visitors included Norman Lourie of Hawthorne Cedar Knolls, Joseph Reid and Helen Hagan from the CWLA, and representatives from the Children's Bureau, the children's unit at Rockland State Hospital in New York, and the Child Study and Treatment Home in New Haven, Connecticut.[155] Visits were especially useful for mental health professionals trying to set up new RTCs. In the process of founding the Vista Del Mar Child Care Service in Los Angeles, executive director Joseph Bonapart traveled all over the country to learn how other RTCs operated, visiting the Southard School, the Orthogenic School, Bellefaire, and Hawthorne Cedar Knolls, among others.[156] In 1958, Pioneer House founder Fritz Redl came to Wiltwyck to advise its leaders about how to organize the living quarters for counselors and children.[157] It was also common for staff members to move among many RTCs in the course of a single career. Child psychiatrist Stanislaus Szurek, for example, began his career at the children's ward of the Illinois Neuropsychiatric Institute and later became the director of the children's ward at the Langley Porter Clinic at the University of California, San Francisco.[158] The travels of RTC professionals strengthened the idea that there was such a thing as "residential treatment" and that it was a common project engaged in by a varied group of professionals across the country.

During the 1950s, residential treatment expanded rapidly. By 1962, the Children's Bureau counted some sixty-one hundred children in RTCs.[159] But some mental health professionals were troubled by what they viewed as a rush to claim the fashionable title of residential treatment center, even when many institutions were not true RTCs. "Any setting today can become a residential treatment facility by overprinting current letterheads with the phrase 'A Residential Treatment Facility for Children,'" worried one psychologist in 1956.[160] Joseph Reid of the CWLA observed that "so many people tack on a façade of 'treatment' without either understanding or caring about what is involved in the development of a sound program."[161] To these professionals, the desirable label of residential treatment center was being watered down by institutions that neither espoused the philosophies nor practiced the care of this small but powerful movement. Whether or not this phenomenon was a real threat, their concerns showed that the RTC label had become desirable and even fashionable.

To RTC professionals, residential treatment was a solution to the growing problem of emotionally disturbed children. Growing efforts to place dependent children in homes rather than institutions and mental hygienists' efforts to locate troubled children for early intervention had identified a leftover population of troubled children who could not be helped in the community. In truth, many of these children were the same delinquent children who might otherwise have been sent to training schools, though others were not. But by focusing on behavior as a symptom of errant family life and creating programs and places characterized by intensive psychosocial intervention, RTC professionals would create the emotionally disturbed child, a new kind of person their institutions were designed to help.

INTERLUDE

The Road to Residential

Children arrived at RTCs in a number of ways. At large state mental hospitals within embedded RTCs, many children were referred from juvenile courts, where they were seen after committing status offenses like truanting, petty crimes, and more serious offenses. At the Napa State Hospital in northern California, 57 percent of the children there in 1949 had been referred by a juvenile court. At the Camarillo State Hospital Children's Unit, the only other RTC in the state, the majority of children there had been sent by a juvenile court.[1] The private Hawthorne Cedar Knolls, with its training school legacy, continued to admit more than half of its children through juvenile courts in the late 1940s and early 1950s.[2] Even when a child might have been admitted voluntarily by a parent, some parents were persuaded to commit their children as delinquents so that the state or local government would cover the cost of their care.[3]

The line between disturbed and delinquent in these situations was fuzzy. On the one hand, some children deemed delinquent by juvenile courts were simply being rerouted to RTCs instead of being sent to detention centers or training schools. On the other, some were only being classified as delinquents in the first place because it was a way of getting a child into an RTC and making sure their stay was paid for. As Norman Lourie, Hawthorne's director from 1946 to 1951, remembered, "one of the big jobs . . . was the business of how do you talk the parents into making a juvenile delinquency charge against their children in order to get a child committed as a delinquent so City and State would pay. . . . You could get paid for juvenile delinquents but you couldn't get paid in a private institution for disturbed children. And we had all these disturbed children but we used to call them delinquents."[4] For administrators at Hawthorne, labeling children delinquent was critical to obtaining reimbursement for their expensive care. This process of reidentifying the same children makes it difficult to estimate exactly what percentage of children at RTCs were delinquent. However, this depended significantly on the RTC, as those like Hawthorne were well integrated into the juvenile justice system. In any case, RTCs, small in size and number, were only able to care for a minority of children labeled delinquent.

At most RTCs in the United States, children were referred from a wide variety of places, including local child welfare agencies, physicians, and their own families. At Seattle's Ryther Child Center in 1947, one-quarter of the children had been referred by social agencies, juvenile courts, relatives, and a mix of schools and physicians; by 1950, 44 percent of children admitted were brought by their own families.[5] Because the center's funding largely came from the Seattle Community Chest and other local agencies, parents were not under the same pressure to commit children as delinquents as parents whose children were treated at Hawthorne Cedar Knolls.[6] Those treatment centers in academic settings, like Langley Porter in San Francisco, Bradley Hospital in Providence, and the Neuropsychiatric Hospital at the University of Michigan, depended largely on physician referrals, contributing to a more socioeconomically advantaged patient population at these institutions.[7]

In general, RTC populations were small, reflecting their selectivity. Of the twelve institutions the CWLA sampled in 1950 and 1951, the average inpatient population was forty-five children, an artificially high number because of the large populations of Hawthorne Cedar Knolls and Bellefaire, which housed 198 and ninety-one children, respectively. Without these two institutions, the average number of children was reduced to 25.2. The ages of the children ranged widely, though most RTCs hoped to admit children fewer than ten years apart; the average age was 11.2 years. Although a few centers admitted children up to the age of nineteen or twenty, most limited admissions to children in their middle teen years.[8]

Not every child in need of residential treatment could be admitted. Children who were intellectually disabled (often referred to as "feebleminded") and those whose conditions were attributable to organic, or physical, causes were typically excluded, as RTCs hoped to focus specifically on children of average intelligence with purely emotional troubles.[9] Race, ethnicity, and religion were usually not restricting factors, at least in theory. Religion was typically not a qualification for admission, except in the case of Jewish institutions like Bellefaire or Hawthorne Cedar Knolls, where only a few non-Jewish children were accepted.[10]

Race was not a criterion for exclusion, at least not theoretically. Of twenty-nine RTCs described by the United States Children's Bureau in a 1953 directory, eighteen had policies specifically welcoming children of all races, while eight limited their admissions to white children, and three did not comment on the issue.[11] Despite the race-blind admissions policies of many RTCs, few treated African American children. For example, the Menninger Children's Division welcomed children of all races but by 1956 still had never had an African American child in residence.[12] At the Children's Service Center of Wyoming Valley in Pennsylvania, African American children were theoretically welcomed, but as of 1951, none had been accepted "because it is thought they would not be able to adjust in the school and community."[13] The gap between theory and practice was reflected in a 1960 study of twenty-one RTCs, which found that 85 percent of children in residential treatment were white and 13 percent were black (the remaining 2 percent comprised Puerto Rican, American Indian, Asian, and mixed-race children).[14]

Some RTCs tried to address this discrepancy. At the Evanston Receiving Home outside Chicago, the admission of its first two African American children was a major step involving a great deal of planning and discussion. The administrative committee admitted that "it has been of some concern to us as well as to the community, especially the Community Fund, that we have not been able to admit Negro children before."[15] Staff planned to study the "experiment" in detail "in order for us to answer the question as to whether or not it is possible to administer an inter-racial residential treatment program."[16] The experiment was such a success that community leaders took note. In 1956, the director of the Welfare Council of Metropolitan Chicago wrote to the president of the Illinois Children's Home and Aid Society (which ran the Evanston Receiving Home) to applaud the group's "thoughtful and creative decision" to accept African American children, which he argued "not only helps meet a genuine community need but . . . also encourages other agencies to review their intake policies."[17] The director responded with appreciation, explaining that "including Negro children at the Evanston Receiving Home is merely a logical extension of our basic policy of non-discrimination. Had staff and money been available we would probably have started it sooner."[18] It is unclear exactly what he meant by this, although a 1955 internal document describes the need to hire an African American housemother to work with the new children, suggesting the administration felt that the children ought not to have a racially incongruous institutional "family."[19] A few RTCs had large numbers of African American children, such as Bellevue, with approximately one-third of its children being African American, and Wiltwyck in

Esopus, New York, which specifically courted children of a variety of racial and ethnic backgrounds.[20]

Admissions policies typically excluded the most severely ill children, who would not be able to handle an open, unlocked setting or who might pose a danger to other children or staff members.[21] Even the University of Michigan's child unit, which was open to "firesetters, chronic truants, childhood schizophrenics, suicidal and homicidal children," deemed "grossly psychotic and deteriorated children" inappropriate and sent them to state mental hospitals.[22] At Wiltwyck, staff members fretted over how to deal with children who set fires. A new policy in 1956 stated that boys who had set fires could not be admitted. On the one hand, safety was paramount. On the other, fourteen of the nineteen boys currently living at Wiltwyck who had set fires prior to admission had not done so since. "Wiltwyck would like to take all whom it believes it can treat," the board of directors explained, "the only exclusionary consideration being the extent of the risk to other children."[23] The director, social worker Ernst Papanek, urged the board not to exclude boys simply because they had set a fire in the past, while not admitting "boys with a compulsive pathology of fire-setting."[24] This discussion illustrated the tension staff members felt between accepting the children no one else would take and maintaining a safe environment.

One factor many centers used in making admissions decisions had nothing to do with the children themselves. Instead, parents' willingness to be involved in their child's treatment was taken into account. At the Cincinnati Child Guidance Home, for example, parents were required to come to regular interviews with their child's caseworker and have their children come home every weekend.[25] For many parents, being a regular part of their child's treatment was simply not possible, especially if they lived too far away to visit regularly or were in institutions themselves.[26] New York child psychiatrist Earl Loomis Jr. suggested that RTCs were too judgmental in labeling parents unavailable to treatment. Just because parents were not able to "meet the nice standardized needs of one interview a week, or a nice conventional case work interview" did not mean they should be deemed "inaccessible" and their children denied admission.[27]

Even if a child met an RTC's admission standards, there was no way every appropriate child could be accommodated. In 1952, there were only thirty-six RTCs.[28] In the 1960s, federally compiled Child Welfare Statistics estimated that only a small number of children were cared for in RTCs. In 1962, this number was 6,100, with 3,800 in publicly run centers and 2,300 in private institutions. Another 5,500 lived in institutions for delinquent children, the report likely referring to training or industrial schools. These children comprised only a small proportion of the overall number of institutionalized children; over 79,000 were estimated to reside in institutions for dependent and neglected children.[29] Even though orphanages were on the decline, a significant number of children still lived in these custodial institutions—some of whom would likely have been considered emotionally disturbed. By 1966, the number of children estimated in RTCs had increased to 6,900.[30] However, this was still an extremely small number, highlighting the discrepancy between the outsized publicity of the work done at RTCs and their ability to care for America's troubled children.

The Big Day

For a child, being admitted to an RTC was a complicated process. Most centers had caps on the number of children they could take at any one time.[31] Others tried to space new children several weeks apart, aware that every new arrival could be stressful for the children already there.[32] Before the new child actually arrived, many RTCs felt it was important to prepare the other children, who would have to share their space and staff with the new arrival. At Southard, the child's room, placement in a group, and even "a specific place at the dining room table" were decided before he or she was admitted.[33] At the Cincinnati Child Guidance Home, staff told the children already living there the name and age of the new child, described his or her appearance, and answered any questions the children had. Because many were concerned that a new child would divert their therapist's attention away from them, staff members would "tell the group which psychiatrist the new child will have and reassure those children who have the same doctor that they will not lose their own time with him."[34] It wasn't a perfect solution, but it did reduce anxieties somewhat. In one instance at Hawthorne Cedar Knolls, a boy who had murdered a relative was about to be admitted and a group of boys who were already there had read about him in the newspapers and did not want him to live among them. As a result, staff members met with the group and explained that the boy's actions were due to an emotional disturbance, after which "they readily agreed that he needed the kind of help *they* were getting" and "said they would do everything to make his experience at the institution as constructive as possible."[35] In these cases, it was important to have the allegiance of the other children, who had the power to shape the institutional atmosphere by making a child feel welcomed or excluded.

For children, arriving at an RTC could be lonely and scary. Thirteen-year-old Josephine remembered that, "when I first arrived at Bellefaire, it was something strange and new to me . . . I felt homesick and not wanted. I ran to my caseworker almost every day."[36] Life at an RTC was full of new people, new rules, and a new daily routine, all of which new children struggled to absorb and adapt to. A group of children who arrived at the Children's Village in Westchester County, New York, in the summer in 1954 wondered about serious matters like how long they would have to stay and whether they would be beaten for bad behavior and also wondered about more mundane things like whether they could have snacks before they went to bed.[37] Others tried to think of every possible excuse for avoiding admission. A thirteen-year-old boy about to be admitted to the Children's Service Center of Wyoming Valley protested, "Oh, my stomach hurts! I won't be able to eat! I'm sure my parents won't make me stay here. I can't believe they would do this to me. . . . I can behave at home. . . . Why can't we all go home and be happy?"[38] To be sure, regardless of how friendly staff members and other children were, coming to an RTC still meant leaving home for an unfamiliar and unusual environment.

The arrival of a new child could be threatening to the children who were already there, who might try to make the "new kid" feel excluded or unwelcome. Eight-year-old Bob was already worried about how his dormitory group perceived him at the Orthogenic School in Chicago. When ten-year-old Paul arrived, Bob felt threatened by the newcomer, whom he believed might threaten the group's social hierarchy. As Bruno Bettelheim, the school's director, remembered it, "He tried from the beginning to put Paul 'in his place.' In a superior tone, he asked Paul if he had brought his ice skates along since the children planned to go skating after the party. Paul was taken aback and felt badly about not having ice skates, or about not knowing how to skate, or both."[39] New kids could be scary or unfriendly too. When nine-year-old Mary arrived at the Orthogenic School, Grace tried to make her feel comfortable by asking her questions about herself and telling her that the school was a good place. In response, "Mary replied with high glee and a nasty smile that she had once hit a girl over the head so badly that many stitches had to be taken in the child's head . . . and that the children here had better watch out and not cross her."[40] Mary's message was clear enough and the children immediately left her alone.

In less emotionally charged situations, children tried to be sympathetic and help one another adjust to their new living environment. When thirteen-year-old Flora came to Bellefaire, her cottage-mate Jean wrote in the *Bellefaire Bulletin* that "Cottage 11 seems to be big to Flora, and I can't say it didn't seem the same to me when I came."[41] A pamphlet written by

Bellefaire children in the late 1940s introduced the center to new children in detail. Called *So You'll Know All about . . . Bellefaire,* it was organized by the Campus Council and offered information about things like food, rules, school, and cottage life. Carrie told newcomers, "Maybe you're a little worried about coming to this place," but assured them that the children in their cottage were expecting them, and would "all try to make you feel at home."[42] Adjustment was gradual but was easier for some children than for others. Jean had a smooth transition; she quickly joined the Stamp Club, was elected homeroom president in school, and made many friends. "I think differently now about Bellefaire," she reflected. "I feel more at ease in the things I do and am much happier than I had been."[43] Staff members tried hard to understand what made children like Jean tick, hoping better understanding would lead to better treatment. Ultimately, they hoped all children would turn out like Jean, happy and comfortable with themselves. In the process of diagnosis and treatment, they would create an entirely new kind of child who commanded new scholarship and significant resources and wielded significant political power.

TWO

Disturbed Children, Disturbing Children

In January 1949, nine-year-old Betty stepped through the doors of the Cincinnati Child Guidance Home. For the next two years, the home would attempt to treat her severe emotional and behavioral problems. After four years of child welfare and child guidance interventions, the home was a last resort. When she was three, Betty's "promiscuous" mother deserted the family. Her father, an alcoholic, was gone most of the time, and the house was so messy that the family was evicted repeatedly. Two foster homes later, Betty arrived at a local child guidance clinic, where the staff noted her "extreme stubbornness, destructive behavior, vomiting, soiling, and diurnal and nocturnal enuresis," or bedwetting.[1] Betty's third foster mother resented having to care for this "defective" child. She regularly beat Betty, who had blank staring spells and skipped school. Fed up with this behavior, the foster mother begged a child guidance clinic to admit the girl to a psychiatric hospital. Instead, Betty was admitted to the home to undergo residential treatment.[2]

The emergence of RTCs like the Cincinnati Child Guidance Home was integral to and indeed inseparable from the identification of a new kind of person: the emotionally disturbed child.[3] This child arose from a unique child welfare landscape with no room for severely troubled children and was defined by her spectrum of diagnoses and by the dysfunctional home environment from which she came. Residential treatment centers arose during a time of intense child mental health reform, meeting a need for treatment that could not occur in the community. In particular, emotionally disturbed children like Betty were defined as children who could not be treated in the child guidance centers that formed the core of community mental health care for children.

In order to further define this new population, RTC professionals sought to classify it. But they did not use strict diagnostic categories, the likes of which were starting to appear in adult psychiatry. Using psychoanalytic language they had adopted for their own purposes, they loosely categorized children according to their behavior patterns. According to their highly variable system, children were either aggressive and acting out or withdrawn and anxious, labels that the popular media attached to boys and girls, respectively. Although this gendered interpretation did not accurately reflect the children treated in RTCs, it reflected broader cultural concerns about juvenile delinquency, gender norms, and the importance of conformity to cultural expectations.

Emotionally disturbed children were also defined by their origin, as RTC professionals invariably traced the etiology of emotional disturbance to disruptions in a child's home environment. Typically, staff members identified pathological family relationships at the root of emotional disturbance, drawing on psychoanalytic concepts and terminology to do so. In the process of choosing, classifying, and seeking to understand this new group of children, psychiatrists, psychologists, and social workers at RTCs made visible, and indeed invented, a new patient population. Children like Betty had certainly existed before the emergence of residential treatment, but RTCs gave them a label—emotionally disturbed—an explanation for their troubles, and a place to go to solve them.

In their discussions about classification and etiology, RTC professionals articulated a vision of the ideal American family and responded to larger cultural tensions about the healthy nuclear family in postwar America. Although suburbanization, the baby boom, and the return of many women to the home after wartime work did contribute to the rise of the nuclear family led by a breadwinning father and homemaking mother, historians such as Elaine Tyler May and Stephanie Coontz have shown that there was no such thing as the perfect 1950s family that we often remember with nostalgia. Rather, image was everything; from popular culture to psychological experts, the companionate, loving, family supported by parents who fulfilled separate, standardized gender roles became a cultural ideal, if not a reality.[4] It was this domestic ideal with which RTC professionals grappled as they described how defective family environments had given rise to emotional disturbance.

Misbehaving Minors

When Bernice Crumpacker, a social work student at Smith College, arrived at the Child Guidance Home of Cincinnati in 1949, the children she met were a mixed bunch. Eight-year-old Peter tried to provoke the people around him, shouting, "nobody likes me," and threatening to jump in front of cars.[5] Eight-year-old Aqua, who had chosen her new name, lived in a fantasy world and told others she was an Indian or a cat.[6] Six-year-old Robin liked to pretend he was a cowboy or Superman. He had a history of skipping school, lying, and stealing and "passed through the house like a tornado and had a temper tantrum and screamed at the slightest provocation."[7] This variety of behaviors was not uncommon at RTCs, where children were alike not in the specifics of their actions but by the fact that their behavior was socially unacceptable and disturbing to others. As child psychiatrist Donald Bloch reflected, "While they are *disturbed* children, they are also *disturbing* children."[8]

Symptomatic behavior could be distressing to parents, teachers, and residential treatment staff. But it was likely just as distressing, if not more so, to the children themselves. Described one Menninger pamphlet, "The children themselves are often miserable, suffering from fears, depressions, alarms, inhibitions, and the consequences of their misbehavior."[9] One does not need to infer the children's feelings from the observations of staff members, because their words were often recorded verbatim. Children in residential treatment made very astute observations about why they were there. Eleven-year-old Linda told her residential worker at the Children's Service Center of Wyoming Valley her life story in just a few moments: "My daddy didn't want me. I didn't like my daddy. I reported him to the police, and he was in jail for robbing a gasoline station. I hate him. He used to pick me up by the ear. He used to throw me downstairs . . . I didn't behave myself. I used to do everything. That's why I'm here. They say I teach the other kids, too. Part of my problem is running away. I ran away here. . . . There isn't anything about me that I like. I hate myself."[10] In that brief statement, Linda explained a series of events: she had been physically abused by her father, whom she resented and she had come to the Children's Service Center because of her bad behavior. She also revealed her awareness of how others perceived her: she was a threat because she helped other children misbehave. And finally, Linda told the worker how she perceived herself. Like Linda, many children knew when to ask for help and were able to verbalize how adults saw them in the process. When one little boy at the Cincinnati Child Guidance Home began to choke another boy with whom he was angry, a residential worker pulled him aside and told him he lacked self-control. The boy "cried penitently and said, 'I do want my self 'batrol,' I is trying to get it—I don't know how to get it. You help me.'"[11] Like this boy, many children were desperate for help and looked to staff members for assistance.

On a basic level, children in residential treatment had failed to adhere to social norms. They failed "to function as socialized members of the community," as one social work student explained, and "had difficulty in subordinating [their] wishes to those of the group," commented two social workers at Hawthorne Cedar Knolls.[12] As a result, they had been rejected by every arena of life: school, home, and community.[13] Administrators from the Illinois Children's Home and Aid Society described their target child as "the child who wears out one foster-home after another."[14] Bradley Hospital in Providence was "a final protective wall" for the child whose "parents, physician, social agencies, and child guidance clinics all have been unsuccessful in drawing him back into a normal path of life."[15] For these children, residential treatment was a last resort. Their deviance became particularly worrisome in the decades after World War II, as residential treatment grew remarkably. As Anna Creadick has argued, normality was an aspirational ideal for Americans recovering from the disruption of war. For children at RTCs, being defined as abnormal made them almost un-American.[16]

Sorting Children

Yet *how* their abnormality was defined was inconsistent and frankly confusing at times. Rather than dividing children into strict diagnostic categories, RTC professionals loosely categorized their behavior and then used psychoanalytic terms to describe it. In most cases, diagnosis was used to describe and understand, rather than classify, their behavior.

RTC professionals divided emotionally disturbed children into two groups: aggressive and acting-out children, and withdrawn or anxious ones. When fourteen-year-old Bobby arrived at the Ryther Child Center in Seattle in 1936, he had been relentlessly shuffled from place to place, moving among his maternal grandparents' home, two foster homes, two boys' preparatory schools, and two children's institutions.[17] He finally arrived at Ryther after his stepfather kicked him out of the house, where he had destroyed furniture and set a fire in the basement.[18] Stories like Bobby's were not uncommon. At the Illinois Neuropsychiatric Institute in the late 1940s, about half of the children "showed aggressive or asocial behavior such as fighting, stealing, temper displays, and destructiveness."[19] At Hawthorne Cedar Knolls, most of the children manifested "aggressive, defiant behavior."[20]

Some children in the first category had committed drastic acts. Jerry came to the Ryther Child Center in Seattle after setting his house on fire and cutting up his stepmother's shoes. Eric was a fourteen-year-old boy who arrived at the children's unit of the Camarillo State Hospital in California after shooting and killing his mother.[21] More commonly, children who "acted out" had truanted from school, stolen, lied, or physically attacked others. Raymond, committed to Camarillo at age eight, had attacked a neighboring child at the age of four and "was very aggressive, bit and kicked others," and "would stab at others with sharp instruments."[22]

Another group of children in residential treatment were withdrawn and exhibited strange behaviors. Physical habits like bedwetting were common among these children, as was the tendency to withdraw from others. At the Illinois Neuropsychiatric Institute, these children comprised a full half of the population and "exhibited varying degrees and types of neurotic behavior such as tics, nailbiting, enuresis, infantile speech, feeding problems, and seclusiveness."[23] As opposed to acting-out or aggressive children, these children were described as passive and withdrawn.[24] Bert, an eight-year-old boy admitted to Camarillo in 1952, "seemed to 'retreat into a shell'" after his little brother was born and was "living in a world of his own," speaking to others only by copying them. Bert's behavior caused his dismissal from two schools and continued at Camarillo, where he was "remote, giggling, in poor contact, incontinent of urine and feces, and [requiring] intermittent spoon feeding."[25] Withdrawn behavior could be bizarre like Bert's, but it could also be quietly distant. Tommy, a ten-year-old boy at the Southard School in Topeka, tended to isolate himself from others. "He played by himself with his toys, and never clung or cuddled when held," described his social worker.[26] A daydreamer, he also seemed depressed and frequently threatened to kill himself.[27] This inwardly directed behavior was believed to be just as dangerous—and perhaps even more so—than that of aggressive children.

Although residential treatment professionals often used the binary of aggressive/withdrawn or external/internal behavior to describe their children, plenty of children did not easily fit this mold. Tommy could change in the blink of an eye: "At one moment his voice can be striden [*sic*], harsh with anger, and next soft, warm and thoughtful."[28] He had "explosive temper tantrums" and could be "stormy and tyrannical" toward his parents, who were often forced to stop interacting in order to appease him.[29] Whether their behavior was directed more toward or away from others, children in residential treatment were there because something was awry in their ability to relate to people around them. While pediatricians and adolescent medicine specialists were trying to normalize difficult behavior as developmentally appropriate, RTC professionals pathologized the more severe misbehavior, which they treated as psychiatric illness requiring inpatient treatment.[30]

While it was children's behavior that largely got them admitted to RTCs, it was their underlying emotional troubles that most concerned the professionals who treated them. According to RTC professionals, behavior was an outward expression of a deeper disturbance, and it was this disturbance that they hoped to treat.[31] In making this distinction between emotions and behavior, these professionals urged their colleagues to withhold judgment on the behavior of the children they treated. One child psychiatrist reminded the readers of the *American Journal of Psychiatry* that "troublesome behavior must be accepted as an expression of the child's difficulty and of what he is able to be at the time," rather than as an indication of his essential self.[32] At Southard School, staff members were instructed to abide by this standard. Their *Child Care Handbook* encouraged residential workers to regard "behavior of children . . . as symptomatic of inner disturbances, and the basic attitude toward the child is a non-judgmental one. There is no 'naughty' or 'bad' behavior, only symptomatic."[33] While misbehavior was pathologic, RTC professionals warned that it was not deserving of blame.

The Diagnostic Dilemma

Although RTC professionals embraced the idea that behavior symbolized deeper suffering, observable actions remained essential to sorting children. The process of diagnosis at residential treatment centers involved using psychoanalytic language to describe a child's behavior. The result was a binary of the aggressive child and the withdrawn child as two representative types onto which both physicians and the popular press mapped assumptions about gender and misbehavior.

It was no accident that analytic language became essential to residential treatment. Psychoanalysis, based in large part on Freudian concepts, had become central to American psychiatry in the first two decades of the twentieth century. Its influence on American psychiatry and culture was both pervasive and eclectic. The actual implementation of analytic thought and practice in America was a hodgepodge of different approaches, few of them classically adherent to one school of thought.[34] During World War II, mental health professionals and trainees had assembled in unprecedented numbers to aid the large number of men who were rejected from the military because of mental illness or who developed psychiatric disturbances as a result of their service. Psychoanalysis, already closely tied to the psychiatric profession, grew in stature as analysts were uniquely equipped to treat cases of war neurosis. Their stature only grew after the war, as the popular press documented a high prevalence of mental illness within the civilian population, prompting unprecedented numbers of Americans to seek out psychoanalysts to treat their troubles. Psychoanalytic concepts, though no longer strictly Freudian, infiltrated popular culture through film, literature, and popular discourse and dominated psychiatry, psychology, and the growing profession of psychiatric social work.[35] As Eli Zaretsky has argued, American psychiatrists after the war fundamentally viewed psychoanalysis as an opportunity for professional and societal reform. As such, a pragmatic approach, rather than an orthodox one, was necessary.[36]

Psychoanalysis had become integral to child mental hygiene in the United States soon after its earliest application to children in Europe. In Vienna and London, Anna Freud and Melanie Klein had begun separately to write about and practice psychoanalysis on young children, albeit taking fundamentally different approaches to the same patient population.[37] By the 1930s, most child guidance professionals were operating within a psychodynamic, or modified psychoanalytic, context.[38] This included social workers, whose training and practice had come to embrace psychodynamic theories, especially an emphasis on the mother-child relationship.[39] Although they remained peripheral to the core analytic community, they became central to the child guidance enterprise.

The application of psychoanalytic concepts to children influenced residential treatment as well. Most RTC professionals had been trained in child guidance clinics and brought this basic worldview with them as they created new programs for severely disturbed children. In the process, they used analytic language and concepts that helped them make sense of the children, typically in a practical manner without attention to formal psychoanalytic theory. For instance, they frequently used the term "maladjustment" to describe a child who was not behaving in accordance with societal standards and "adjustment" to describe a therapeutic success—a child who could conform to cultural expectations and was ready to be discharged home.

The appropriation of psychoanalytic terminology for diagnosis was both logical and paradoxical. On the one hand, psychoanalytic language in psychiatry had been common parlance in psychiatry since at least the Second World War and was institutionalized by the publication of the *Diagnostic and Statistical Manual of Mental Disorders* in 1952.[40] On the other hand, much of this language described a person's internal emotions rather than his or her observable behavior. Furthermore, other than identifying congenital conditions, the diagnostic manual did not discuss children at all.[41] In describing emotional disturbance, RTC professionals appropriated and adapted this language to describe children's external, observable behaviors.

At RTCs, the diagnostic categories of behavior disorder and neurosis or psychosis were linked to clinical descriptions of acting-out and withdrawn behavior. "In the primary behavior disorder," explained Herschel Alt of Hawthorne Cedar Knolls, "the child discharges his conflicts through aggressive behavior. In the psychoneurotic the conflict produces anxiety which remains bound up and expresses itself indirectly through a variety of neurotic symptoms."[42] A label of neurosis often indicated a child's tendency to withdraw from social interactions as well.[43] Psychosis, perhaps the most severe diagnosis bestowed on withdrawn children at RTCs, was a label applied to children who were detached from reality.

This tendency to sort children into one of these two categories is starkly evident in a mid-1950s fundraising pamphlet for the Southard School, which introduced potential donors to the kinds of children they might find there. The first two pages described the (likely imaginary) characters of Dick and Nancy, each of whom needed the school's services for different reasons.

First we meet Dick:

> "Lick him!"
> "Send him to Sunday School."
> "Put him to work!"
> "Oh, he'll outgrow it."
>
> And Dick might have gone on:
>
> to harass neighbors
> to rob a neighborhood store
> to set fire to a garage
> to be sent to a reformatory
> to make crime headlines
>
> But a wise doctor advised his parents:
>
> "The Southard School and Hospital can help disturbed children."[44]

Dick was the prototypical child with a primary behavior disorder, which was marked by delinquent (law-breaking) behavior, aggression, and "a deviation from the accepted code of morals."[45] This diagnosis was the most standard way to describe the acting-out or aggressive child. In the most extreme cases, a child was labeled a "psychopathic personality," which reflected "a chronically perverse adaptation to society."[46] These children had, according to the administrators of Hawthorne Cedar Knolls, a "deficient conscience . . . defective self-control, primitive emotionality, a high degree of impulsivity . . . [and] antisocial attitudes," among many harsh descriptions characterizing them as almost incorrigible.[47]

If Dick was the prototypical acting-out or aggressive child, Nancy was the classic withdrawn child:

> "My, I wish our children were as quiet as she is!"
> "Nancy's always been such a *good* child."
> "No, Nancy would rather sit with us than go out and play."
> "Nancy does not seem able to keep up with the rest of the class."
>
> And Nancy might have gone on:
>
> to a dull apathy
> to a silent withdrawal
> to strange compulsions
> to an inability to talk or to eat
> to physical and mental deterioration
>
> But a wise doctor advised her parents:
>
> "The Southard School and Hospital can help disturbed children."[48]

Not only was Nancy withdrawn, but without immediate assistance, the pamphlet warned, she might also have eventually developed strange behaviors like refusing food and becoming mute. When a withdrawn or anxious (often called "neurotic") child's troubles worsened, he or she might develop schizophrenia, the most extreme variant of neurosis. Childhood schizophrenia was a fairly new diagnosis; it had first been described in the 1930s and 1940s by child psychiatrists who described a group of children with similar behaviors.[49] These children were uninterested in the environment around them or in other people; some lived in private fantasy worlds. Children with schizophrenia seemed to have blunted emotions, and they often spoke incoherently or not at all. Many had delusions or hallucinations and evidenced "bizarre," "primitive" behavior like playing with feces and eating garbage or strange motor tendencies like facial grimaces or catatonia.[50] One such child, Cindy, was an eight-year-old girl referred to the Children's Hospital of Cincinnati in 1950 when she began to talk "in a confused manner" and "heard her grandmother, who was in another city, talking to her."[51] At the hospital, she said that her grandmother, who was not present, was talking to her and that the doctor had three eyes. She also seemed catatonic with "a waxy flexibility and fluidity of movement."[52] She was admitted to the Child Guidance Home in Cincinnati several months later, with a diagnosis of hysterical psychosis, a variant of schizophrenia.[53]

In the twentieth century, the terms "childhood schizophrenia" and "autism" were often used interchangeably to describe withdrawn or strange children. In the 1930s and 1940s, researchers like Lauretta Bender at Bellevue and J. Louise Despert at the New York Psychiatric Institute studied the syndrome of childhood schizophrenia, which they identified as a disorder affecting a child at all levels of functioning and affecting his or her contact with reality. At times, these researchers used the terms "autism" or "autistic" to describe a child whose behavior was directed inward, ignoring the outside world. Leo Kanner first used the word "autism" in 1943 to describe a new disorder of withdrawn and repetitive behavior in the setting of normal intelligence, which he believed represented an early manifestation of schizophrenia.[54] Others who became dominant in the study of autism, like Bruno Bettelheim, shared this view.[55] However, many—including medical journal editors—used the terms interchangeably.[56]

While discrete diagnoses like primary behavior disorder and schizophrenia did exist, it was much more common to use a combination of diagnostic phrases to describe a child. A brief examination of children at the Cincinnati Child Guidance Home in 1950 illustrates this pattern. For example, eight-year-old Peter, the child who tried to get attention by threatening to jump in front of a car, was diagnosed as having "neurotic behavior disorder with marked feelings of anxiety and possible suicidal features," a label that drew on many diagnostic concepts (neurosis, behavior disorder), an emotion (anxiety), and a behavioral observation (suicidal).[57] Stanley, a nine-year-old boy who had been a client of the juvenile court for stealing and truanting, had a "primary behavior disorder with aggressive tendencies," a diagnosis that used a description ("aggressive") to further classify the behavior disorder, likely related to his delinquent behavior of stealing and truanting.[58]

Labels like schizophrenic or neurotic were not static. They might fluctuate several times throughout a child's stay. At Hawthorne Cedar Knolls, a diagnosis was considered "a frame of reference or a working hypothesis."[59] Of twenty-five children admitted there between January 1943 and June 1944, thirteen children were counted as "Diagnosis Certain from Outset," while three had their diagnoses changed during the process of referral and nine were listed as "Diagnosis Tentative."[60] Twenty-two complex diagnostic categories described the children, from "P.B.D. [primary behavior disorder], Neurotic Traits, Oedipal" to "Neurotic Tendencies with Behavior Disorder" and "Psychopathic Personality with Schizoid Features."[61] By the time the children had been at Hawthorne long enough to "adjust" (according to staff members), only four had "indefinite" diagnoses and the number of diagnoses used to describe the children had been reduced to seven.[62]

Diagnostic categories were inconsistent from center to center. In Reid and Hagan's 1952 study of twelve RTCs, the authors presented the centers' own diagnostic classifications rather than trying to reconcile twelve different systems and warned their readers that these systems were "only roughly comparable."[63] While centers used similar terms like "neurosis," "psychosis," and "behavior disorder," it was difficult if not impossible to determine what characteristics comprised a given diagnosis. Furthermore, their lists of children involved different sets of corresponding diagnoses. Bellefaire's eighty-one children had twenty-four different diagnoses, most commonly "neurotic with marked fears and symptoms of withdrawal" and "neurotic with acting-out symptoms," while at Hawthorne Cedar Knolls the most popular diagnoses were schizophrenia, psychoneurosis, and character neurosis.[64]

RTC professionals insisted that "the diagnosis determines the treatment plan," as one social work student at Hawthorne Cedar Knolls explained.[65] At Hawthorne, director Herschel Alt recommended a "flexible, low-pressure environment for the deeply disturbed, sensitive child" and "a clearly defined, more rigidly organized environment for the acting-out, aggressive child, who needs help in controlling his impulses."[66] At the University of Michigan's Neuropsychiatric Hospital, staff members employed theoretical and practical approaches in their management of different categories of children. For example, children's unit director Ralph Rabinovitch employed psychoanalytic models for treatment. "The neurotic child," he explained, "requires corrective relationships and an opportunity for direct psychotherapy often of an interpretative type," whereas "the schizophrenic child with his basic dysidentity and amorphousness of ego boundaries requires repeated reiteration of simple identities and a program of the most clear-cut type."[67] These theoretical explanations had practical consequences, as the unit's occupational therapist, Ann Martin Edelman, explained using more plain language. Neurotic children needed to "[form] positive relationships on the ward to offset previous traumatic relationships," and this could be done by showing children that you like them, giving them responsibility, and setting clear limits, like giving time-outs for aggressive behavior.[68] Schizophrenic children, whom she described as "desperately anxious, unsure of [their] own identity," needed circumscribed projects like woodwork, tile beads, and weaving.[69] Still, the extent to which a child's diagnosis truly influenced his or her treatment remains unclear.

Bad Boys and Quiet Girls

Was it an accident that "Dick" was an aggressive, delinquent boy and "Nancy" was a quiet, good girl? Probably not. For example, a social work student at Ryther in Seattle suggested that "our culture demands greater conformity of girls than boys," and a Massachusetts RTC psychiatrist observed that boys displayed "socially obnoxious and aggressive behavior," while girls were more likely to have behavior "of a rather passive character."[70] These characterizations were part of a long history of gendering behavior and mental illness and reflected new ideas about juvenile delinquency in popular culture.[71]

In the popular literature on residential treatment, delinquent boys were common protagonists. When *Life* magazine wrote about the Ryther Child Center in 1947, it chose to profile seven-year-old Butch, who had started setting fires in his foster home. The accompanying photo essay, consisting of re-created incidents during Butch's stay, showed the boy kicking staff members, running naked through the hallways, running away, being brought back to the center sedated, and ripping up a pair of pajamas.[72] Eleven years later, a feature story in *Harper's Magazine* titled "The Case of the Furious Children" described the children living at the National Institutes of Health's child psychiatric unit. Even the title shocked the reader, who was told that "the 'acting-out' child . . . is an island of wild emotion in a hostile world . . . Every impulse, however fantastic, must be gratified immediately and violently. . . . Two dark roads stretch before him—disastrous mental illness or delinquency blending into adult crime."[73] Certainly, many of the boys there had committed arson and had attacked others, but alarmist statements like this exaggerated their threat to society and made residential treatment seem like a life-saving, compassionate measure.[74]

Other articles were less blatant but similarly equated delinquency with boys and inwardly directed pathology with girls. In her 1950 story on Hawthorne Cedar Knolls in the *New York Times*, Gertrude Samuels consistently used "he" and "his" to describe the arrival of a typical "delinquent" child and presented two boys as representative case studies.[75] Two *Parents* magazine articles about the Ryther Child Center presented models of passive girls: Martha was a fiercely independent little girl who didn't want to interact with others and teenage Ann was self-involved and obsessed with her appearance.[76] In a *Chicago Tribune* feature on the University of Michigan's child psychiatry unit, the author described Bobby, "who made a habit of stealing big trucks"; Jackie (a boy), a fire setter; Joe, the child who had chopped down several cottages with an ax; and "little Roberta, who turned her frustrations inward until her disturbed emotions resulted in severe ulcerative colitis."[77] Articles like these further reinforced the public perception that boys in residential treatment were "bad" and girls were more quietly, inwardly disturbed.

In part, this division was emblematic of the cultural power of traditional gender norms in the mid-twentieth century.[78] But concerns about bad boys also reflected broader concerns about delinquent boys, which were at an all-time high in the 1950s. Movies like *Rebel without a Cause, The Wild One,* and *Blackboard Jungle* suggested that teenage male delinquency was everywhere and could strike innocent victims at any time.[79] These fears were made more legitimate by several decades of study of the adolescent as a developmentally unique entity and the development of a strong consumer-oriented teen culture.[80] Although many boys in residential treatment were not yet teenagers like the characters in these movies, delinquency was so strongly gendered in postwar American culture that journalists' bias toward covering bad boys (at the expense of their quiet or bizarre counterparts) is understandable. In contrast, the Academy Award–nominated 1956 film *The Bad Seed,* based on the bestselling novel and Broadway play, depicted emotional disturbance hiding beneath a calm exterior. In the film, a loving mother gradually realizes that her sweet, seemingly perfect daughter Rhoda has secretly murdered a classmate who beat her in a school penmanship competition. Over the course of the movie, Rhoda seems happy and untroubled by her classmate's death, suggesting that deep disturbance could exist beneath a veneer of absolute normality.[81] Given this cultural attention to the dangerous potential of the acting-out boy and his more quietly disturbed female counterpart, it is not surprising that journalists focused on these types of children in their coverage of residential treatment.

Of course, the relationships among clinical practice, popular media coverage of residential treatment, and cultural depictions of bad boys and quiet girls were not straightforward. After all, Dick and Nancy appeared in a publication by Southard School. Even if their two types were not necessarily representative of RTC populations, administrators were likely aware of their strong cultural valence for potential donors. Even *The Bad Seed*'s Rhoda Penmark had an aggressive, violent core underlying her placid appearance. Indeed, a closer look at children in residential treatment suggests that stereotypes and gender ratios do not tell the whole story. In my review of over sixty case studies from the medical literature, archival materials, and social work theses, withdrawn boys were described as much as aggressive or delinquent boys (as characterized by the authors), as were withdrawn and aggressive girls.[82] Yet for Americans reading mainstream newspapers and magazines, the gendered nature of emotional disturbance was hard to miss.

A third kind of child was by definition neither the bad boy nor the quiet girl. This child so brazenly defied gender norms that even if he or she exhibited other symptoms, this form of cultural defiance garnered the bulk of clinical attention. Wilma was depressed, assaulted other children in her detention home, and had "uncontrollable temper outbursts."[83] It was not these symptoms, however, that the University of Michigan child psychiatry unit focused on but her decidedly unfeminine behavior. On the ward, "she refused to wear girl's clothes, and for the most part remained unkempt. The male attendants reported that her behavior was particularly bizarre and unpredictable in their presence."[84] That the staff members focused on these observations, particularly the nuanced latter, illustrates the great attention RTC staff paid to gender nonconformity. It was not Wilma's violent assaults on other children that they worried about but her distaste for dresses and good grooming.

The popular media loved the gender-nonconforming child. In 1955, *Time* featured the story of Jim, a fifteen-year-old boy who had been sent to Ryther Child Center by a juvenile court after an arrest for indecent exposure in which he was found in women's clothing.[85] In Cleveland, local television station WNBK broadcast the fictional "Portrait of Elaine," which depicted the workings of Bellefaire.[86] "Elaine" was a teenage girl who refused to talk to the boys at Bellefaire and whose personal hygiene and behavior were so poor that it "deliberately seemed to destroy her chances for dating with the boys on or off campus."[87] She seemed to defend her boyish image, pelting a snowball with a rock inside it at one boy who asked her why she wore pants all the time.[88] Going beyond the quiet boy or aggressive girl, children like Jim and the fictional Elaine so blatantly defied gender norms that their gendered behavior in itself constituted their emotional disturbance.[89] Featured in popular media, their transgressions only served to reinforce traditional gender norms in children's behavior.

Broken Homes, Broken Children?

After describing and classifying disturbed children, the next task for RTC professionals was to explain how they became disturbed in the first place. One prime suspect was what RTC professionals (and Americans, more generally) referred to as a "broken home." This vague, all-encompassing term could refer to any aspect of family dysfunction, but child welfare professionals largely employed it to describe families affected by physical dislocation, divorce, desertion, illness, or death. By the postwar period, the pathological potential of these homes was a well-accepted fact.[90] Popular culture references to broken homes and the troubled children they produced were plentiful. Comic book superheroes of the 1940s and 1950s were internally tormented and driven to fight crime after their intact homes had been destroyed. Superman was an orphan with unlimited strength—except when kryptonite made him completely vulnerable. Batman's rage derived from seeing his parents murdered by a mugger when he was a young boy, and Spiderman's angst-ridden sense of "great responsibility" was formed after a criminal he had let go murdered his Uncle Ben.[91]

Children from all kinds of broken homes comprised a large proportion of RTC populations. In 1947, the director of Seattle's Ryther Child Center estimated that 85 percent of their children came from "homes broken by divorce, separation, death or institutional commitment," while 75 percent of Bellefaire's children were estimated to come from similar backgrounds in the same year.[92] These "broken homes," explained Eva Burmeister of the Lakeside Children's Center in Milwaukee, were "marked by strain, tension and anxiety. . . . All this makes for an emotional disturbance."[93] The absence of one or both parents, these professionals believed, caused a fundamental instability that could lead to emotional disturbance in the worst cases.

At the extreme end of this spectrum was Karl, an impulsive, fire-setting boy at Pioneer House in Detroit whose mother had experienced a series of failed marriages during which she had dragged the boy far and wide. Her second husband—Karl's father—was a circus acrobat with whom she traveled around the country, leaving the boy at home with "good friends."[94] The two adults then took Karl to live in the South Pacific, where he was largely raised by women in the local community. They ultimately returned to the United States and divorced, after which Karl's mother married and divorced an alcoholic man who physically abused her. By the time Karl arrived at Pioneer House, his mother had married once more to another alcoholic. That a social work student had presented each of these movements in detail was no accident. The implication was clear: Karl's constant movement and lack of a stable, two-parent home had contributed to, if not caused, his antisocial behavior.[95]

Whether or not two healthy parents were present, finances strained the stability of many homes. At Bellevue, so-called broken homes and poverty often went hand in hand. In her study of seven schizophrenic children in the early 1940s, social work student Edna Baer described children whose unstable immigrant families were all on welfare. Francis's parents were unmarried, and his mother's new husband was in jail.[96] Harry's father had died, and his mother was unable to care for her children at home despite receiving financial relief.[97] Joseph's father was in a state mental hospital, and his mother had unsuccessfully attempted to abort her pregnancy with him using ergot and castor oil because she was too poor to afford a professional abortion.[98]

Despite the prevalence of poverty among children treated at RTCs, it was often difficult to draw clear connections between economic security and a child's behavioral problems. Lillian Johnson, the director of the Ryther Child Center, admitted that many of the children the center treated came from "lower income families. . . . But we believe it is the interaction of these disturbed parents that accounts for the high rate of emotional disturbance and delinquency rather than the factor of poverty itself."[99] As more residential treatment centers became established in the 1950s, RTC professionals noticed that their patients were increasingly coming from across the socioeconomic spectrum. In 1949, the chairman of Hawthorne Cedar Knolls told the *New York Times*, "We still get products of the slums, but also we see more of the youngster who comes from families suffering little, if any unusual economic deprivation."[100] In this population, the relationship between poverty and emotional disturbance was becoming less clear.

For RTC professionals, the relationship between socioeconomic status, broken homes, and emotional disturbance was not straightforward. Nevertheless, the language of broken homes displayed professionals' implicit judgments about which kinds of homes were unhealthy and, by proxy, which kinds of homes gave rise to well-adjusted children. The ideal home, they believed, had two married parents living under the same roof. This ideal was plainly visible in studies of children in residential treatment. Reid and Hagan's study measured the percentage of children at each center whose parents were married and living together.[101] Donald Bloch's study of children referred for residential treatment in New York State similarly calculated the percentages of parents married, parents living together, and children living in the same home all their lives.[102] Children whose families deviated from this norm, professionals were arguing, were most in danger of emotional disturbance. This middle-class family ideal would drive many aspects of residential treatment, from the physical setting of RTCs to the rationale of the milieu treatment they provided.

The concept of the ideal American family embraced by RTC professionals reflected larger cultural tensions about the healthy nuclear family in postwar America. During the war, politicians and advertisers had called on Americans to fight on the front lines and the home front for the sake of democracy and the American family.[103] This discourse only intensified during the Cold War, when the nuclear family was called on to be a tool of domestic containment against Communism.[104] The companionate, loving, family supported by parents who fulfilled separate, standardized gender roles became a cultural ideal, if not a reality.[105] Musicals and films like the 1961 film *The Parent Trap*, the 1959 musical and 1965 film *The Sound of Music*, and the 1949 musical and 1958 movie *South Pacific* showed that true happiness could be achieved only when a family was made intact.[106] The power of this cultural ideal influenced professionals at RTCs, who assessed children based on the "intactness" of their homes and ultimately sought to repair broken families.

Disturbed Families Make Disturbed Children

While broken homes might contribute to a child's problems, RTC professionals believed that the real trouble could be found only by examining the interactions among family members. Reflecting on the first ten years of Ryther Child Center's existence in 1947, executive director Lillian Johnson and social worker Joseph Reid acknowledged that as many as 85 percent of the children the center treated were from broken homes. These homes, they argued, were not the primary cause of emotional disturbance. Rather, it was broken relationships that had created broken homes, damaging the children who lived there in the process.[107] For example, they explained, a home broken by divorce had been a pathological environment long before the actual divorce. A child growing up in that home "probably had not lived in an atmosphere of happiness and contentment prior to the divorce," and it was that atmosphere that had contributed to the child's problems.[108] In their efforts to understand the etiology of emotional disturbance, RTC professionals pointed to pathological family relationships, especially those involving the parent(s)-child dyad (or triad), as the most common inciting cause. Rather than pointing to a child's disturbed mind or character, RTC professionals placed the deviant, disturbed child at the center of a dynamic relational web.

This approach moved beyond the individual pathology of the child and looked toward the family as a pathological object. In this way, residential treatment was closely related to family therapy, which began to emerge in the 1950s. Family therapists, most of whom had been trained as psychoanalysts, pointed to dysfunctional family interactions, rather than specific individuals, as the source of mental illness; to them, the family was itself the patient.[109] RTC professionals made no such claims; the child was still their patient. But their etiological models of emotional disturbance focused on family interactions, suggesting that individual children were not inherently pathological.

In the most common type of pathology, the parents' own emotional troubles influenced their behavior toward their child. The head of Hawthorne Cedar Knolls' parent organization described this process in which "parental tension . . . is transmitted by a kind of contagion to the child . . . a disturbed parent imposes his particular problem on the child as a kind of self-treatment."[110] These "contagious" problems might include troubles like marital dissatisfaction, unplanned pregnancies, poor relationships with their own parents, and, among fathers, a lack of "stimulating and expanding work or play outlets for themselves."[111] According to this model of emotional disturbance, the parents' childhood relationships with their own parents would simply play out in their own parenting, and on and on.

If any child owed her disturbance to contagious parental troubles, it was Darlene, a nine-year-old girl admitted to Bellefaire in 1954. A "tense, anxious child," Darlene suffered from bedwetting, nightmares, and had "severe temper tantrums when did she did not have her way."[112] A look at her parents explained it all. Darlene's father, "a cold, reserved man," stayed away from his daughter and left the childrearing to his wife. She, in turn, "began to resent her marriage and the sacrifice of her career. She unconsciously looked on Darlene, her first-born, as the symbolic cause of it all," interpreted the Bellefaire staff.[113] The lack of love from her father and resentment from her mother, the article continued, made Darlene hate her parents, believe she was simply "no good," and behave poorly.[114]

The contagion model was especially prominent in the case of children who blatantly transgressed traditional gender boundaries. Jim, who as mentioned earlier had been arrested in Seattle for indecent exposure and wearing women's clothes, was described by *Time* magazine as a product of his parents' own atypical gender behavior: "Jim's mother was a heavyset, masculine woman who ran the household, even to repairing the plumbing; his father was a light-boned, slightly effeminate weakling who talked in a high-pitched voice."[115] These patterns of gender transgression, coupled with his mother's wish that he had been a girl, were presented as the explanations for Jim's feminine behavior. According to the author, Jim's parents had merely "transferred" their own gender nonconformity and his mother's wish for a daughter onto him. Similarly, television viewers learned that the fictional Elaine, who tore up her friends' party dresses and maintained her ugliness, had a father who had always wanted a son and nicknamed his daughter "Butch." [116] Thus, viewers were led to believe that Elaine was merely trying to live up to her father's expectations with her masculine behavior. The stories of Jim and Elaine suggested that children whose behavior seemed to defy gender norms were merely echoing their parents' own problems.

The idea that a parent's own emotional troubles and early life experiences could directly influence his or her child's behavior was reflective of the strong psychoanalytic character of residential treatment. As Stanislaus Szurek, director of the Langley Porter children's unit, explained, "The idea was that perhaps . . . all forms of mental disorder in childhood had not only their genesis, but also their maintenance, in the child's early and continuing experience with . . . the parents. These conflicts of parents stemmed from *their own* early childhood experience" (emphasis mine).[117] One social work student at the Child Guidance Home of Cincinnati even placed diagnostic labels on the parents of the children she saw. The fathers, she determined, were overwhelmingly psychoneurotic, which she ascribed to their own parental relationships: "Fears of inadequacy and of masculinity are marked in these men who have yet to resolve their feelings towards their own fathers."[118] At the heart of emotional disturbance was the fundamentally analytic centrality of the parent-child relationship.

Sadly, social workers and psychiatrists described how a parent trying to deal with his or her own problems too often could inflict actual trauma on a child. Samuel, a "noisy, hyperactive, aggressive" twelve-year-old boy from Des Moines, was referred to Bellefaire in 1942. Samuel's mother had not wanted any children, and as a result, "she [was] reported to have beaten him almost daily, to have threatened at various times to disown him, to put him into a reform school, or even kill him."[119] This heartbreaking description of Samuel's background is particularly revealing because it is grounded in an assumption that the mother's abuse was caused by her disinterest in having children.

Although parental pathology could be the impetus for physical or emotional abuse, RTC professionals were careful to explain that it was the interaction between parent and child that resulted in a child's ensuing disturbance. Kevin, a boy at Pioneer House who was preoccupied with "carnage and slaughter," came from a home where he had been "beaten, threatened with a shotgun, booted, thrown into the drainage ditch behind the house, and locked in the woodshed for long intervals without food" by his stepfather.[120] Kevin lived in "abject terror" of the man and told a camp counselor that he hated his stepfather.[121] Vera Kare, the social work student who analyzed his case, concluded that Kevin's behavior was an unconscious response to his abuse: "Terrorized by the stepfather, yet powerless, Kevin evidently sought an avenue of partial escapade [*sic*] by attempting to remain an infant."[122] Although the abuse emanated from a parent, Kare was arguing that it was Kevin's reaction to the abuse that resulted in his symptoms. Emotional disturbance was rarely a one-way road; instead, RTC professionals believed, it resulted from the dynamic interplay of parents and child.

Deprived of a Normal Upbringing

Disturbance could also result from a lack of interaction between parent and child, a state that child mental hygiene professionals called deprivation. As child psychoanalysis grew in the 1940s, leaders in the field focused their attention on the relationships between mothers and children and their effects on children's emotional development. During her work at the Hampstead Nurseries in rural England during World War II, where children had been taken from their parents to ensure their safety, Anna Freud observed that children seemed to regress developmentally without their mothers.[123] In 1951, British psychiatrist and psychoanalyst John Bowlby declared in his report for the World Health Organization, *Maternal Care and Mental Health,* that maternal love and caregiving early in life were critical for a child's lifelong emotional health.[124] The converse of maternal attachment, of course, was maternal deprivation, which had the potential to jeopardize a child's natural development. In the United States, psychoanalysts David Levy and Margaret Ribble used analogies to vitamins and food to describe the physical and emotional sustenance that children needed from their mothers to develop properly.[125] In contrast, they used metaphors derived from nutritional deficiency diseases to describe the catastrophic effects of deficiencies of parental nurturing.[126]

RTC professionals employed these metaphors as well. As early as 1937, Bellevue's Lauretta Bender argued that "the essential needs of any normal child are food, clothing, warmth, support (from falling until they have learned to walk), protection from an aggressive world, and demonstrations of love from the persons who give them these things."[127] To her, parental nurturance was as important for survival as the provision of food and clothing. Similarly, Hopkins's Barbara Betz described her inpatients as having "a deficiency of some of the essential emotional 'vitamins,'" and social worker Helen Hagan described children in residential treatment as those who have "not had the emotional sustenance necessary . . . to develop a healthy personality."[128] This deficiency produced emotional disturbance as the child attempted to cope with a lack of love "in ways that are detrimental to himself and to society."[129] Ultimately, experts believed, it would hinder healthy personality development.

Ten-year-old Brian presented a classic case of deprivation. His mother worried about hurting her "frail," colicky infant son, who was so difficult to toilet train that she became "disgusted and couldn't bear to touch him."[130] When his baby sister was born, his mother began to ignore him completely. Brian had such difficulty expressing himself and relating to others that his nursery school deemed him intellectually disabled. When he was admitted to the Cincinnati Child Guidance Home in 1951, Brian became upset when he had to share a staff member's attention and gave orders like "don't tuck me in" and "don't kiss me goodnight."[131] In analyzing his behavior, social work student Angela Baird focused almost entirely on the deprivation she believed Brian had suffered. His "attempts to obtain affection, attention and recognition," she explained, "[indicate] the amazing extent to which he sought dependency gratification which had previously been withheld."[132] As Baird saw it, Brian was merely trying to reclaim the attention he had never been given by his mother.

Arrested Development

The final theoretical framework used by many RTC professionals to explain emotional disturbance defined disturbance as a consequence of interrupted normal development. Because of strife in the family, this theory argued, a child's development could be prematurely halted, resulting in behaviors that were inappropriately young for the child's age.[133] As a fundraising pamphlet for the Menninger Children's Division explained, "The emotionally ill child is not able to make the sort of emotional growth which is necessary to progress from the very dependent infant to the independent adult."[134] The developmental framework overlapped closely with other etiological models of emotional disturbance, as in the case of Martha, a four-year-old girl admitted to the Ryther Child Center in the late 1940s for a strange case of severe eczema that seemed to worsen at stressful times. The little girl was fiercely independent, refusing all help from adults, and was covered in bandages to prevent her from scratching the eczema. Ryther director Lillian Johnson described her case in detail for the readers of *Parents* magazine.[135]

Martha's early background was one of deprivation caused by her mother's own parental issues. When Martha's mother was in the hospital giving birth to her, her own mother died. Psychologically unable to breast-feed or care for her newborn, she stayed in the hospital for an extra month receiving nursing help. Reasoned Johnson, "Her own bottled-up emotion cut off from the youngster the love and warmth she should have had."[136] The result was unintentional deprivation: "There was no cruelty, no neglect. There was simply a lack of that vital nourishment in the way of love which is so essential to a child's growth."[137]

At first, Martha stayed away from the staff members and other children. But one day after lunch, she walked over to the staff table and leaned against the knee of a female staff member, which they took as a sign that she was reaching out for affection. Soon afterward, Martha began to act like a toddler, sucking her thumb, sitting in the laps of staff members, and eating in a high chair.[138] She demanded that staff members help her take baths and get dressed, prompting one staff person to comment, "Sometimes it is nice to be a baby again, isn't it, Martha?"[139] When her parents came to visit, they were baffled by this infantile behavior. But as the staff explained to them, it was perfectly normal: "Patiently we explained to them that you cannot skip periods in life's development, that this child had never had normal babyhood and that now she was going back to relive what she should have had at the age of one or two, that this was a part of therapy and that they must trust us."[140] Because Martha's development had halted quite early, it was essential that she go back and reexperience each developmental stage in order to fix her stunted personality. Gradually, Martha returned to behavior more appropriate for a four-year-old, her eczema cleared, and her family reunited happily. Martha's story illustrates how deprivation, a parent's own troubles, and stagnated development could all come together to create emotional disturbance. The only solution was to reverse these troubles to restore normal affection and development. For readers of Martha's story, the damaging effects of deprivation were clear, but so was the potential of treatment to undo them. Even for the most troubled children, the article implied, a happy home life was within reach.

The Dangers of Blame

Johnson took care to state that Martha's deprivation was not due to any intentional actions by her parents. Although she acknowledged that parents were often the cause of emotional disturbance, she warned against placing blame on them: "Blame is a queer word. . . . Intentionally they would never have injured anyone. But out of the complexity and hurt of their own lives they failed to meet the needs of their child."[141] This might have been a surprising statement for the readers of *Parents* magazine, who were used to hearing about mothers who were to blame for their children's problems.[142] Historians have given much attention to the emergence and persistence of often vicious "mother blame" in the 1940s and 1950s.[143] However, residential treatment professionals went out of their way to warn the public and other mental health professionals against the dangers of mother blame and parent blame more generally. Even if disturbance originated in the parent-child relationship, they argued, identifying this relationship as a causal factor need not be associated with blame.[144] Their efforts to acquit mothers and focus on troubled relationships flew directly in the face of a prevalent, often vitriolic cultural discourse about bad mothers and instead sought to involve both parents in a more productive, forward-looking conversation about what might be done to restore healthy family relationships.

Blame, RTC professionals argued, was counterproductive to treatment. Ralph Rabinovitch of the University of Michigan's child psychiatry unit advised in the *New York Times* that "simply to blame and threaten parents is not only useless, it tends to discourage parents from seeking the help they often need desperately."[145] Frequently, parents already felt very guilty and believed they had caused their children's problems. In a Bellevue group for parents of schizophrenic children, parents were overheard blaming themselves for their children's problems, saying things like "I should never have been a father," "I guess we didn't prepare him for reality," "we never know what we're really doing to our children," and "maybe we're mentally sick ourselves."[146] The three psychiatrists who ran the group reflected that "these parents feel responsible for the child's illness and are overwhelmed with anxiety. . . . Sometimes professional advice they have received has tended to confirm or intensify their guilt feelings. Some relate having been told that the child's maladjustment results from their own neurosis and that they are the ones who need treatment."[147] With perceptions such as these, it is understandable why parents would be hesitant to seek care for their children, knowing that professionals might augment the shame they already felt.

Navigating around blame could be tricky. Langley Porter's director suggested that the parent be told: "I have a hunch that all or much of your child's difficulty is in some way connected with some difficulties you are experiencing" and that the professional offer to help with the parent's own problem, which would likely help the child as well.[148] A social work student at the Cincinnati Child Guidance Home suggested being sympathetic to these parents, who "are in a vulnerable position" because "popular education—the magazines, P.T.A. speakers and others—point to the parents as the root of all children's ills."[149] Regardless of professionals' attempts to tread carefully, many parents likely felt blamed for their children's disturbances. But it is telling that RTC professionals, who took care of the most disturbed children, cautioned against the use of unilateral parent blame. At the very least, it suggests that they were aware of the predominant mother-blaming thread in psychiatry and popular culture and sought to characterize themselves as an enlightened alternative.

Residential treatment centers offered a safe haven for children so troubled that they had been rejected by their schools, communities, and even their own parents. The emergence of a new place—the RTC—was inseparable from the creation of a new kind of person: the emotionally disturbed child. While child mental hygiene professionals had served and identified troublesome children in child guidance clinics, RTCs were created to meet the needs of children too ill to be managed in the community.

Children's deviant behavior was categorized by RTC professionals according to the binary of aggressive and acting out or quiet and withdrawn, categories that mapped loosely onto the psychoanalytic concepts of neurosis and behavior disorder. Although journalists tended to describe boys in RTCs as bad and girls as quiet, images that circulated more broadly in popular culture, in reality these categories were far less gendered. Betty is a perfect example of the shortcomings of this model. Her truancy and aggression, typical of the delinquent boy embraced by the popular media, did not correspond to her classic "neurotic" tendencies to wet the bed or stare into space. Despite its imperfections, this diagnostic system helped residential treatment professionals sort children by their patterns of behavior, which they then hoped to trace back to dysfunctional patterns of family interaction.

As for Betty, the girl's troubles were traced back to "severe emotional deprivation in early life" from both her negligent parents and her unkind foster mother.[150] For over two years, the staff worked to teach the girl that she was loved and accepted. The close relationships with staff members like her "docie" Dr. Krug and "Crumy," her social worker Bernice Crumpacker, were a critical element of the process. Sorting out which staff members did what, though, could be difficult for children. Betty often asked, "'Who does what around here?' and seemed to have difficulties accepting somewhat different relationships with staff members."[151] As we will see in the next chapter, RTC professionals themselves often had trouble making the same determinations. Thrown together in a new kind of mental hygiene experiment, many would find themselves playing roles somewhat different from what they had imagined.

THREE

Playing by Ear

Looking back on his years as the head childcare worker at Southard School from 1949 to 1952, Ed Love reflected that "it was a very upbeat time at the school. The staff worked well together and we all felt like we could conquer the world."[1] William Goldfarb, a psychiatrist at the inpatient Henry Ittleson Center for Child Research in New York City, similarly remembered that the 1950s were "a period when there was a kind of elated feeling that the residence could cure the psychotic child."[2] These nostalgic sentiments mirrored statements RTC professionals had made in the early days of residential treatment as well. At the 1954 annual meeting of the American Orthopsychiatric Association, Bellefaire's director went so far as to label optimism "the essence of residential treatment itself."[3] And yet, some professionals argued that this unbridled optimism ought to be tempered by caution. While residential treatment seemed to provide a new solution for children previously deemed untreatable, Hawthorne Cedar Knolls' former director Herschel Alt warned in 1960 that "we are in a romantic mood about its possibilities, and do not recognize the limits of treatability of some children, even with the best methods at our disposal."[4] Even though residential treatment offered new hope, Alt worried that RTC professionals had begun to ascribe "almost magical qualities" to it and would lose sight of the fact that some children were simply incurable.[5]

Alt's concerns reflected just how essential optimism was to the identity of RTC staff members, who felt that they were embarking on a new venture that demanded flexibility and a willingness to experiment. Child guidance clinics had depended on the triad of psychiatrist, psychologist, and social worker, each of whom operated within strictly prescribed roles, usually with the psychiatrist as the leader.[6] At RTCs, these roles became less defined and hierarchical as social workers expanded their roles and often became

RTC directors and psychotherapists. Completely new to the team were residential workers, a set of staff members whose only training occurred onsite yet who spent more time with the children than any clinical staff member. Low salaries and challenging work made the job unappealing, and clinical staff members struggled with the possibility of professionalizing these workers in order to create a more qualified and unified staff. Many formal and informal methods of communication were instituted to facilitate the integration of RTC staff members, from didactic conferences to record keeping and informal mingling. However, tensions between professional and nonprofessional employees remained. Residential workers felt unappreciated by psychiatrists and social workers who ignored their hard work and made impractical suggestions. Despite these tensions, a sense of team spirit pervaded many RTCs, where staff members felt determined to confront the challenge of treating severely emotionally disturbed children.

For the sake of clarity, I will use the term "RTC professionals" to refer to those with graduate training, including psychiatrists, psychologists, nurses, and social workers. "Staff members" is a more inclusive term that will represent both RTC professionals and "residential workers," the nonprofessional individuals who cared for children around the clock. Finally, "employees" will refer to all individuals who worked at an RTC, including ancillary workers like plumbers and gardeners.

Must Work Well with Children

The professional environment of an RTC was predicated on the notion that every staff member played an important therapeutic role, regardless of his or her educational background or previous experience.[7] "There are no individuals on our staff whose roles are considered ancillary or adjunctive—the very words being forbidden," explained Southard's director, psychiatrist Robert E. Switzer.[8] Instead, administrators generally believed that any staff member had the potential to interact with a child therapeutically. "At times the ward secretary or handy man may play a valuable therapeutic role," noted members of the University of Michigan's child psychiatry inpatient unit.[9] Typically, observed one psychiatrist, children understood very well who was in charge but nevertheless formed close relationships with whomever they related to best, whether it was the elevator operator or the kitchen maid.[10]

Administrators worked hard to cultivate these relationships.[11] At the Lakeside Children's Center in Milwaukee, the director strove to keep the population of children under forty-five so that staff members, including "the case workers, the house mothers, the cooks, Jim Nelson, the maintenance man, and me" could get to know them well enough to "develop meaningful relationships" with them.[12] These efforts were also reflected in hiring practices. In one particularly detailed social work thesis, Hipolito Bravo studied the roles and desirable qualities of every staff member at Hawthorne Cedar Knolls, from the director to the supply supervisor, porter, carpenter, and chef. While he predictably described training qualifications for positions like psychiatrist, psychologist, and social worker, Bravo also specified that the laundry worker "must be able to relate well and work satisfactorily with children" and that the chef "must be emotionally mature and be able to handle and work with boys."[13] Bravo also noted that the chef worked with children in the kitchen and that the carpenter was responsible for leading boys in a workshop, giving these employees an opportunity for direct interaction with the children.[14] This kind of detail, which Bravo collected from Hawthorne administrators, suggests that every staff member, no matter how minor, was considered therapeutic. These relationships had such high stakes, explained Bradley superintendent and psychiatrist Arthur Ruggles, that they could have detrimental effects on a child's progress as well: "Why, we even worry about the carpenters and electricians who work around the school. . . . A painter in a corridor can say the wrong thing in the wrong way to a child and undo months of work."[15] Such comments appear today as exaggerated but reflected the earnest belief many administrators shared that all staff members had the potential to play a therapeutic role.

In some cases, people playing seemingly minor roles could become beloved and valued community members. In 1952, the Bellefaire newsletter interviewed the institution's head seamstress, Margaret Schwartz, who had emigrated from Nazi-occupied Austria, where she had escaped death by sewing army uniforms. Schwartz explained that she enjoyed her job because she loved children and had none of her own.[16] As a seamstress, the article explained, Schwartz did more than sew on buttons. When a boy stole some clothing from the supply room, she did not accept his subsequent apology, telling him, "You didn't hurt me by stealing. You hurt yourself."[17] Instances like these allowed Schwartz to engage with children in a meaningful way and made her one of the most popular people on the campus. "Through this close contact with every youngster," the article explained, "Mrs. Schwartz' desk drawers are overflowing with letters and pictures from children who have left the campus. They all address her as 'Ma.' She probably knows more about these children than anyone at Bellefaire."[18] Not all plumbers, chefs, and seamstresses were like Mrs. Schwartz. This article was written for a newsletter that was sent to community members, donors, and potential donors and probably does not reflect the relationships most children had with staff members in ancillary positions. Still, it suggests that for some children, the most important people in their lives were not those with the most training or experience but those in seemingly minor or supportive roles.

Who Are All These People?

In a booklet to welcome new children, written by children on the Bellefaire Campus Council, a child named Mignon introduced the staff members: "Cottage parents, caseworkers, group workers, dieticians, maintenance, staff, sewing room people, resident director, cooks, librarian, office staff, psychiatrists, psychologist!!! Who are all these people? What do they have to do with you when you come to Bellefaire?"[19] In February of 1952, there were forty-one clinical staff members for the eighty-one children living at Bellefaire.[20] Similarly large staff to child ratios existed at RTCs of all types.[21] During their stays, children at RTCs would gradually come to meet the large, varied cast of characters who would be caring for them over the next several months or even years.

Directors of RTCs, whom many children would come to know quite well, were typically psychiatrists or social workers. The two were about equally likely to serve in this position, but each institution tended to appoint one kind of professional, typically driven by its history and sources of funding. For example, child psychiatry units at academic medical centers like Langley Porter (part of the University of California at San Francisco) or the University of Michigan were directed by psychiatrists, whereas those run by philanthropic organizations, like Hawthorne Cedar Knolls, Bellefaire, and the Evanston Receiving Home, were directed by social workers.[22] Professionals disagreed about who was best suited to run an RTC. Predictably, the predominantly psychiatrist participants at the 1956 American Psychiatric Association conference concluded that they were most qualified for the job.[23]

Social worker and CWLA executive director Joseph Reid suggested that RTC leadership ought to be shaped by an institution's character. Since social workers took a more pragmatic approach to administration and treatment, he argued, they should be in charge of programs that emphasized treatment. Psychiatrists, with their specialized training, could then take the lead in RTCs that emphasized research and training.[24] In reality, this reflected how RTC directors were actually distributed. At Hawthorne Cedar

Knolls, funded by the Jewish Children's Bureau of New York City, the emphasis was on service to the local community and the director was a social worker. At Southard School, part of the highly regarded academic training and research center the Menninger Clinic, the director was a psychiatrist. This division of labor reflected each profession's distinct goals. Because child psychiatry was still a relatively new profession, training was largely focused on producing leaders who would use research to move the field forward. In comparison, social workers had always framed their profession as one that provided service to the community.

In the child guidance clinic, the triad of psychiatrist, psychologist, and social worker was revered as the standard unit of professional service.[25] Each had a prescribed role, "with the psychiatrists examining the child doing a mental status [exam], with psychologists testing the child, and the social worker evaluating the family," as Bradley director Maurice Laufer remembered.[26] At RTCs, staff members arrived from a wide variety of backgrounds, not all of which included child guidance. Furthermore, they worked together in larger, more flexible teams. Still, this professional trinity played a central role at every RTC.

The close relationship between the residential treatment and child guidance movements was evidenced by the large number of RTC psychiatrists who had previously worked in child guidance clinics. Two consecutive Southard directors had worked or trained at the Denver Child Guidance and Mental Hygiene Clinic before moving to Topeka.[27] Reynold Jensen and Spafford Ackerly, who founded RTCs at the University of Minnesota and the University of Louisville, respectively, had spent more than a decade working at child guidance clinics they had founded at those same universities.[28] Before that, Ackerly had done research with William Healy and Augusta Bronner, the founders of the child guidance movement, and Jensen had spent a year at their Judge Baker Child Guidance Clinic.[29] For Jensen, the impetus to start the inpatient Children's Psychiatric Hospital came from failed attempts to work with children who were too sick to be treated at the outpatient child guidance clinic.[30]

Other RTC psychiatrists arrived from a variety of practice settings. Lauretta Bender and Frank Curran both trained in adult psychiatry and neurology before arriving at Bellevue to work with children, and Spafford Ackerly had even spent several years as clinical director of Worcester State Hospital in Massachusetts, where there was no children's ward.[31] Others had spent time on the staffs of other RTCs; the University of Michigan's Ralph Rabinovitch and his wife, Sara Dubo, had both trained with Lauretta Bender at Bellevue, and Salvador Minuchin had trained at Bellevue and subsequently worked at Hawthorne Cedar Knolls and Wiltwyck in Esopus, New York.[32] Notably, few RTC psychiatrists came from training schools.[33] This is not surprising, because RTC professionals saw their project as developing in direct opposition to the punitive, custodial tradition of training schools and aligning more with the psychiatrically minded, progressive approach of child guidance.

Psychiatrists at RTCs typically participated in at least one of three tasks: administration (as directors), psychotherapy, or part-time consulting.[34] Frequently, female psychiatrists like Othilda Krug of the Cincinnati Child Guidance Home and Lauretta Bender of the child psychiatry unit at Bellevue Hospital served as RTC directors.[35] This reflected the strong presence of women in the developing field of child psychiatry. In 1956, women comprised 31 percent of the membership of the American Association of Child Psychiatry—a sizable proportion compared to the less than 9 percent of American psychiatrists and 6.1 percent of American physicians who were women.[36] It is especially impressive that these women were not only physicians but had also assumed leadership roles in many cases, a situation made possible by the newness of residential treatment as a professional venture.

Surprisingly, pediatricians did not usually work alongside psychiatrists at RTCs. There were some exceptions; Bradley Hospital's director, Maurice Laufer, was a pediatrician who was simultaneously training to be a child psychiatrist, and Reynold Jensen trained in both pediatrics and psychiatry.[37] But pediatricians were usually part-time consultants who only cared for children at RTCs when they became physically ill. Their absence from staff rosters might seem peculiar because pediatrics and child psychiatry had much in common, at least in theory. By the mid-twentieth century, pediatrics had matured as a profession and pediatricians were increasingly concerned with the emotional aspects of their patients' lives.[38] Perhaps the most famous example of this cross-fertilization was Benjamin Spock, whose 1946 *Common Sense Book of Baby and Child Care* reflected the pediatrician's psychoanalytic training in its attention to both physical and emotional health.[39] But the two specialties had emerged separately, pediatrics from concerns about infant mortality and infectious disease, and child psychiatry from the community-oriented mental hygiene movement. There existed palpable tension between the two as some pediatricians perceived the new profession as encroaching on their specialty.[40] Explained Reynold Jensen, "The pediatrician, whether appropriate or not, had assumed the child was his exclusive territory, mental, physical, and all."[41] But child psychiatry was getting stronger. By the late 1950s, it had become a defined medical specialty. Its professional association, the American Academy of Child Psychiatry, was founded in 1952, and in 1959, the American Board of Psychiatry and Neurology created a specialty board certification for new trainees.[42]

Psychologists played a much more limited role than did psychiatrists in RTCs. They were never directors, and their role was typically limited to the same kinds of psychological testing they employed in child guidance clinics.[43] Testing might be used to understand a child's emotional state, assess his or her intelligence, or determine which occupations he or she was best suited for.[44] RTC psychologists had either a master's degree or a PhD in psychology but had little else in common with one another. Some had worked in child guidance clinics, but others had experience in other children's institutions, hospitals, camps, child welfare agencies, or even as group workers or recreational therapists in RTCs.[45]

The staff members with the most wide-ranging roles were social workers. Alternately referred to as caseworkers, psychiatric caseworkers, or psychiatric social workers, social workers at RTCs had a multitude of overlapping roles, including administrator, treatment coordinator, and individual caseworker for children and parents. As RTC administrators, social workers were in positions of authority, as opposed to their subservient or ancillary positions in child guidance clinics and psychopathic hospitals.[46] Although the profession had been largely female in its first several decades, RTC social workers were not always women. Bellefaire, Hawthorne Cedar Knolls, and High Meadows were all directed by male social workers in the 1950s.[47] As treatment coordinators, social workers regularly communicated with a child's referring agency, psychiatrist, psychologist, cottage parents or residential workers, and parents to coordinate treatment.[48] In this capacity, the social worker could inform parents about the results of their child's psychological testing, report on a child's school progress to his cottage parents, or update the psychiatrist on any pertinent changes in parental attitudes toward treatment. His or her paperwork was endless. After one Bellefaire board member spent two days at the RTC learning about the role of the caseworker there, she reported that "records are never finished, they are always added to. They require approximately one fourth of the time of the worker."[49] As Andrew Abbott has observed, social workers like these have traditionally functioned in the interstices of multiple roles, coordinating the work of many other professionals.[50]

In the role of caseworker, social workers combined aspects of psychotherapy with a more practical, problem-solving approach in their interactions with individual children and parents. On the practical side, a social worker might send update letters to parents, plan visits, or help a child who was being picked on.[51] But that same social worker could also help parents examine their attitudes toward their child and understand how their parenting styles had fostered their child's problems, as we will see in chapter 4. In some cases, they might even conduct full-fledged psychotherapy with children.

"Casework," a term whose meaning was vague and whose practice was fluid, was central to the professional identity of social workers in the mid-twentieth century. In the first two decades of the century, social work was a profession in formation, largely concerned with environmental and social forces and interested in issues of poverty and charity. During the 1910s, this focus moved away from the environment and toward the individual. Standardized in part by social worker Mary Richmond in her 1917 work *Social Diagnosis*, the new practice of casework used the medical model of diagnosis and treatment to help individual clients. Although Richmond herself continued to address social and environmental forces, two additional phenomena influenced the profession's trajectory. During World War I, social workers served alongside psychiatrists and psychologists, adopting their individualized approach. After the war, as psychoanalysis became a dominant ideology, they adopted analytic theories to better understand the individual personality. By the 1920s, casework defined the consolidated profession of social work, which had come to emphasize individualized treatment over broader social problems.[52]

Casework, however vaguely defined, was central to social workers' professional identity. Throughout these changes, social work had remained a fundamentally female enterprise. But with casework, social workers disavowed their previous identity as mere charity workers, believing they had adopted a scientific methodology that defined them as professionals.[53] Yet while casework established social work's professional identity, it simultaneously threatened that identity. By the 1930s, some social workers worried that casework, with its psychoanalytic basis, made their work indistinct from that of psychiatrists. Many argued that they had relinquished their expertise on poverty and social welfare to become psychiatry's handmaidens.[54] Others fought to distinguish casework from psychotherapy, often relying on semantic definitions of the two.[55]

Casework was a double-edged sword for social workers. Its closeness to psychiatric practice threatened its uniqueness, but its vague yet elastic definition permitted social workers new opportunities to flex their clinical muscles in RTCs. As Abbott has suggested, professions are better defined by their dynamic boundaries and attempts to define their "turf" than by their training requirements, organizational structures, and certification procedures.[56] In the case of social work, its contested boundaries were critical to its developing identity as a profession. Because of the experimental nature of residential treatment, formerly lower-ranking professionals like social workers had more latitude in how they defined their roles. No longer were they mere coordinators of care. At RTCs, they could be therapists for children and parents and could even be directors.

Like their psychiatric colleagues, social workers at RTCs came from a broad range of professional backgrounds. Child guidance clinics and general child welfare agencies, unsurprisingly, were frequently represented.[57] But other social workers followed a more circuitous route to residential treatment. Norman Lourie, Hawthorne's clinical director, was the first man to enroll at Cornell's College of Home Economics, where he took courses on child development and lived in a campus-area settlement house. Graduate work in education and then social work followed, after which he received individual psychoanalytic training. Finally, Lourie joined the army during World War II, where he was trained as a clinical psychologist and served as chief of social work, training nonprofessionals to care for psychiatrically ill soldiers. It was only after the war that Lourie found his way to Hawthorne Cedar Knolls, after an army contact helped him get a job at Hawthorne's parent agency, the New York Jewish Board of Guardians.[58] Other paths included running a state training school, doing research for the U.S. Children's Bureau, working at general hospitals, and working at other institutions for children.[59] These paths were so numerous that the participants of the American Psychiatric Association's 1956 conference on residential treatment had difficulty defining the ideal background for an RTC social worker. General experience in the child welfare field should be required, participants argued, with outpatient child psychiatric clinic experience "desirable" but able to be substituted by more general casework experience in a family or children's agency.[60] Simply put, clinical experience with children was required.

Training a New Generation

Residential treatment centers were themselves becoming fertile training grounds for social work students. Students typically spent between several months and an entire year doing field work in a clinical setting to gain practical experience, and starting in the 1940s, many started to do their field work at RTCs. Students who chose this option were more likely to be women, representing the profession's gender bias, and came from just a few schools.[61] At the end of their time, they were required to produce an original thesis, typically involving statistical or observational research based on individual case records. After graduation, it was uncommon for students to subsequently seek permanent positions at RTCs.[62] However, their exposure to this model of treatment no doubt influenced their subsequent careers and likely helped RTCs gain professional exposure.

Residential treatment centers were also a training ground for other kinds of child mental hygiene workers. Many centers prided themselves on their educational programs, hoping that their relatively small institutions would produce a new generation of professionals who could found new RTCs and work with emotionally disturbed children throughout the country. The University of Michigan's Child Psychiatric Hospital trained psychiatrists, psychiatric nurses, occupational therapists, and remedial education specialists, among others, boasting that they provided "the state . . . with a facility for training the many professional workers who are necessary to enable the state to meet its total need for caring for mentally and emotionally disturbed children."[63] Southard School's goals were even loftier, linked to the identity of the Menninger Clinic as a nationally renowned research and training center: "Southard School would be the ideal setting for training of highly skilled personnel who would in time eventually go into administrative and supervisory positions in other residential treatment centers throughout the country," explained a document listing the center's future plans.[64] While RTCs may have been small, their administrators intended for their training programs to staff a new generation of progressively oriented mental hygiene professionals.

Most RTCs also participated in constant in-service training for existing staff members. Because residential treatment was such a new venture, staff members attended frequent conferences and seminars to learn more about the children they treated and reflect on the most effective ways to help them.[65] These experiences required all staff members to participate and to accept the fact that, regardless of their previous training, they all had a lot to learn. At Bradley Hospital, all staff members were required to take part in a three-month training course to acquaint themselves with the institution's particular approach, no matter their professional background.[66] Activities like these reinforced the notion that residential treatment was experimental and even the most experienced professionals needed additional training to learn the tools of the trade.

Residential Workers and the Challenge of in Loco Parentis

For a large subset of RTC employees, in-service training comprised their entire introduction to residential treatment. These men and women had many titles, depending on the particular center at which they worked. As Hawthorne's Herschel Alt explained, RTCs that were former training schools for delinquent children called these workers cottage parents. In hospitals, they were nurses or nurse attendants. Elsewhere, their titles could include "counselor, group leader, group therapist, and residential worker."[67] They were united by the fact that they spent most of the day working alongside children, as opposed to a psychiatrist or social worker, who might see each child for only a few hours each week.[68] Although they typically had no professional training (except for nurses, whom I will discuss later), these residential workers spent significantly more time with the children than any psychiatrist, psychologist, or social worker. Many even lived on the center grounds. Their duties were specific to each institution and ranged from the practical, like setting behavioral limits and instilling good habits, to the abstract, like helping children establish positive relationships with adults and acting as substitute parents.[69]

These amorphous yet important members of the RTC staff baffled the professionals who worked alongside them, even at the fundamental level of labeling their role. The working group on personnel at the 1956 American Psychiatric Association conference could not agree on a common title, arguing that the term "child care worker" was inaccurate for those who worked with adolescents and might "imply to the worker that he should care for the child as if the child were a baby."[70] Some participants simply referred to these staff members as occupying a "fourth discipline," apart from psychiatry, psychology, and social work.[71] Their proper role in treatment was also a topic of debate. "At one extreme," explained two social workers, "they are thought of as custodians; at the other, as substitute parents."[72] Few RTC professionals took the former view, but several specified important differences between the work of a residential worker and that of a therapist. Child psychiatrist J. Franklin Robinson described the residential worker as someone with practical, rather than emotional, concerns: "His concern is not to help the child express and examine his feeling, but to help him act in relation to living requirements."[73] Othilda Krug, also a child psychiatrist, distinguished the two by the depth of their concerns. The residential worker, she explained, dealt with a child's smaller, daily needs, while the psychiatrist treated her internal strife.[74]

Although the residential worker's role remained a point of contention, many RTC professionals regularly acknowledged the important role residential workers played in the treatment process. Social workers Joseph Reid and Helen Hagan described them as "the major single therapeutic force of the entire residential treatment effort," and Bellefaire psychiatrist Oscar Markey told the institution's trustees that "the smallest amount of service comes from the psychiatrist. The greatest amount comes from the resident staff and case workers. They have learned how to care for the children in the way that the psychiatrist might have done 15 years ago."[75] In essence, those with the least training were charged with making the biggest difference.

The individuals comprising the fourth discipline had very little in common besides a lack of professional training. One 1959–60 study of American RTCs found that 62 percent of residential workers had completed college, but only 11 percent had done graduate work, compared to 98 percent of the clinical staff (psychiatrists, psychologists, and social workers).[76] Individual RTCs had different educational requirements for residential workers. At Langley Porter and Hawthorne, only a high school education was required, but at the Children's Service Center of Wyoming Valley and Southard School, a college degree was necessary.[77] Residential workers had typically sought out their jobs for one of a few reasons. While some wanted to be helpful and work with children, others hoped to rectify their troubled childhood experiences or simply make a living.[78] At Southard, most of the residential workers hoped to one day enter the child welfare professions. Lillabelle Stahl, who was a recreational therapist there from 1941 to 1943, was recruited to Southard from a psychology class at Washburn University alongside her friend Donna Testerman.[79] Stahl would stay at the Menninger Clinic as a secretary for the rest of her career, while Testerman went on to a career in social work.[80]

For most of these men and women, training would begin on their first day of work, differentiating them from the professional staff members who had completed several years of postgraduate work. For new residential workers, the world of an RTC probably seemed very confusing and full of new and unusual rules and philosophies. One 1960 episode of the CBS docudrama television series *Armstrong Circle Theatre* followed the experiences of the fictional Martie Clyde, a new counselor at Bruno Bettelheim's Orthogenic School in Chicago. When Clyde first arrives at the school, fresh from college but recognized by the director as having "great potential," she is nervous and has no idea what to expect. Her apprenticeship experience, the narrative explains, will be four months long and will require her to adjust her own behavior and expectations to match those of the school. Her first jolt comes early, when a shy, mostly mute boy named Wally realizes his mother has left him at the school without saying goodbye. When he shouts "Mama!" and tries to run for the door, Martie's first impulse is to hold him tightly and comfort him. Another counselor quickly breaks the two apart as Bettelheim explains to the boy that his mother is gone but that he is welcome to go confirm her departure for himself. After the boy runs off, Bettelheim explains to Martie that Wally's outburst provided an important opportunity to show him that the staff trusted him to go look on his own.[81] Martie is not expected to know this already; instead, it is assumed that she will observe how the school's particular milieu functions and adapt her behavior appropriately.

Although lessons like these could only be learned by experience, RTCs also provided intensive didactic curricula to teach new employees the practical and theoretical aspects of their new jobs. This in-service training might include seminars on psychology or psychotherapy, case conferences in which a single child was discussed by clinical staff members, and one-on-one consultations with clinicians.[82] In addition to working directly with children at the Orthogenic School in the *Armstrong* episode, Martie also attends a conference in which the entire staff discusses treatment plans for individual children. When Martie suggests that it might be time to separate the mute, inwardly directed Evelyn from her doll, which she clutches all day long, Bettelheim warns her that doing so right now will just make Evelyn hate Martie and will have limited therapeutic benefit.[83] In interactions like these, new workers could test out their ideas among more experienced staff members and learn skills for working with this challenging population. In these more didactic elements of training, practical competence was an important goal, but so was gaining a basic grasp of the psychoanalytic theory that underlay the approach of most RTCs.[84] This scene also establishes a clear hierarchy; it is the professionals who create and interpret the rules of the milieu, and the residential workers who are expected to follow them. Although actors portrayed Martie, Bruno Bettelheim, and the other staff members and children, the real Bettelheim delivered a short on-screen message at the end explaining that the school hoped to help children "live at peace with themselves" even if they could not achieve complete normality. Bettelheim probably served in a consulting capacity with the producers, making the episode a fairly accurate, though dramatized, representation of life at an RTC.

Although there existed no standard professional training for these workers, RTC professionals had elaborate wish lists of qualities they hoped residential workers would embody. Administrators at Hawthorne Cedar Knolls, for example, looked for candidates with "considerable experience with children" who were patient and "not afraid" of the most disturbed youngsters.[85] Applicants were evaluated on "their intelligence, warmth and understanding, their desire to help children, and their ability and willingness to learn."[86] One Hawthorne administrator even specified that an ideal residential worker "has achieved a set of personal values about which he has deep convictions but, hopefully, he does not insist on them too rigidly."[87] Ultimately, argued Bellefaire's residential director, personal characteristics mattered far more than any formal training in making a residential worker an effective team member.[88]

As much as administrators might have had these ideals in mind, residential workers who met these qualifications were not easy to find. Since residential work was not a recognized profession, there was no clear pool from which centers could identify suitable candidates.[89] More importantly, the job offered too few benefits to be appealing to many people. Wages were so low at Southard School, argued a psychologist charged with evaluating its program, "that selection of qualified persons is impossible."[90] In 1949, residential workers there earned fifty cents per hour, above the national minimum wage of forty cents but far from the seventy-five cents that would be made federal law in January 1950. By 1954, their salaries had doubled to one dollar per hour, advancing workers beyond the maids who earned only seventy-five cents while remaining relatively low.[91] At the children's psychiatric ward of Bellevue Hospital, nurses' aides (their equivalent of residential workers) earned $2,680 per year in 1956, much lower than the national average wage of $3,532.36 and far below the salaries of social workers and junior staff psychiatrists, who earned $4,500–5,900 and $7,100–8,900, respectively.[92] Added to low wages were long hours, the task of caring for extremely troubled and often difficult-to-manage children, and little or no privacy for those living in the center itself.[93]

Given these conditions, it was no wonder turnover was alarmingly high.[94] Even the best cottage parents at Bellefaire, residential director Morris Mayer observed, could only last three or four years "without losing something in their own lives and happiness."[95] The situation at Southard was even direr. In the 1940s and early 1950s, most residential workers stayed for just a few months or a year at most.[96] At Bellefaire in 1950, five cottage parents were so frustrated by their circumstances that they approached the Bellefaire Board of Trustees to discuss their salaries. Explained cottage mother Mrs. Goodman, "A cottage mother's job is most difficult. We are expected to be adequate in understanding the problems of the children as well as in housekeeping. Our starting salary is $48.86 a week. $18 is deducted for maintenance. We put in 55 to 60 hours a week."[97] At best,

Mrs. Goodman was earning eighty-nine cents per hour; the national minimum wage was seventy-five cents an hour.[98]

At Hawthorne Cedar Knolls, frustration among residential workers boiled over into a strike on February 16, 1962, when sixteen cottage parents and twenty other employees including social workers, nurses, maintenance workers and a psychologist staged a walkout. Among their complaints were "overwork, inadequate pay and dangerous conditions."[99] Although the strike ended after ten days, the administration considered closing down the center and had already moved twelve children to another RTC in the meantime.[100] A similar strike followed in March of 1964, and administrators resorted to using drugs to tranquilize the children, whom they charged were incredibly anxious and felt that they were being deserted by their parents (cottage parents in this case) once again.[101] Despite these circumstances, many residential workers remained extremely devoted to the children in their care. Remarked Southard School director John Geisel in 1946, "The income of housemothers, teachers, recreation therapists, and companions is still so small as would seem to work against the unselfish devotion that characterizes their service."[102] How could RTCs retain these workers, so critical to their vision of a therapeutic milieu but so overworked and underpaid?

The Promise of Professionalization

Administrators at RTCs were extremely concerned about this situation. Aware that they were employing a workforce of untrained individuals to perform the bulk of daily care, they suggested improvements such as increased pay, shorter hours, more thorough training, and better supervision.[103] They also debated a more fundamental question: What was the optimal role of the residential worker? At the heart of the debate was uncertainty about what, exactly, defined a professional. For some participants, the term implied a more active role in planning treatment and less subservience to the existing members of the clinical staff. For others, professionalizing residential workers required implementing standardized education and training, like the kind psychiatrists, social workers, and psychologist had undergone before joining the staff of an RTC.[104]

A few RTCs believed that residential workers were already professionals. At the Ryther Child Center in Seattle, wrote one social work student, "The house staff members are considered a part of the professional staff."[105] Child psychiatrist J. Franklin Robinson, who directed the Children's Service Center of Wyoming Valley in Pennsylvania, also included residential workers among his professional staff. Explained Robinson, "A profession is defined, in part, as a pursuit which requires study and training. . . . As we have progressed in our understanding of the technical competence required by the resident worker, we have introduced the designation resident professional worker."[106] For Robinson, being a residential worker required special training and skills, making the position deserving of a professional designation.

But for most RTC administrators, the prospect of professionalizing residential workers involved making many changes, not all of them good. Residential workers ought to be more involved in planning and executing treatment, many believed, but might this make the drudgery of small, daily tasks less appealing?[107] Surely helping children brush their teeth and make their beds would seem demeaning to individuals who were also discussing these same children's home lives and helping plan for their discharges. And if rigorous, standardized education and training were implemented, they worried, "not many people would be attracted to this field, especially with present salary levels."[108] Finally, if these newly professionalized workers kept detailed observational records like other staff members, this work "might rob their relationship with the child of some of the naturalness which is so essential for the continuous day-by-day relationships."[109] How best could the needs of residential workers and RTCs be balanced?

Residential treatment centers took two main approaches in response to this quandary, adjusting the role of the residential worker to bring it into line with that of the other staff members and implementing formal training programs for new and continuing residential workers. On a daily and weekly basis, some RTC administrators began to include residential workers in staff conferences, inviting them to share their observations and impressions of the children they spent more time with than anyone else.[110] Others stressed the importance of giving residential workers more guidance on the nuances of working with emotionally disturbed children. Staff members from the University of Pittsburgh's Children's Residential Treatment Service told the story of Mr. W., a childcare worker who had been placing a child in isolation night after night because of his relentless temper tantrums at bedtime. When the center implemented more formalized in-service training for residential workers, Mr. W. was assigned a supervisor who gave him one-on-one guidance and encouraged him to move beyond considering the "surface behavior" of the children in his care.[111] As a result, Mr. W. started to wonder why the boy was having tantrums in the first place and learned that if he let the boy wander off for a few minutes at bedtime, he would eventually return without having any tantrums at all.

"Such an 'experiment,' as Mr. W. called it, was a source of great satisfaction to him," the authors explained. "It marked his demonstrated transition from seeing himself as caretaker to that of an aware and responsible child care worker.'"[112] The key to this transition had been supervision and a scientific outlook, which the authors emphasized by referring to Mr. W's "experiment" with the young boy.

Redefining the residential worker's role was also a symbolic process, involving elevating his or her status. Simply put, the other clinical staff members had to see this new worker as their colleague, not their subordinate. "He is no longer simply a caretaker, companion, or recreation worker," the University of Pittsburgh team explained. "He has to define his role as a therapeutic agent and a central figure in the child's residential life."[113] At Bellefaire, social worker and head residential worker Morris Mayer reported in 1945 that cottage parents were the "hub of the institution."[114] Explained Mayer, "We no longer see the cottage parent as being merely a housekeeper. We see her as a person who can develop an atmosphere in which each child in the living group can blossom and grow [to] the ultimate of his potentialities."[115] Such proclamations sounded almost too good to be true; it is likely that many or most residential workers still felt overworked, underpaid, and underappreciated. Still, statements like these signified that the trinity of child guidance—the psychiatrist, psychologist, and social worker with their designated roles and internal hierarchy—was being reconstituted as a more flexible team in the residential setting.

Starting in the 1950s, a few agencies and institutions began offering formal training programs for residential workers. At the University of Pittsburgh, psychiatrist Henry Maier and his colleagues founded a training program that ultimately offered a master's degree in childcare and development through the University's School of Social Work.[116] Other programs were offered on a more short-term basis. In April and May of 1955, the University of Chicago's School of Social Service Administration and the Welfare Council of Metropolitan Chicago offered a five-week class titled Training Course for House Parents of Children's Institutions. Classes covered practical topics like techniques for working with groups of children and keeping them physically healthy, as well as a more theoretical course called "Understanding the Individual Child," taught by psychoanalyst Esther Schour. In this course, participants would learn about children's behavior and development in "unfavorable" home conditions, likely within a psychoanalytic framework.[117] Professionalizing residential workers necessitated not only providing practical training but also introducing them to the theoretical context used by the other clinical staff members.

Nurses: The Other Residential Workers

The role of nurses at RTCs was similarly in flux. At centers that were part of a hospital, nurses tended to play the role of residential worker.[118] Unlike most residential workers, nurses had established themselves as professionals since the early twentieth century. Yet as round-the-clock caregivers at RTCs like Bellevue, Langley Porter, and the Illinois Neuropsychiatric Institute, nurses were expected to draw on the same feminine nurturing qualities on which their predecessors had drawn as they formed a new profession.[119] Essentially, they were expected to act as substitute mothers during a child's stay.[120] This made for excellent press. One *Chicago Tribune* feature on the University of Michigan Children's Psychiatric Unit depicted the ward as a homey, inviting place for troubled youngsters where "the psychiatric nurses never wear uniforms, often curl up on the patients' beds for a night time story and a bit of mothering, or help with fudge making and corn popping at impromptu evening parties in the snack kitchen."[121] The image of nurses in a locked psychiatry ward making fudge and popcorn made RTCs out to be the anti-institution. Americans, journalists were implicitly arguing, took care of their children.

This marked a major change for many nurses. At the Illinois Neuropsychiatric Institute, nurses exchanged their uniforms for street clothes and began sharing meals with the children.[122] As two psychiatrists there warned, nurses at hospital-based RTCs had to adjust to a more flexible professional hierarchy. Specifically, they now had more discretion to act independently. "Ordinarily nurses are trained primarily to carry out orders," they explained, "but as therapists they must be free to react more spontaneously. They cannot wait for a doctor's orders when a child is threatening to run away."[123] At times, their role, atypical as it was, came into conflict with other staff members. At the Illinois Neuropsychiatric Institute, nurses initially clashed with recreational and educational therapists (the latter term likely referring to men and women who served as teachers on the ward), with whom their duties overlapped. In fact, tension was so high among these groups at one point that one nurse commented that the "lack of collaboration has resulted in such undesirable situations as competitiveness, sabotage, discouragement, and frustration."[124] In response, ward administrators worked hard to democratize the professional structure on the unit and move away from "a professional caste system where everyone is in competition with everyone else to prove his worth."[125] Nurses in particular were encouraged to record formal observations on a child's behavior and present these alongside their psychiatrist colleagues at ward meetings.

The result, explained one nurse, was improved morale and decreased staff attrition.[126]

Notably, both this nurse and another nurse colleague who wrote about the same issue likely served as both nurses and administrators on the ward as they both wrote articles in medical journals about their experiences.[127] In fact, RTC professionals wondered whether nurses should play supervisory roles. As Susan Reverby has demonstrated, the historical split between rank-and-file nurses and those who took on administrative roles was class based and contributed to dissention within the profession about what nursing was at its core.[128] Nurses who did not play supervisory roles likely did not publish their experiences in the medical literature, leaving questions about their experience in a two-tiered system.

Drawing outside the Lines

With an expanded staff that might include residential workers, nurses, group workers, recreational workers, teachers, and custodial workers and a novel therapeutic environment, RTCs were both able and required to establish a more fluid professional structure than that of the child guidance clinic. In the RTC, the traditional division of labor used in the child guidance clinic was insufficient for caring for more severely disturbed children around the clock. To meet these new challenges, staff members were forced to improvise, taking on new responsibilities and ceding others. Because residential treatment was an altogether new venture, one that staff members frequently referred to as "experimental," improvisation was necessary.[129] The result was a professional flexibility in which "roles kind of blended into each other," comprising "a rather shifting team [in which] membership [was] not static."[130] In 1972, former Southard School director and child psychiatrist Edward Greenwood reflected that "child psychiatry as I see it, led the way for the expanded use of personnel at all levels."[131] Indeed, it was this unique, experimental environment that allowed staff members to develop new skills and contribute to the development of modern child mental health as an interdisciplinary, team-oriented field.[132]

This flexibility became particularly important in the provision of individual therapy. At Bellefaire in the 1940s and 1950s, financial limitations meant that there were never enough psychiatrists to administer individual therapy to all the children who needed it. As a result, social workers took the reins, conducting the bulk of psychotherapy with guidance from staff psychiatrists.[133] At some RTCs, psychotherapists included clinical psychologists as well.[134] Similarly, there was also some overlap among traditionally professionalized staff members and nonprofessional residential workers. At Bellefaire, some social workers physically moved their offices inside the cottages where the children lived so they could offer "on-the-spot help to children and cottage parents."[135] This helped build closer relationships between caseworkers and cottage parents and between cottage parents and the children they supervised.[136] In the process, the social worker had become a quasi-residential worker, living alongside children for much of the day.

An especially dramatic upending of the traditional hierarchy occurred at High Meadows in Hamden, Connecticut, when Bob Evans became program director. Evans's background was atypical of RTC administrators. As a conscientious objector during World War II, he had worked for two years with convalescing children at the Children's Center in New Haven. Evans then worked at a juvenile court and at the Institute of Living, a psychoanalytically oriented psychiatric hospital where he worked with homicidal youngsters. He had no formal training in social work or any other discipline. Social worker and High Meadows superintendent Charles Leonard was so impressed by Evans's ability to take charge of the chaotic center that he sent him to a one-week seminar on directing inpatient treatment centers and subsequently appointed him program director.[137] The flexibility of staff roles at RTCs spurred some experts to declare all employees fundamentally equal. "No one is of necessity more important than the others," declared psychiatrist Charles Bradley.[138] But despite such proclamations, stark differences remained among clinical and nonclinical staff members with respect to status and salary. Though child guidance expert Abraham Simon decreed that "the worth of all staff members is potentially equal" at an RTC, he also warned that salaries did not necessarily correlate with worth.[139] These discrepancies would not go unnoticed by either party.

United but Divided

Ideally, RTC administrators hoped to integrate their heterogeneous staff into a seamless whole. In a variety of settings, RTC staff members wrote about the importance of using teamwork to integrate the institution's many functions. One social work student described the Ryther Children's Center as embracing an "integrated concept of treatment," and a Southard School manual titled *Handbook for Parents* explained that group living, psychotherapy, and education at the school were "not separate entities, but one integrated process . . . brought together . . . by trained and skilled staff who are simultaneously and consistently acting together as a team."[140]

This theoretical team-based ethos was so strong that two psychiatrists attributed the emergence of team-based medical treatment to the work done in RTCs.[141]

Attempts to integrate the work of staff members took place on many levels, some more formal than others. In a 1961 talk, Southard director Robert Switzer enumerated forty-one different ways staff members interacted, from conferences and seminars to record-keeping, discussions over coffee and in hallways, and "psychiatrist visits with kitchen, housekeeping and maintenance staff."[142] Most RTCs relied on similar, albeit less documented, methods. Some encouraged staff members to circulate beyond their typical physical locations. Just as social workers moved their offices into Bellefaire cottages in the early 1950s, psychiatrists at the University of Michigan's child psychiatry unit made a point of being a regular presence on the ward. Two Hawthorne administrators advised staff members who were also acting as individual therapists to become part of the child's environment on a daily basis. "Treatment in an institution setting," they suggested, "offers the therapist an opportunity to become integrated in the child's world, to become a part of his reality."[143] Informal communications were also important for sharing information and cultivating good relationships among staff members. High Meadows superintendent Charles Leonard remembered trying to persuade staff psychiatrists that they could only be successful if they cooperated with the cottage parents. "Play pinochle with them. Drink coffee with them. Have a beer in town with them," he advised. "Let them know you're a real guy . . . and you will have access to the kids . . . in a way that you'll never get sitting in your office."[144] Otherwise, Leonard was implying, psychiatrists would remain firmly ensconced in a supervisory position. If integration was to be successful, the traditional hierarchy of professional over nonprofessional staff members had to be flattened, at least somewhat.

More formally, large numbers of conferences brought staff members together to share information and formulate unified plans of treatment for individual children. At Bradley Hospital, Wednesdays were reserved for reviewing the progress and treatment plans for continuing patients, followed by discussion of a single child who had been there for six weeks or was about to be discharged. In both conferences, all staff members caring for children, including the residential workers, were present. These meetings were supplemented by teaching conferences, intake conferences for new children, and psychotherapy seminars.[145] Conferences were nothing new; the novelty was in the sheer number of them and their inclusion of nonclinical staff. When Norman Lourie arrived at Hawthorne in the late 1940s, the institution was in the process of transitioning from a training school to an RTC. Conferences were limited to psychiatrists, psychologists, and social workers; residential workers and teachers were not included. One of Lourie's first actions as director was to include these staff members in conferences. "You had to have particularly the people who lived with the children, they had to be present at case conferences," he recalled.[146] Even if they were present, they most likely played a less active role than psychiatrists or social workers, who were charged with making major decisions about a child's care. Still, Lourie's inclusion of residential workers and teachers spoke to his goal of creating a more inclusive, democratic working environment.

Written records also offered a means of conveying information, especially among staff members working at different times of day.[147] At Southard, childcare workers kept a logbook in which they summarized the events of the previous shift for the workers replacing them. If a child had been particularly difficult, the worker taking over responsibility for the child would be warned, even if the two workers did not have the opportunity to communicate in person.[148] Childcare workers also posted written notes in the library to alert therapists to important developments in a child's behavior.[149] Although a total of three sets of records were kept on the children, information did not circulate freely. Childcare workers communicated their observations to therapists in writing, but a child's psychotherapy record was only visible to therapists, their supervisors, social workers, and psychologists.[150] Despite efforts to promote integration, some hierarchy remained.

Despite attempts to integrate the many functions of an RTC into something greater than its parts, many barriers remained, from high staff turnover and a high proportion of part-time employees to an unclear sense of who was in charge and tensions among staff members.[151] Even with the abundance of conferences, coffee breaks, and record taking at Southard, administrators there remained unhappy with what they perceived as a paucity of interaction across disciplines. Director Edward Greenwood complained that "what is said or done by a child or for a child frequently is not communicated in writing or by a telephone call, or face to face, with other members [of the staff]."[152] The silence between clinical staff and residential workers was especially problematic. One psychiatrist visiting Southard reported that "the child care workers were almost pathetically grateful for being told something in conference about what was going on in therapy. . . . Some of them had the feeling . . . that the communication was strictly a one-way affair."[153] These gaps in communication made it difficult to connect a child's life in the milieu with his progress in individual psychotherapy—a connection that RTC professionals felt was critical to each child's success.

Unfortunately, tensions between residential workers and clinical staff members were common. Oftentimes, staff performing psychotherapy embraced their position at the top of the totem pole in ways that frustrated their colleagues, particularly when they believed "they [were] a cut above the other staff" and only gave "lip service to the value of milieu therapy," believing that individual therapy was what really contributed to a child's progress.[154] The divergent responsibilities of clinical and nonclinical staff also fomented conflict. When a child acted out in particularly destructive ways, residential workers might have recommended that the child be discharged, whereas the child's psychotherapist was more likely to justify the child's behavior as a means of working through deeper psychological issues.[155] One psychiatrist observed that psychiatrists and caseworkers, who saw children less frequently than residential workers, were liable to make suggestions that were "utterly impractical in the group situation," making their colleagues "suspicious and resentful."[156] Meanwhile, the residential workers who were charged with laying down the rules often felt like the children saw them as the bad guys "while the clinical staff are fairy godmothers and godfathers."[157] These tensions were at least in part due to the differential in training, prestige, and pay between residential workers and professionalized staff members.

RTC professionals recognized that the children in their care were not naive about professional discord. When staff cooperated and behaved consistently in similar situations, Krug observed, the children felt more secure.[158] Krug recalled the story of Mary, a nine-year-old girl who told her psychiatrist (likely Krug) that she felt confused "like two different malted milks in the same shaker at the same time."[159] Mary was worried that the residential worker she was closest to would be "angry or lonesome" if she spent time with the psychiatrist, a pattern the staff linked to the parental discord Mary had been exposed to at home. When the psychiatrist and residential worker convinced Mary "that neither would be lonely or angry when she was with the other," the girl told her caretakers she trusted them. Ultimately, explained Krug, she learned that it was safe to love both parents, even if they had disagreements. Although in this case the animosity between psychiatrist and social worker was imagined, real professional distrust in the RTC could affect children directly. As social worker Gisela Konopka warned, "Only if we have genuine respect for each other's competence . . . can we expect children to regain trust and respect for an adult world around them."[160] Even if there existed legitimate discord among staff members, was it fair for adults to expect troubled children to cooperate if they could not manage to do so themselves?

In the 1940s and 1950s, RTCs were exciting and challenging places to work. Their experimental nature forced professionals and nonprofessionals to come together in often-makeshift ways that resulted in both tension and collaboration. Professional discord at RTCs primarily arose between professionals and so-called residential workers, who spent the most time with the children despite their relative lack of training and experience and were paid very little for their troubles. Even with these tensions, many RTC administrators specifically noted the high morale of their employees. At Bellevue, director Lauretta Bender reported that "our general feeling is one of unity and collaboration," and at Bellefaire Morris Mayer reported that "there is a close feeling between the members of the cottage parent, casework, recreational and other professional groups[,] a feeling that we are all pulling together on the same string."[161] Even with its many growing pains, the professional atmosphere of the RTC laid the groundwork for child mental health to become an integrated, interdisciplinary field. This would become especially important as staff members tried to integrate the traditional therapy hour with what RTC professionals would later call "the other 23 hours" of the day—life in the therapeutic milieu.

INTERLUDE

Therapeutics in Residential Treatment

Lenny was not a good kid by any measure. At the age of eleven, he had begun stealing mail and committing burglaries. He then progressed to stealing cars, getting into gang fights, and robbing local businesses. At school, he got into fights with other students and slept through class—when he showed up at all. Home was not a safe haven either. Lenny was constantly shuffled between relatives, his mother was an inconstant presence in his life, and his grandmother yelled at him so much that on one occasion he even threatened her with a knife. When he was found with a stolen car containing a gun, the juvenile court agreed to send him out of state to live with relatives. When that failed and the by-then fourteen-year-old was found once again with a stolen car, the juvenile court sent him to Hawthorne Cedar Knolls in Westchester County, New York, for treatment of his "psychopathic" personality.[1]

When Lenny arrived at Hawthorne, the staff created a detailed therapeutic plan for him, taking into account his behavior and the internal turmoil that likely accompanied it. The plan was twofold: "a well-defined and limiting environmental situation with consistent, non-retaliatory handling by adults . . . coupled with vigorous psychotherapeutic effort directed at his character defenses."[2] Using individual therapy to address Lenny's internal emotional problems and a structured environment with well-defined boundaries, the staff hoped "to stimulate conflict in the boy about his behavior and his ideals, with the ultimate aim [of bringing] about [an] increase in self-control and positive change in personality structure."[3] At Hawthorne and other RTCs, a child's behavior and emotions were closely linked and treated simultaneously. As Lenny came to understand the motivations for his behavior in individual therapy, Hawthorne staff members hoped, he would also learn to adjust his behavior to group norms in his cottage, changes that would ideally be mutually reinforcing.

Lenny's treatment plan illustrates how professionals were justifying and planning treatment in RTCs throughout the country. At its most basic level, RTC professionals believed, residential treatment should offer three components: individual psychotherapy with the child, social work with his or her parents, and a therapeutic milieu, or environment, in which the child would live.[4] The three would be integrated, so that each element informed the others: "In individual psychotherapy . . . each child is helped . . . to resolve internal conflicts and anxieties. . . . At the same time, their parents are being helped by psychiatric caseworkers or psychiatrists to understand themselves, their children and their problems together. . . . To this traditional collaborative is added the unique and most important aspect of in-patient treatment, that is, 'the therapeutic atmosphere and milieu or the corrective living experience.'"[5] To most RTC professionals, these three elements formed the foundation of residential treatment.[6]

The following three chapters explore the heart of residential treatment: the treatment itself. Chapter 4 explores the role of individual therapy with children and their parents. Therapy provided a unique space for children to discuss their worries and empowered them to negotiate for their needs with the adults caring for them. For their parents, individual casework with social workers was an opportunity to address their parenting skills and the sadness and frustration of living with a troubled child. Chapters 5 and 6 focus on the therapeutic atmosphere, or milieu, which most starkly separated residential treatment centers from their outpatient counterpart, child guidance clinics. Instead of relegating treatment to a few hours each week, RTCs provided an environment for children that was itself therapeutic, so children would receive treatment around the clock. In the milieu, children would theoretically learn to function successfully in a world of social relationships so they could ultimately return to their community and to a family environment, healed by social work with their parents.

Rationalizing Therapy

Though no two RTCs were the same, etiology largely guided therapy; that is, RTC professionals structured their treatment approaches based on how they believed emotional disturbances arose in the first place. The first principle was the simplest. Since emotional disturbance was rooted in pathological family relationships, residential treatment would temporarily sever these relationships by removing a child from his home environment. As

Othilda Krug of the Cincinnati Child Guidance Home explained, "Both need a period of relief from the tension of seriously disturbed family relationships."[7] Social work student Bernice Crumpacker made a more blatant analogy to organic illness: "The placement of a child in a residential setting is comparable to removing the source of infection in order to treat a physical disease."[8] But removal and treatment of the child was not enough. Despite their physical separation, RTC professionals believed that the child remained "an integral part of his family."[9] Treating the child alone would not solve his problems entirely, because they had originated in family relationships. Instead, treatment had to involve the whole family.

At Langley Porter in San Francisco, the children's unit director believed that psychotherapy with parents "offers very often an additional therapeutic lever which may be of critical importance" and warned that even a child who had made great individual progress was likely to relapse if he returned to a home where his parents had not changed at all.[10] Hopes of treating parents were not unique to private or academic RTCs. The director of Napa State Hospital's children's unit explained in plain words that "the treatment program might be summed up as preparation of the child for an adjusted environment to be followed by provision of the adjusted environment; and if either half of the program fails the entire effort breaks down."[11] Of course, this was not always possible. Some parents were not involved in their child's life at all, troubled themselves, or unable to take time away from their jobs to participate in therapy. In situations where it was not possible to treat the parents, RTC professionals hoped to "vaccinate" the child against an unchanged, potentially harmful home environment. At the Southard School, the readjusted goal "may be to strengthen and assist him so that he can tolerate and endure some of the tensions and anxieties he previously suffered in the parent-child relationship."[12] For many children, this approach would have to suffice.

In explaining their therapeutic rationale to the public, RTC professionals stressed the importance of reversing the effects of childhood traumas. Bellefaire's spring 1958 newsletter explained that instead of teaching the three R's (reading, 'riting, and 'rithmetic), the center hoped to engage in one R—"righting," to right "the psychological wrongs that have happened to them throughout all their young lives."[13] The idea that each child had an emotional scar, visible or invisible, and that therapy should aim to discover and heal it, was rooted in the etiological notion that trauma could directly cause emotional disturbance.

Similarly, the etiological theory that disturbances could stall a child's development guided the therapeutic rationale of residential treatment. If physical and emotional development had halted or somehow proceeded out of order, residential treatment would put it back on track. Some professionals vaguely referred to the idea of helping a child develop normally or "move along a path of growth."[14] Others specifically hoped to artificially guide children through normal development from infancy onward in order to correct any gaps or wrong turns. These professionals described this process as "recapitulated" development, using an evolutionary term to describe how these deficiencies might be rectified.[15]

Although RTC professionals explained and justified their therapeutic approach based on their etiological model of emotional disturbance, in practice much of what they did was grounded in practicality. As one *Reader's Digest* article noted of the Southard School's approach in 1939, "The Southard remedy is psychiatric science, plus a kind of calm, detached common sense."[16] Theoretical models were useful to a point, but children in residential treatment were a brand new population, defined by their resistance to treatment. Much of residential treatment was guided by common sense and the employment of a broad range of treatments in the hopes that something might work. With little tradition to guide them and an especially challenging group of clients to treat, RTC staff members linked theory with practicality to create a novel therapeutic tradition.

Mind over Matter: Residential Treatment and Somatic Therapies

During the 1930s and 1940s, many psychiatrists working with adults hoped to cure the mind by treating the body using a variety of methods they called somatic therapies. These therapies initially included hydrotherapy, insulin coma therapy, psychosurgery or lobotomy, and electroconvulsive therapy.[17] In addition, a variety of new pharmaceuticals were introduced in the 1950s and 1960s to treat psychiatric problems like depression, anxiety, and psychosis.[18] All were used on the basis of the belief that treating the body could help treat the mind.

Although these treatments were widely used in large, overcrowded mental hospitals, in part to manage the behavior of severely ill adults, somatic therapies were rarely used at RTCs, with some exceptions. In the 1930s, Charles Bradley had performed pioneering work at the Emma Pendleton Bradley Home (no relation) using amphetamines to treat children with disordered behavior and restore social adjustment, wherein children behaved according to accepted social standards.[19] However, Bradley's work remained an isolated experiment. Lauretta Bender, who strongly believed in an organic component of emotional disturbance and became known for her experimentation with somatic therapies in the pediatric population, used electroconvulsive therapy to treat more than a hundred children at Bellevue in the 1940s and conducted experiments using LSD to treat children with childhood schizophrenia in the 1960s at Creedmoore State Hospital.[20] A few other RTCs employed somatic therapies, although to a limited extent. For example, in the late 1940s, the University of Michigan children's unit was using electroconvulsive therapy and insulin coma therapy and Brisbane had employed electroconvulsive therapy for four schizophrenic children.[21]

When RTC professionals convened in Washington in 1957 for the American Psychiatric Association conference on residential treatment, a unified sense of caution pervaded the discussion of somatic therapies. Frank Curran, the director of the Charlottesville Children's Service Center and formerly of Bellevue's adolescent psychiatry ward, called the use of somatic therapies "one of the most controversial aspects of therapy in working with children."[22] Even Lauretta Bender declared, "I think we are getting away from that a good deal. That was four or five years ago."[23] In preparation for the meeting, Bellevue child psychiatrist Archie Silver had compiled a detailed summary of which somatic therapies were being used at RTCs and why. The picture he painted was one of restraint and targeted use. First, he concluded that only six RTCs currently employed somatic treatments, and all did so only as one element of a larger treatment plan. Because these centers believed "that behavior is the resultant of the reciprocal interaction of biological, psychological and environmental forces," it made sense to use all three as therapeutic targets.[24] The limited, specific use of somatic therapies in RTCs was an important marker separating them from their adult counterparts, such as mental hospitals. Just as mental hospital superintendents were employing these therapies to empty their hospitals, RTC professionals were building new institutions that purposefully kept their distance from their colleagues' attitudes and approaches. Instead, RTCs would come to depend on a very different therapeutic armamentarium, anchored by individual psychotherapy and the so-called therapeutic milieu.

Defining the Endgame

Residential treatment offered an optimistic future for children who might otherwise have been sent to punitive reform or training schools. Fundamentally, RTCs aimed to restore a child to his family and "community," the latter a vague term that referred to a minimum of living in a home and attending public school.[25] Theoretically, a child would return not just to the same home he had left but to "a more stable, happier family group."[26] This was, of course, not always possible. Some children had come from foster homes or other institutions, and their parents were not part of their lives. In other cases, their families had not evolved at all. In these cases, RTC professionals focused on returning the child to "*a* family in the general community," even if it was not *their* family (emphasis mine).[27] At the 1956 American Psychiatric Association conference on residential treatment, social worker Arthur Mandelbaum reflected, "I think it is an overgeneralization to say that the goal of in-patient treatment is to return the child to his family. . . . To return him to the community, is a far better way of putting it."[28] This reasoning was adopted by the American Psychiatric Association, which declared in the published conference proceedings that residential treatment "is designed to return the child to his family, or at least to the community."[29] Realistically, many RTC professionals acknowledged that it would not always be possible for a child to resume life in his or her original family—the community would have to do.

At most RTCs, successful reintegration into the community had specific prerequisites. First, the child would abide by social norms, a goal referred to as "social adjustment."[30] RTC professionals hoped that the children they treated would go on to be "respectable, self-supporting and law-abiding citizens."[31] The first step was attending public school. Several RTCs sent most or all of their children to local public schools right away, while others gradually moved children into public schools as their behavior improved.[32] Another milestone was the ability to keep a job. Bellefaire helped children work toward this goal by giving them paid on-campus jobs in places like the sewing room, maintenance shop, or switchboard.[33] As staff members at the Evanston Receiving Home believed, the goal of residential treatment was for "the children [to] take their places as normal citizens of the community and make a contribution to it."[34] In this sense, RTCs aimed to support the Cold War notion that productive citizens could and should be bulwarks of democracy.

Beyond the practical goals of returning children to their homes and communities, RTC professionals hoped to help their children achieve a set of less tangible milestones. As Bellefaire's executive director reflected, "If we can help the boys and girls to become normal and happy children, we have experienced a fine return on the investment we are making."[35] The seemingly simple goal of producing happy children echoed throughout the writings of many professionals and was an easy message for the public to digest.[36] An article about Bellefaire in the Jewish publication *B'nai*

Brith Woman's World explained that emotionally disturbed children "basically . . . are unhappy children. And the problem for Bellefaire . . . is to make them happy again."[37] Health and happiness went hand in hand.

Despite these cheery proclamations, happiness was a complex goal requiring profound internal change. Change was specific to an individual child and might include developing self-acceptance or confidence or even learning that life was worth living.[38] "Self-identity and self-acceptance are considered basic to any positive change in a child's behavior," explained a former Ryther assistant director. Instead of aiming for an "unrealistic" cure, "the best that treatment can do for most cases is to buttress their personality, nurture their ego to the degree that they are better able to meet adverse situations and cope with reasonable success."[39] Similarly, the Southard staff measured internal change by a child's level of self-acceptance. Through establishing healthy relationships with staff members, they believed that "a child can gradually learn to live with his problems" and gain "a sense of dependable acceptance of himself as an individual regardless of his level of deviation from the norm." [40] Amid the flowery language of the Ryther and Menninger staff were two contentions: first, that the children would never be completely normal and, second, that children had to experience fundamental internal changes to improve. The first was sobering and perhaps disheartening, but admitting that the children might always be somehow different allowed staff members to focus on improving and strengthening the children rather than helping them to approximate some vague external norm.

Children at RTCs adopted the language of self-improvement and internal change too. One young girl being discharged from Bellefaire reflected that "Bellefaire helps the kids have confidence in themselves." She recalled her first days at the campus school, when she believed she had no academic promise. After she received an A on her first English paper, "I decided to see if I could get another. I did and then I knew I could do it. Now I Have [*sic*] so much confidence in myself."[41] Certainly this girl's optimism was not universal, but it is telling that her main reflection on her stay is not her changed behavior but her changed feelings about herself. Internal changes like these were crucial, but they were also difficult to attain and difficult to measure. Since such changes were individualized, a one-size-fits-all approach to therapy would not work. Instead, treatments would have to be personalized to meet the needs of each individual child, an approach that would prove demanding on a center's time and resources.

FOUR

The Special Relationship

Tommy, whom we first met in chapter 2, was a picture of contradiction. On the one hand, he was a lonely, severely asthmatic, isolated nine-year-old boy afraid of himself and the world around him. He did not interact with other children and preferred to play alone. When he first arrived at Southard School in 1949, he refused to engage with anyone besides his designated adult companions, whom he did not even allow to enter his bedroom but were instructed to stand outside and keep guard for him. He was so scared of the world around him that he was unable to cross the street separating Southard's two buildings by himself, and he so feared the consequences of his own turbulent emotions that he frequently threatened to kill himself. But Tommy was also "irritable" and had frequent temper tantrums to the extent that his parents had to stop talking to one another at all for long periods to avert a tantrum. "The parents seemed completely enslaved by the child," noted the chief social worker.[1]

Tommy's parents espoused a hands-off approach to their son, neglecting to interact with him with physical closeness for fear of damaging him. His social worker and therapist, Dorothy Wright, described them as "conscientious, intellectual, without spontaneity, shy, cool, compulsive, and at the same time eager to help their only child."[2] Their parenting skills seemed lacking, but Wright determined that they were not to blame, as "they could hardly be described as 'rejecting.'"[3] Tommy disagreed, having "come to think of his parents as being cold, critical, inescapably demanding and punishing," according to psychologist Dorothy Fuller.[4] Most notably, Tommy did not live on Earth. He told Wright that he was a Martian general, "commanded countless space ships, was out to destroy the world, sailed to faraway regions of space, destroyed stars and invaded different solar systems."[5] Rudolf Ekstein, Wright's supervising psychoanalyst, collaborated with her in several medical journals and offered his own analysis of Tommy's case as well, referring to the boy as the "Space Child."

For the next three years, Tommy would engage in intensive psychotherapy at Southard, aimed at bringing him back to Earth and mending his fear, isolation, and distrust of others. As we have seen, RTC professionals hoped to incite internal personality changes among the children they treated and foster happiness, confidence, and self-acceptance. Individual sessions with children and their parents were critical to making these changes. For children, individual therapy provided a unique space in which children and their adult therapists could interact, each interpreting the other's words and actions and, at times, manipulating the other person for his own gain. Therapists hoped to change their charges' behavior and underlying personality, while children might use therapy to express their emotions, understand and work through their problems, or exercise authority over adults.

Simultaneously, many centers hoped to engage in individual therapy (often called casework) with a child's parents. This work was intended to help parents understand their child's behavior and make practical changes to their parenting styles and attitudes so that she would return to a healthier home environment. Out of necessity, these sessions often led to discussing parents' own emotional troubles, which were inextricably linked to their children's. Although child guidance clinics had long worked with both children and their parents, RTCs hoped to heal families even when parents and children were physically separated. Although this lofty goal often remained unfulfilled, it reflected RTC professionals' determination to heal families, not just individual children.

One-on-One Time

For RTC professionals, individual psychotherapy or casework was central to inciting both behavioral and personality change.[6] Two large studies of residential treatment in the 1950s found that all of the centers examined did some form of individual therapy.[7] Therapy was performed by a variety of professionals, including child psychiatrists, psychiatry and child psychiatry trainees, social workers, and psychologists, and was generally psychodynamically oriented (based on analytic concepts).[8] This was in contrast to child guidance clinics, where psychiatrists did the majority of individual therapy with children. Among the twenty-one centers examined in one Child Welfare League of America (CWLA) study, twelve primarily used social workers as therapists, six used psychiatrists, and three used a combination of professionals including psychologists.[9] When social workers were the primary therapists, they were typically supervised by psychiatrists.[10]

Individual therapy did not look the same at any two RTCs. Children at Bellefaire spent half an hour each week talking with a caseworker.[11] Children at Langley Porter met with a psychiatrist two or three times a week for thirty to sixty minutes.[12] Children at the Illinois Neuropsychiatric Institute worked with a psychiatrist, psychologist, or social worker between one and four hours per week in a different building from the one where they ate, slept, and attended school.[13] The content of therapy also varied greatly. At the Evanston Children's Home, children engaged in traditional psychoanalytic psychotherapy in which they primarily talked with their therapist.[14] Other RTCs offered children the option of talking or playing (fig. 4.1). Since the 1920s, analysts like Anna Freud and Melanie Klein had used play to gain children's trust or help them work through feelings that

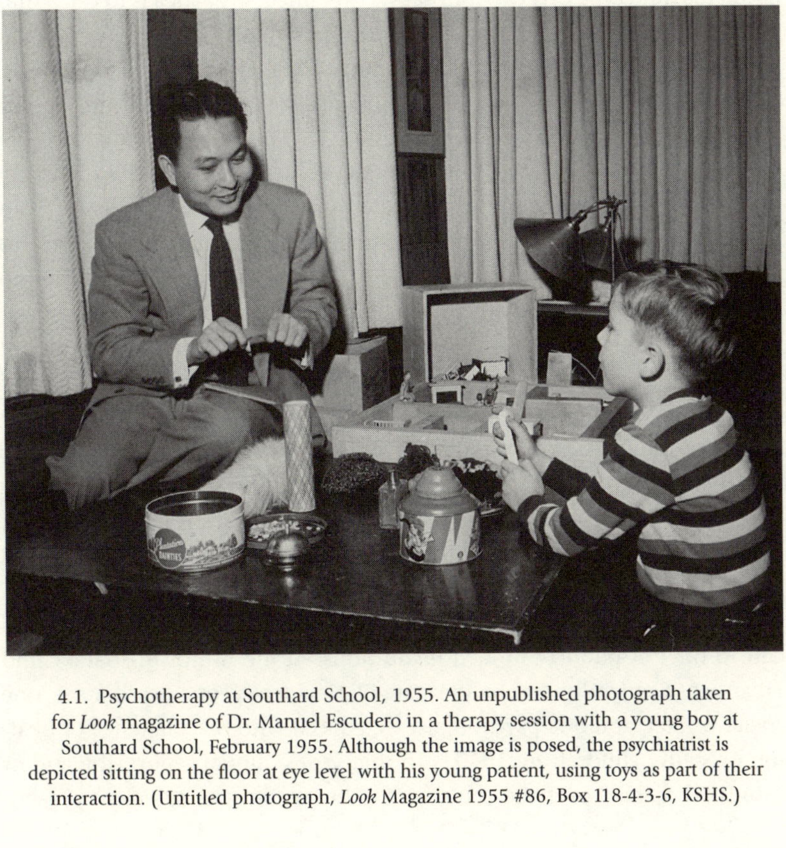

4.1. Psychotherapy at Southard School, 1955. An unpublished photograph taken for *Look* magazine of Dr. Manuel Escudero in a therapy session with a young boy at Southard School, February 1955. Although the image is posed, the psychiatrist is depicted sitting on the floor at eye level with his young patient, using toys as part of their interaction. (Untitled photograph, *Look* Magazine 1955 #86, Box 118-4-3-6, KSHS.)

were difficult to explain with words.[15] At the New York State Psychiatric Institute, the interview room was "equipped with a large variety of toys and plastic materials."[16] The psychiatry resident might talk about the child's fantasies, dreams, or even address her problems directly, but typically the child played with materials like "clay, finger paints, drawing materials [and] toy soldiers" or might even play board games with the therapist. Rather than discussing the child's problems directly, the residents hoped to use "the child's activity and comments at play . . . to understand the child's difficulties, to discuss the child's difficulties with him."[17] Playing or doing other activities of the child's choice, they believed, offered a back door to his or her emotional struggles.

Therapy might take other, nontraditional forms. At Pioneer House and later at the National Institutes of Health, Fritz Redl promoted what he called the "life-space interview," in which a child having a problem was immediately approached by a therapist or other RTC staff member to talk about his difficulties. As two journalists explained, "The idea is to catch him when he's 'hot' and able to talk freely about what he feels."[18] As National Institutes of Health (NIH) unit psychiatrist Earle Silber later remembered, the life-space interview "was an effort to really turn incidents into opportunities for therapeutic work with a child. . . . That is, if a fight ensued between two children, it wasn't just a matter of interceding, but really trying to sit down and provide some understanding of what had happened."[19] In one instance, a boy named Albert had gotten so upset that he was trying to hit, kick, and bite counselors, who had to restrain him. As Albert and group worker Joel Vernick sat quietly playing cards after the incident, Vernick "was wondering out loud what was bothering him, why he threw things and hit me when he wasn't even angry with me." Albert then revealed that he had been hiding a pocketknife. He and Vernick discussed his reasons for being upset and hiding the knife, and together returned it to the nurses' station.[20] The life-space interview took traditional psychotherapy out of the office and into the playroom, taking advantage of the child's residence to insert the individual therapeutic relationship into his daily life. This approach would be more broadly interpreted in the milieu therapy approach as well.

Individual psychotherapy was taxing on an RTC's resources and difficult to offer at publicly funded institutions. At the Arthur Brisbane Child Treatment Center, funded by the state of New Jersey, one psychiatrist, one social worker, and one psychologist were faced with the challenge of treating over fifty children by 1950.[21] In that year's annual report, the author expressed dismay over the center's inability to provide sufficient psychotherapy to meet the Children's Bureau's recommendation of three hours per week for each child.[22] It was especially difficult for the social worker to provide individual therapy, because she regularly traveled all over the state to work with parents and local child welfare agencies.[23] By October 1951, only five of the twenty-six children at Brisbane were receiving individual therapy.[24] At the Camarillo State Hospital children's unit, there was only one full-time psychiatrist who was also the unit director. Because she had so little time to do individual therapy herself, she began "to assign as many children as possible for individual therapy [to others], using social workers, psychologists, chaplains, and others as therapists."[25] Even for some private RTCs, individual therapy was very costly, and administrators used social workers instead of psychiatrists because they were more plentiful and cheaper.[26]

Individual therapy in a residential treatment center was different from what a child might receive in an outpatient, child guidance setting. At an RTC, it was just one part of a larger treatment plan, and the therapist was directly integrated with the child's daily life. A child could discuss her daily experiences with a therapist and likewise bring her insights and emotions from therapy to bear on her interactions with staff members and other children. Two Hawthorne Cedar Knolls administrators argued that "treatment in an institutional setting offers the therapist an opportunity to become integrated in the child's world, to become a part of his reality."[27] At the Illinois Neuropsychiatric Institute, children saw their therapists on the way to activities and "frequently . . . stop[ped] in the office of their therapist to sell or give her cookies they have made or to show off costumes for a play."[28] Therapists could also be a formal component of the therapeutic milieu. At the Orthogenic School, a child's therapist was often the same counselor who spent the day with his or her peer group of children.[29] At the University of Michigan children's unit, therapists spent a significant amount of time on the ward in addition to office-based therapy sessions, observing "the child in school, in shop, at meals and in play activities."[30] This informal arrangement gave them the opportunity to see how children behaved in a variety of settings, as well as a chance to get to know them outside the constraints of the office.

The unusual entanglement of a therapist with her client's daily life at RTCs could pose unexpected problems. Charles Bradley lamented the paradoxical difficulty of getting children to talk about their problems because they were relatively happy in the therapeutic environment. When they were in outpatient treatment, they arrived from their home and school environments with ample material for discussion, but when they came to his office from their groups at Bradley Hospital, they seemed to be a world apart from their troubles.[31]

Another perplexing aspect of residentially based individual therapy was the potential to break the traditionally confidential relationship between patient and therapist. This relationship was already quite different in the case of children and their therapists. In 1960, the Group for the Advancement of Psychiatry, an analytically oriented organization that researched major issues in the field and issued recommendations to colleagues, suggested that the relationship between patient and therapist be akin to that of a lawyer and his client, with confidence broken only in extreme crises like a psychotic break.[32] But in the case of children, the group argued, a parent's right to know enough "to provide for the health, welfare, and best interests of the child" had to be balanced with preserving enough confidentiality to create a comfortable therapeutic environment. As the report concluded, "The child rightfully may feel betrayed if his every thought is transmitted indiscriminately to the parents."[33] Remaining aligned with both a child and his or her parents was an ongoing challenge.

In RTCs, an additional layer of complexity arose from the involvement of many different individuals in a child's treatment. In 1956, Menninger social worker Arthur Mandelbaum described the tension between respecting a child's trust and interpreting her implicit hope that her words might be transmitted to the residential workers who cared for her on a daily basis.[34] A handbook for Menninger residential workers one year later attempted to solve this conundrum by tiptoeing around the issue of confidentiality: "The child needs the security of knowing that his deepest thoughts remain private when revealed to the psychotherapist. The therapist conveys not the confidential material, nor the content of the material itself, but the meaning of the problems and the essential implications of the child's conflicts."[35] But how could the therapist talk about the general issues that arose in therapy without betraying its substance? And would doing so preserve any level of confidentiality between the child and his therapist? In an external evaluation of Southard, one psychiatrist argued that keeping up the charade of confidentiality was naive: "My own opinion is that it is unrealistic . . . for the therapists to maintain a traditional attitude of the inviolability and complete confidentiality of all that transpires in a psychotherapeutic session."[36] Conflicts like these demonstrate how individual psychotherapy in the residential treatment setting posed new challenges, even as it created new opportunities for integrating formal therapy and daily life.

Self-Expression and Self-Knowledge

Individual therapy was predicated not on extinguishing a child's undesirable behavior but on fomenting "inner change."[37] This change could not happen unless the child felt free to express himself. In therapy, a child had an opportunity to express his emotions "in his own world," or on his own terms, through conversation or play.[38] Betty, whose story we explored in chapter 2, used individual therapy to indirectly tell her psychiatrist how much she hated her foster mother (according to Dr. Krug) when she pointed to a drawing of the foster mother and said, "She looks mean, doesn't she?"[39] Stephen Eliot, who chronicled his childhood at the Orthogenic School thirty years later, played with his therapist's dollhouse during his interview hour before he was comfortable enough to initiate conversation. "In much of my play with the dolls," he remembered, "the mother doll was vain and preoccupied, fed her children with a bottle of glue, and often chopped their heads off with a room divider in the dollhouse that was loose on one side, so I could swing it up and down, thus making it a guillotine. The father doll could use the guillotine, too."[40] To Eliot, these actions represented his feelings toward his mother. But just as words could be interpreted in many ways, so could play. In her notes on Eliot's therapy session, analyst Margaret Carey described the mother figure as "not mean to the children, she was just somewhat indifferent."[41] Just because a child was expressing himself did not necessarily mean the therapist understood what he was saying.

Self-expression could also take the form of behavior or comments that would otherwise be socially inappropriate. Betty called Dr. Krug a "dirty rat" and a "bitch," and told her, "You don't like me because I hate you. All the women can go to hell."[42] Richard, jealous that his therapist had begun to treat another boy at the Orthogenic School, tested the limits of the therapist's patience by throwing candy wrappers all over the floor of her office and stomping on her coat.[43] Because testing a therapist's limits was considered part of a child's natural response to therapy, residential treatment experts advised therapists to remain neutral and merely try to understand the child's behavior.[44] Instead of getting angry, Richard's therapist commented, "I wish you'd tell me what you're angry about. You're stepping on my coat but I can't tell from that what's really the matter."[45] As Richard's therapist demonstrated, self-expression was always mediated through the therapist, who would interpret the child's behaviors and comments as they emerged. As one social work student explained, "The worker may carry on a monologue suggesting how the child might feel, thus giving the child permission to express and feel his own ideas and fears."[46] This narrative would ideally both describe what the child was doing and empower him or her to discuss the behavior in question.

Through these verbal and nonverbal exchanges, therapists hoped to help children sort out their unconscious conflicts and gain insight into their own feelings and behavior. They hoped that therapy would help children learn to examine their own feelings critically, understand the motivations for their behavior, and observe the effects of both on their relationships with other people.[47] A 1950s handbook for parents of children at Southard School explained the process in simple terms: "As the child plays or talks, he comes to feel that he is understood in a unique and special way. This understanding is used by the therapist to help the child know himself better, to learn the origins of his feelings, the meaning of these feelings, the connections between his feelings and his behavior, and most of all to experience emotional relief which gradually leads to the possibility of healthy change."[48] The therapist served as a guide to the child's journey toward better self-understanding.

When Lenny, the law-breaking fourteen-year-old boy at Hawthorne, began individual therapy, he gave the impression that everything was fine. He regularly did his chores in the cottage, had a good relationship with his cottage mother, was performing well in school, and even played on the school's football team. But his therapist knew Lenny was not telling the whole story, and was aware of the boy's long history of rule-breaking behavior and fractured family life.[49] As former Hawthorne director Herschel Alt reflected, he exemplified the "'operator' who played all the angles,'" putting on a front of perfect conformity so the staff would discharge him as soon as possible. What Lenny didn't know was that while good behavior was important, it was not enough: "Change, as well as good behavior, is required."[50] He would have to make a good faith effort to become a better person, not just act like one.

After one year of stalemate, Lenny's female therapist left the institution and was replaced by a male therapist who decided to take a more straightforward approach to Lenny's attempts at manipulation. One day, the therapist remarked that the boy tended to smile throughout therapy and suggested he might be smiling to appear compliant and avoid thinking about his real problems. Lenny, perhaps suprisingly, admitted the therapist was right, saying "he smiled so that the worker should not know what he was thinking." He spoke of "weak" and "strong" fronts that he used to interact with adults. "When he was with adults he used the weak one—ingratiation and compliance—so that they would think he was a nice guy; when he was with his peers, he used the tough front."[51] Only after Lenny had acknowledged his tactics (or defense mechanism, in the language of his treaters) was he able to make significant progress at Hawthorne. He stopped trying to act tough in front of his friends, opened up about his feelings of helplessness, and reined in his behavior so much that he was discharged and sent home, where he successfully attended school and found a job. These changes were not easy—personal uncertainty about whether to move in with his mother and the nagging responsibility to check in with his social worker once a week remained hurdles. But the staff felt that Lenny's progress would not have been possible had not his therapist pointed out his defense mechanism and had Lenny not acknowledged it.[52]

As in Lenny's case, therapists had well-defined goals for individual psychotherapy, but could not accomplish them without the child's cooperation. Staff members expected children to take responsibility for attending their appointments.[53] At the Orthogenic School, group counselors would remind children about their appointments the first few times, but then expected children to remember and attend therapy by themselves. For children who could not tell time, counselors might draw a clock face indicating the appropriate therapy time. "Either attending or avoiding the individual sessions remains the responsibility and the privilege of the child," explained Orthogenic School director Bruno Bettelheim. "Even our most disturbed six-year-olds are well able to come on time if they really want to . . . it is always up to the child whether he wishes to go or not."[54] Southard School took this responsibility to an extreme, waiting to commence therapy until a child asked for it.[55] But sometimes, children simply failed to show up. At the Evanston Children's Home, some avoided therapy by dawdling on the way home from school.[56] At the Bradley Hospital, breaking appointments was common, but therapists tried to talk with children to determine why they had skipped the appointment.[57] To account for this lack of predictability, therapists had to be flexible, keeping the child's hour open even if he or she arrived late, or seeing a child at a different time if he or she requested it.[58] This approach to therapy characterized the larger philosophy of residential treatment: children were autonomous human beings who should be given the same respect and consideration as adults. Rather than judging or punishing children who skipped their appointments, therapists expected them to take responsibility for their own treatment.

Psychiatrists at the National Institutes of Health's child psychiatry unit learned about the process of negotiating with their therapy clients the hard way.[59] The first children on the unit arrived for short diagnostic stays of three to eight months, and therapy initially seemed impossible because the psychiatrists were busy dealing with runaways and children who were physically attacking one another. When the psychiatrists started to bring the children to their offices for thrice weekly interviews, the children refused to come. First, the psychiatrists assumed the children were just too delinquent for therapy but gradually realized the children did not trust them because they were only there for short periods of time and they worried that the psychiatrists, who were also administrators, might "tell on them" to their family or the other ward staff. To partly resolve this issue, the psychiatrists abandoned their administrative roles in favor of purely therapeutic ones, but the struggle was hardly over. When the second group of children arrived on the unit, also for short stays, therapy was moved to one predetermined hour after lunch to not interfere with other activities. Still, children resisted therapy. Two unit psychiatrists remembered: "On some days the appearance on the ward of three to five therapists at the beginning of Therapy Hour became a signal for the group of youngsters to hide. Not infrequently the whole therapy hour was spent in a teasing hide-and-go-seek. . . . Sometimes four or five children were giving their therapists the run-around in and out of bedrooms, down the corridors, or in the dayroom. It became part of the group code [among the children] that 'you just don't go off alone with your therapist.'"[60] The milieu of RTCs not only helped adults collaborate with children in nontraditional ways; it also enabled children to bond with one another and avoid the grownups, if they wanted to.

When the third group of children arrived for longer-term treatment in the fall of 1954, the psychiatrists had playrooms built specifically intended for therapy. They assigned three hours of the day to individual therapy and had group counselors escort individual children to and from the playrooms. They observed with relief that the children "have expressed themselves with surprising freedom in the playroom, in their use of competitive games, with plastic art materials, in doll play and histrionic make-believe, and even in words."[61] It also didn't hurt, they believed, that the children knew their stays at the treatment center would be longer and were less hesitant to form a relationship with their therapist. By observing the children's behavior and responses to therapy and through trial and error, the psychiatrists had constructed a treatment plan that the children were excited to engage in. Though they had initially felt completely helpless and deferent to the will of the children, these professionals had regained a sense of control by constructing an environment that enlisted the children's cooperation.

How did children perceive individual therapy? Narratives of their experiences are few, but there was unsurprisingly a range of reactions, from devotion to outright resistance. In the handbook Bellefaire children wrote to welcome new children, they praised their caseworkers: "It is through your regular visits with them that you have a chance to tell all your problems to someone who can help you. Your caseworker is a special person you can always count on."[62] Stephen Eliot's therapy sessions with Dr. Margaret Carey at the Orthogenic School began when he was eleven and gave him "a sense of sanctuary . . . I needed some protection where I could talk without fear of repercussion. I needed space from everyone . . . and Margaret gave it to me."[63]

But while telling another person all his problems was easy for Eliot, it could be strange and difficult for other children. Lee Stringer, an author who reflected on his stay at Hawthorne Cedar Knolls in the early 1960s, remembered that he liked his caseworker, Mrs. Mendelsohn, so much that he didn't want to trouble her with his problems and usually said he felt fine. "I know I'm supposed to tell her stuff," Stringer reflected as if he were reexperiencing his childhood. "She being my caseworker and all. But it's a hard thing for me to do. There are all sorts of things I think when I'm with her. But don't say. You could probably fill a book with them."[64]

Many RTC professionals did fill a book with them—or at least very long case studies in medical journals. Tommy, the boy at Southard who believed he was a Martian general, was the subject of extensive scholarship and debate; he was the subject of three medical journal articles and an interdisciplinary presentation and discussion at an annual board meeting. By taking a close look at one child's experience in psychotherapy, the complex give-and-take between child and therapist and its implications for a child's progress emerge. The professionals who recorded his story preserved a great deal of Tommy's own words and actions from therapy sessions, as well as their own thoughts and reactions at the time and on later reflection, making his story particularly rich.

The Space Child and the Push and Pull of Psychotherapy

Of his space fantasy, psychoanalyst Rudolf Ekstein concluded that "the timid, shy, and asthmatic-ridden youngster could permit himself utmost aggression only in the faraway spaces of the universe."[65] According to this analysis, Tommy's wild fantasy world helped him manage his incapacitating shyness by giving him an (imaginary) place to express himself without fear. As in this example, therapists would use both practical and psychoanalytic explanations to make sense of children's often illogical behavior. Sometimes they would share these insights with the children in order to help them understand their behavior; at other times, their conclusions were relegated to medical texts for their colleagues' edification.

In Tommy's case, his therapist's analyses of his fantasies guided his treatment. Ekstein and Wright's main concern, they explained three years later, "was with the distance between the psychological world of this faraway monster and that of the little fellow who was yearning to be loved and accepted by his parents, by the children and the teachers in the school."[66] This concern would guide Tommy's therapy, which they hoped would bring Tommy back to Earth and "crash [his] autistic defenses."[67] Both practical and psychoanalytic, their plan attacked an internal conflict (his distancing as a defense) and the practical limitations of interacting with a boy so wrapped up in his strange fantasy that he was unable to communicate on any normal level. At first, psychologist Dorothy Wright tried interacting with Tommy as though he was on Earth, but he was uncooperative. Only after she began to talk to him *as* the Martian general did he engage with her. Here, it was necessary for Wright to accept a child's perspective in order to establish any kind of therapeutic relationship with him.[68]

After several months of Martian interaction, Tommy came back to earth in the form of Oscar Pumphandle, who was talking to his therapist in Topeka, and "Tommy," who was doing atomic research in Arizona. The two allegedly did not know about each other.[69] Thus began Dorothy Wright's attempt to present her interpretation of the situation to the boy sitting in her office. First, she privately surmised that Tommy had transferred his aggressive impulses to "Tommy in Arizona," who was content blowing up atomic bombs. She then tested this theory on Tommy, suggesting that Arizona Tommy might be scared of therapy and that perhaps Oscar might quell his fears. Oscar replied that Arizona Tommy, an atomic researcher, was not afraid of anything. Testing him further, Wright suggested that maybe Oscar was afraid of Arizona Tommy (who, in her opinion, represented Tommy's forbidden impulses to act out).

The results were almost catastrophic and Wright felt that she had "loosed the uncontrollable devil."[70] Tommy began to act bizarrely and aggressively inside and outside of therapy: "The child attempted to masturbate openly during psychotherapeutic hours, began to steal and to destroy equipment, blew up car tires, expressed hate for staff members, organized gangs with other children, and turned from a timid youngster into a vicious little monster."[71] Wright did not express moral judgment but refused to allow this behavior to continue indefinitely, telling Tommy "that she would not permit him to be destructive" and that staff members would ensure that he was not a danger to himself.[72] Self-expression was encouraged in therapy, but not without limits. For better or for worse, Wright's provocative testing of the boy had clearly had a major effect on him. The metaphorical "distance" between Tommy's behavior and his destructive impulses had decreased dramatically, and he returned to Earth.[73]

Although Wright was now interacting with Tommy himself, the boy soon developed a new fantastical tool. According to him, he now possessed a time machine that enabled him to travel back to any point in history and change it. At this point in his therapy, he began to interact more with Wright. She was now allowed to travel back in time alongside Tommy, where he saved her from atomic destruction, an act she viewed as an encouraging sign of his growing positive feelings toward her.[74] Wright also believed the time machine represented Tommy's attempt to conquer his fears and anxieties by controlling history. She once again provoked Tommy, suggesting that it might be better to understand the past instead of always trying to change it. He rejected this idea, telling her to "shut up" and "keep on the subject, to make no comments that he did not want to hear, and above all, to make no comments that had to do with problems of therapy."[75] Interactions like this illustrate the extent to which children were "in charge" of therapy. Regardless of a therapist's suggestions or actions, children were free to speak and often act as they wished. Frequently, they made demands that a therapist often had no choice but to obey. For them, therapy became a place where they could manipulate adults and negotiate with them. Tommy set the terms for his therapy, at one point informing Wright that she was stuck in the land of the dead and that she could emerge only by collecting blocks from him. One block would be granted at the end of a "good" therapy session, which "was one in which the therapist would not discuss any painful psychotherapy material."[76] Wright pushed back, saying that she refused to accept his terms, but Tommy stayed his ground, informing her that "if that's the way you feel about it you will just have to stay down there, that is all there is to it."[77] For session after session, Wright engaged in protracted negotiations with her young client.

Even though Tommy seemed to be improving slowly, he still expressed doubts that psychotherapy could help him get better. "You cannot help me," he told Wright one day. "Psychotherapy will never help me. I need a mental hospital forever and ever."[78] Still, he noticed that he was changing and worried that his parents would like the "new" Tommy when they came to visit. In one interview with Wright, he expressed this concern and then said, "Well, let's dramatize that interview. I will be Mrs. W. and you will be Tommy."[79] In the following exchange, which was reprinted in its entirety in a journal article, Tommy both took control of the therapeutic exchange and demonstrated the insight he had come to acquire about his own progress:

TOMMY [*PRETENDING TO BE MRS. WRIGHT*]: Well, why don't you think they will like you as you are?

THERAPIST [*PRETENDING TO BE TOMMY*]: Well, the way I figure it I tried so hard to be the kind of child my parents wanted me to be and I failed and that's why I am sick.

TOMMY: Yes, there is probably something to that. How do you feel about it now?

THERAPIST: Well, I feel I have changed some and I don't know if they will like me as I am now.

TOMMY: But you told me worrying about whether or not they would like you is what made you sick before. Why don't you forget about what kind of boy your parents want and just act like you feel like acting?

THERAPIST: You think if I do that my parents will be upset?

TOMMY: Well, they will understand better when they see the social worker and she can explain to them that it is important for a boy to be himself.

THERAPIST [*PRETENDING THAT SHE WAS CRYING*]: But, Mrs. W., I hardly know my parents.

TOMMY: Of course you don't. It will take a long time for you to know them and they to know you.[80]

In this fascinating exchange, Tommy provided insight into his own problems, reassuring "Tommy" that his newfound change was positive and that his parents would ultimately understand and accept it, even though it might be difficult at first, owing to their past relationship troubles. The conversation is equally significant because it demonstrates how Tommy and Mrs. Wright understood each other's established roles in therapy and were able to change places and anticipate what the other might say. Individual therapy was a peculiar format in which adult and child occupied predictable roles but also participated in constant negotiations. Each could set the terms of discussion, and the limits of socially acceptable behavior were temporarily ignored, making this negotiation possible. Individual therapy thus epitomized the approach of residential therapy, which took children and their point of view very seriously.

Wright and Ekstein sounded deft and sure of themselves in their analyses. But they did not feel that way at the time. As Ekstein remembered in 1989, Tommy was the first case he supervised at Southard School: "'The Space Child' opened a new world for me. In the beginning it was trial and error. . . . I had to live myself into the worlds of both the therapist and the child."[81] Ekstein's comment is a potent reminder that while academic theories and careful planning guided residential treatment and the individual therapy it involved, an atmosphere of perpetual experiment persisted. Writing up case studies for publication or presenting them at national meetings provided avenues for RTC professionals to analyze their work, formulate theories and practical recommendations, and present them to a like-minded audience. When Wright and Ekstein presented Tommy's history at the American Psychiatric Association's national meeting in 1952, prominent child psychiatrist and psychoanalyst J. Louise Despert provided commentary, critiquing Wright's initial hesitancy to engage with Tommy's space fantasy as "unnecessary stalling."[82] This commentary was then published alongside the case history in the *Bulletin of the Menninger Clinic*, which was not intended to serve as a definitive guide to inpatient therapy with schizophrenic children (the authors openly admitted they did not have all the answers and continued to work with Tommy in therapy) but as a practical example from which other practitioners might draw their own conclusions.[83]

Parents as Patients

Archival and published records do not reveal much about Tommy's parents' involvement with Southard School. Ekstein explained several decades later that Tommy's parents lived out of state and that his father committed suicide at some point during Tommy's ten years of psychotherapy with Wright, which must have been a great blow for a boy who already felt so rejected.[84] Most Southard parents were actually quite involved in their child's care. During the 1950s, Southard increasingly asked parents to participate in individual interviews with caseworkers when they came to visit their children. These interviews, staff members hoped, would allow parents to grapple with "such problems as separation from the child, their difficulties in relationship to the child, a review and understanding of the treatment progress, and . . . a thorough exploration of the parents' feelings and ideas regarding having the child at home again."[85] They might also serve two pragmatic purposes: helping a family remain involved during this period of separation and accelerating a child's improvement by demonstrating that her parents were invested in her treatment.[86]

Casework with parents took place at most RTCs. According to a 1959–60 CWLA survey of twenty-one RTCs, staff at two-thirds of the centers regularly saw all parents for interviews, and the remaining third either saw some parents or referred parents for therapy elsewhere, often at the local agency that had originally recommended residential treatment.[87] Both mothers and fathers participated (mothers more so, but not significantly) and both received between twelve and fifteen hours of interviews total, on average.[88] Despite these statistics, the provision of therapeutic or even practical interviews for parents was a controversial issue. A few centers dogmatically insisted that parent interviews were essential to residential treatment. At the Children's Service Center of Wyoming Valley, children were only admitted if parents consented to interviews at least every four weeks, which was notable because most of the children there were not local.[89] Center staff justified this demand because they believed that children only existed as part of a family. Explained director J. Franklin Robinson, "A child is not an independent social unit. It operates in a family group."[90] If children's problems resulted from parental interactions, it was only appropriate that parents be treated as well.[91] Similarly, Langley Porter's director of child psychiatry argued that, because a child's emotional disturbance could always be linked to his parents, treating both in psychotherapy was vital.[92]

Officially, the American Psychiatric Association and American Academy of Child Psychiatry deemed parental involvement important to residential treatment. However, their 1957 joint report on residential treatment also acknowledged the practical difficulties of having regular meetings (therapeutic or practical) with parents "for such reasons as geographical distance, death, desertion, illness, and imprisonment."[93] At the Illinois Neuropsychiatric Institute, thirty-three of forty-one parents sampled in the late 1940s were involved in some sort of interaction with the center—a relatively high proportion.[94] However, these parents were not necessarily engaging in any sort of therapeutic interaction. Many simply spoke with a social worker about where their child might go after treatment, for example.[95] The parents who did not interact with the staff at all, one study found, had practical limitations like job conflicts or other children to take care of at home, were concerned about the stigma of becoming involved, or distrusted the center.[96] Many centers had no regular interactions with parents. At Bradley Hospital and at Bellefaire, most parents lived too far away to visit; at Bellefaire, there were too few caseworkers to have meaningful interactions with many of the parents who were available in any case.[97] At Hawthorne Cedar Knolls, administrators found that many parents were "inaccessible to case work help" and had neglected to make use of social services offered to them in the past.[98]

In the event that parents were able to meet with an RTC staff member (usually a social worker) on a regular or semiregular basis, interviews might include discussion of their role in creating the child's problems, his or her attitude toward the child's treatment, or even the parent's own emotional troubles. Most RTCs tried to keep discussion focused on the child in treatment, helping parents work "through [their] own feelings stemming from the child's engagement in treatment and [their] own involvement in the child's problem."[99] The parents of Claude, a twelve-year-old boy admitted to Langley Porter in 1949, used their interview time to reevaluate how they interacted with their son. At school, Claude bullied other children, and both students and teachers disliked him immensely. When he was admitted to the unit, he was about to be expelled.[100] In his preceding one year of outpatient treatment, his father had met with social workers fourteen times, his mother twice. During Claude's three-week stay on the inpatient ward, his parents' interviews increased in frequency, with eleven visits for his father and five for his mother.[101] Even as they were trying to help parents, social workers could be harsh and judgmental; the social worker described Claude's father as "an exacting, rigid, and punitive person . . . his attitude toward the patient was irritable and accusing."[102] But instead of suggesting analytic explanations for their behavior as they might in sessions with children, they focused on making practical recommendations. This social worker explained to Claude's father that his son's behavior was due to his unhappiness and advised that being strict with him was not a good approach. Over time, the father came to understand his own motivations better, concluding that he was perturbed by his son's similarity to himself and had thus felt compelled to be especially harsh with the boy.[103]

Meanwhile, Claude's mother, whom a social worker described as a "demure, soft-spoken, gentle appearing woman," cried during her interviews and worried about her son's troubles in school. She explained that she often felt her husband's punishing attitude toward the boy was unnecessary but did not want to cross him. Again, the social worker made the practical suggestion that punishing the boy and denying him "deserts and other pleasure [*sic*]" might not be the best approach.[104] On reflection, the mother remembered many moments in the past when Claude had felt "left out and neglected." She resolved to give him more freedom to do activities typical of his age and "became capable of letting him fight with other boys, listen to the radio and even read the funnies—all formerly strictly forbidden."[105] Just as in individual therapy with children, therapists suggested interpretations and hoped that parents would gain insight into their own behavior. But unlike their work with children, their suggestions to parents were less analytic or suggestive and more practical and prescriptive.

In these interviews, parents' own troubles were fair game for discussion, especially as they related to their children. At the Children's Service Center in Pennsylvania, the mother of eight-year-old Charles told a therapist that having her son out of the house was a relief because her two children had fought constantly but also admitted to feeling guilty for having these feelings at all. As this mother sorted out her feelings toward Charles, she began to reflect on the damaging aspects of her own past: "I was never fearful of Charles' aggression until he got older. Then, I got afraid I wouldn't be able to handle him. That's the way I felt about my father, an overpowering fear of his aggressiveness. Now I see it was my father and not Charles I've been afraid of."[106] For this mother, it was impossible to address her feelings toward her son without coming to terms with her own upbringing. These discussions were of great importance to many parents. One mother told the Lakeside Children's Center director, "I thought you'd just take children here. I've got to talk to someone about myself."[107] When she learned that she was welcome to do just that, she altered her work schedule to make sure she could attend every appointment. Another mother reflected, "I've sure changed this last year. Our weekly appointments mean an awful lot."[108]

For Mrs. N., interviews were initially a place to discuss her feelings toward her ten-year-old son Charlie, who had been admitted to the Cincinnati Child Guidance Home for "destructive and defiant behavior, fire-setting, stealing, enuresis, and learning and behavior problems in school."[109] During Charlie's prior outpatient treatment, Mrs. N. had discussed her anger toward her misbehaving son and simultaneous "feelings of utter inadequacy and of guilt" about her own parenting skills.[110] When Charlie entered the home, Mrs. N. initially criticized everything about it, from the food to the way the staff treated the children. But she did admit that things had calmed down at home now that Charlie was gone. As she became used to his absence, she reflected that being apart from him "brought her increased social and work satisfactions, growing independence from her family, and greater understanding of Charlie."[111] By the following year, she had begun to date men and bought her own car in pursuit of further independence. Despite these personal gains, she seemed less interested in Charlie than ever, stating that he was "an albatross" to her.[112] Two years after Charlie's admission, she was hoping to move into her own home, but her feelings toward her son had not changed. Despite Charlie's increased "emotional control" and "decrease in oppositional" behavior, Mrs. N. was still not interested in being part of her son's life.[113] Her caseworker noted with regret, "In summary, Mrs. N. seemed to make slower progress in her relationship with Charlie than she had with the problems relating to her parents."[114] By some measure, therapy had been a success—but not for its intended goal.

Instead, Mrs. N. found herself closer to achieving her own dreams but further away from her role as Charlie's mother.

Keeping the Family Intact

Apart from official interviews, RTCs encouraged parents to visit their children frequently, either on or off campus. Some centers held weekly visiting hours on the weekends, and many encouraged children to visit home as soon as they were ready.[115] For children whose parents lived too far away to visit, staff members encouraged parents to stay in touch with regular letters to their child.[116] These visits and letters played an important role in treating "the whole family" and were an important antidote to fears that institutional care would deprive children of parental love.[117] "Knowing what you are doing and what is going on at home reassures him that he is still a member of the family and that everyone remains interested in him," explained a Menninger handbook for parents.[118] Children at Bellefaire, many of whom came from far away, were apt to experience "fear of abandonment: the fear that his parents and family have completely renounced him and that there *is no one to whom he really belongs* and no one who really cares."[119] Keeping in touch with parents by any means was an an important antidote to these feelings.

Parental contacts were also considered a part of the child's treatment plan. As a child changed away from the home, returning there could be a litmus test. How did his "new self" function in a familiar environment? Had the home environment itself changed? If individual interviews helped parents reevaluate their child's troubles and learn new parenting skills, home visits gave them opportunities to test these skills.[120] For one thirteen-year-old boy with a "severe hysterical tic," treatment was in part intended to help him learn to be independent. When he returned home for a weekend, his mother reported that in one instance "Tom came running into the house complaining that another child hit him. My husband took the attitude of trying to protect him, but I told him that was not the thing to do. Tom had to go out and face the situation for he has to learn to take things and meet his own fear." Her handling of the situation reflected the work she had done in her own interviews. Previously, she might have acted as her husband did. But the social worker had led her to see that she needed to let Tom make his own mistakes. On telling this story to her social worker, Tom's mother reflected, "I think I'm changing too, don't you?"[121] The home visit had served as a test for both mother and child, allowing them to try out new skills and see how far they both had come.

When visits were over, parents and children could report back to staff members on their experiences, which served both as a metric of progress and new material for therapy. For Cindy, whose mother seemed uninterested in caring for her, visiting her formerly estranged father's house was the first step toward joining a new family. Although her mother attended only a few casework sessions, her father and stepmother became very involved in their own interviews and invited Cindy to spend Christmas day at their home. While she was there, "Cindy found her family and . . . learned they had a real interest in her happiness. The entire family was glad to see her and she returned to the Home glowing with her new found [*sic*] acceptance by the people who were important to her."[122] Perhaps more importantly, a subsequent weekend found Cindy unhappy because her father's family now expected her to do chores and behave like the other children in the family. However, the staff of the Cincinnati Child Guidance Home believed this was a sign of improvement on the family's part, as her father had been working with the social worker on being more firm with his daughter and helping the "stepmother set standards of behavior and expectations not only for Cindy but for the other children in the home."[123] At Southard, where most children were from out of state, letters provided a proxy for visits. Staff members censored mail in both directions so they could understand the developing concerns of both parents and children.[124] When social workers wrote biweekly update letters to parents, they would comment on the content of letters between parents and children to help parents "understand better what concerns, problems, or questions they [the parents] might share with the child; and . . . to know what questions, concerns and problems are raised by the child as he writes to the parents."[125] These concerns might serve as fodder for subsequent therapy sessions and treatment planning, as well as a marker of the child's (or parents') improvement.

Visits home might be a valuable part of the treatment process, but they were hardly vacations. "Visits home which we glibly refer to as 'vacations' are 'vacations' only in the sense that they take the youngster away from Bellefaire," commented one internal memo.[126] Instead, a visit was a "highly charged emotional experience" that required children to return to "the scene of his crime," where everything had gone wrong.[127] Home was where many children had experienced their worst problems, from pathological emotional relationships with parents to physical abuse. If home had been a happy place, going there might upset a child who felt he had missed out since being away. Children who had been at an RTC for some time might have built up unrealistic expectations about how wonderful it would be to go home, only to find that their imaginations had run away with them.[128]

On a practical level, home visits threw a wrench into a family routine adjusted to the child's absence. Parents of children at the Cincinnati Child Guidance Home had to agree to have their child at home on the weekends, which they frequently found extremely disruptive. Furthermore, families with more than one child found it difficult to pay attention to their other children during a home visit with a child whose behavior was erratic or troublesome. Siblings felt left out, complaining that the visiting child got extra attention.[129] One father explained to a social work student that "the children's anticipation of Patrick coming home is one of resignation. Patrick is a very demanding child and the others are apt to get left out."[130] And when the "celebrity" child returned home, parents felt a mixture of relief and melancholy. Parent contacts, designed to keep families intact even while children were being treated away from home, helped RTCs treat the whole family. But they also stirred up a mix of emotions for parents, siblings, and children that could be more disruptive than constructive.

Seeking Solace in One Another

Having an emotionally disturbed child was a terrible strain on many parents. One Southard School administrator reflected in 1942 that "many parents would prefer to consider their child 'exceptional' and even retarded rather than to face the fact that he is suffering from a neurosis . . . which is not related to organic deficiencies but to early parental mismanagement."[131] Despite many professionals' attempts to assuage parents that they were not to blame, parents felt guilty for having played a role in their child's problems and angry or embarrassed at their child's socially inappropriate behavior. To deal with these emotions, some parents became involved in support groups where they could share their troubles and receive sympathetic understanding. At Bellefaire, parents from the Cleveland area met once a month "to express their thoughts and feelings about placement, about Bellefaire and about their children." It is not clear if the parents themselves started the group, but the head residential worker reflected that even parents who had been "hostile and inaccessible to any contact" were helped to gain perspective on their child and his stay.[132]

In New York City, two Bellevue psychiatrists created a group for the parents of schizophrenic children, whom they noticed were especially troubled by their children's problems and yet especially reluctant to seek help.[133] In the process of running the group, the psychiatrists learned what it was like to care for a seriously disturbed child at home. Many of these parents had gone from doctor to doctor to find out what was wrong with their children and shared "common feelings of social isolation and hopelessness."[134] They had to constantly negotiate a social environment in which their children might act bizarrely or inappropriately at any time, which was not only embarrassing but infuriating.[135] Feelings like these only aroused more guilt, which was already prominent among these mothers and fathers, who were convinced they had caused their children's problems.[136] Describing their children's common behaviors and symptoms, observed the psychiatrists, proved "liberating" and helped the parents let go of "the sense of the uniqueness and insuperable guilt" they felt.[137] Group members, many of whom attended long after their child had been discharged from the hospital, began to look forward to the future. They discussed tactics for dealing with community members, like openly telling a suspicious neighbor that their child was emotionally disturbed and getting treatment. Many of their concerns had no answers, like their fears that a child would never live independently or that they might have another schizophrenic child.[138] But the group gave them a safe forum to share their feelings and know they were not alone.

Two years after the group had formed, the members began to discuss how they could become actively involved in securing resources for other emotionally disturbed children in their community.[139] These concerns would soon comprise the agenda of a new, larger group for parents, the League for Emotionally Disturbed Children, founded in New York City in 1950 by twenty parents of disturbed children.[140] Concerned by the dearth of treatment facilities for seriously disturbed children, this group of parents enlisted the professional guidance of RTC professionals and other civilian allies to fund research, create more diagnostic and treatment facilities, fund schools, and educate the public about the plight of disturbed children and their need for increased services. The league became a national organization in 1954, and by 1956 boasted a thousand members.[141] Although it is difficult to ascertain exactly who belonged to the league, its board counted prominent mental health experts like Kenneth B. Clark, J. Louise Despert, and Mortimer Sackler among its members, alongside other prominent figures like author Pearl Buck and food magnate Bernard Manischewitz.[142] Its fundraising activities, which included art exhibitions at the Perls Galleries and the Brooklyn Museum and performances at Broadway's Majestic Theatre, point to a wealthy, well-connected leadership.[143]

Echoing the work of parents in support and advocacy groups for intellectually disabled children and the civil rights movement more broadly, members used rights-based language to compare disturbed children to other children with disabilities, arguing that disturbed children "should be given a chance to enjoy the rights and privileges granted to all children in our democracy."[144] The organization achieved national notoriety, as theater fetes and door-to-door campaigns by socialites, performances at Carnegie Hall, and mayor's teas at Gracie Mansion sought to raise money for the children.[145] The league's growth and popularity was evidence not only of increasing public awareness of childhood mental illness but also of parents' creative use of groups to provide emotional support and galvanize social action.[146]

Individual psychotherapy was an integral part of healing emotionally disturbed children and their parents in RTCs. It gave children an opportunity to express their feelings without inhibition or judgment, enacting the child-centered philosophy of RTCs. By giving children a voice and taking them seriously, RTC professionals believed they could earn the trust and cooperation of their young charges. Only when Dorothy Wright chose to take seriously Tommy's fantasies, addressing him as a Martian General, speaking to Oscar Pumphandle, or going on time traveling adventures, did she believe she was able to bring him back to Earth and to his own troubled emotions. Meanwhile, interviews with parents served a complementary role, helping RTC staff members treat the entire family and create an improved environment to which a child could eventually return. Visits home, though often stressful and emotionally draining, helped parents and children test out their new selves and approaches to one another. When the pressure became too much, some parents could turn to each other for support in special groups. For others, private suffering was likely the norm, as many parents struggled to deal with the stigma of childhood emotional disturbance and their own guilt over what they perceived as flawed parenting.

Even intensive individual therapy at an RTC was limited to a few hours each week. From dawn till dusk, children spent their days in a new kind of institutional environment, the therapeutic milieu. In this specialized atmosphere, they had a chance to implement the insights they had gained in therapy and attempt to apply them to the real world. For many children, learning to play well with others would prove the most challenging task of all. But for Tommy, it was individual therapy rather than the therapeutic milieu that was critical to mastering his inner demons. After three years of treatment, he became more engaged in group activities, learning to ride a bicycle, play football, and swim. He even wrote and starred in a short play at summer camp about an "inter-planetary costume party." Commented one caseworker, "It was interesting to see how Tommy and others could laugh about space ships, rockets, martian men, etc.," the very concepts that had once symbolized his detachment from the world around him.[147] Although his final summer was one of upheaval—he went home for two weeks, went to camp, saw his room at Southard renovated, and was about to start public school at Topeka High—he displayed a new confidence, telling Wright, "Look Dorothy, I can handle all of these and I'm going to take them one at a time."[148] While Wright admitted he was still a "very timid anxious youngster," she concluded with pride that "he is less unhappy and more at peace with himself because he has spent the last three years at Southard School."[149] To Wright, her journeys to Mars and back had been worthwhile.

FIVE

A New Home

Although individual therapy was probably the most essential part of Tommy's treatment at Southard School, his therapist Mrs. Wright was not the only staff member who had played an important role in his care. A recreation worker seemed to genuinely like and accept the boy, and with his encouragement, Tommy began participating in group activities and interacting with other children.[1] When his new housemother arrived, Tommy "tried to scare her by asking if she had ever worked in a 'mental institution' before," telling her that the Southard kids behaved horribly and asking her if she thought she would be able to handle them. But she did not take Tommy's bait, instead explaining "that she would like to try to make a life for the children that [was] pleasant and home-like."[2] Her explanation reflected the staff's strong belief that the milieu, or environment in which the children lived, should be warm and homey.

Although individual therapy played an important role in residential treatment, the most important aspect of RTC life was the time a child spent in the milieu, a carefully planned environment where he or she ate, slept, played, and went to school. RTC professionals went to great lengths to make the milieu warm and welcoming, developing and describing the environment they created in direct opposition to what they characterized as the punitive, cold atmosphere of training schools. In theory, the milieu was meant to make the RTC a "noninstitutional institution." In practice, the milieu was an unusual environment where adults did not assume traditional authoritarian roles but allowed children to take charge of their own lives and behavior. Permissiveness reigned, and children were encouraged to express themselves freely without fear of judgment or punishment. If it functioned correctly, RTC professionals hoped the milieu would provide a kind of protective bubble for these damaged young minds. Stephen Eliot recalled that he and his friends at the Orthogenic School in Chicago "would refer to the 'outside world' because all of us, kids and staff, lived in a place that was a world unto itself, with its own laws, customs, mores, and culture."[3]

Whether the children were consciously aware of it, their caretakers intended the milieu to serve as a powerful therapeutic tool that would not only treat their emotional struggles and behavioral symptoms but also impart unto them some sense of normality. By approximating the physical and emotional atmosphere of a "typical," white, middle-class American home, RTC professionals aimed to provide normative experiences to correct the pathological ones that had brought children there in the first place. This chapter considers both the rhetorical and physical aspects of the milieu. How did RTC professionals explain the way it worked? Why was it important for them to differentiate the RTC environment from other institutional environments and how did they do so? Finally, why did administrators go to great lengths to approximate the atmosphere of a white, middle-class American home? The following chapter considers the practice of milieu therapy, exploring the daily texture of RTC life and examining the ways in which staff members engineered activities to help children approximate or achieve "normality."

Being "Normal" in Postwar America

Historians have debated just how conformist postwar American society was. While Cold War anxieties found their way into American mass culture, from films to high school textbooks, their subtler influences on daily life are more difficult to categorize.[4] In the 1950s, some liberal intellectuals feared that Americans were becoming one homogeneous, unthinking mass.[5] Just how true was this perception? While our nostalgic view of the postwar era as one of bland conformity is skewed, historians have also convincingly demonstrated the intense pressure American men and women felt to conform to certain cultural norms, particularly around gender and sexuality.[6] Cultural pressures to achieve normality emerged in a postwar America weary of conflict, eager for sameness, and overwhelmed by prescriptive literature and academic discourse about how to achieve "American-ness." Although normality was by definition an unachievable ideal, Americans spent much political, emotional, and financial capital worrying about how they could best fit in.[7]

In postwar America, "normal" was explicitly and implicitly white and middle class. After World War II, a combination of factors including population growth, economic prosperity, and physical dislocation contributed to increased social mobility for many Americans. Being middle class became an ideal. In fact, an enormous, heterogeneous swath of Americans claimed membership in this group, from blue-collar workers to gray flannel suit–wearing organization men.[8] In some ways, the term "middle class" became devoid of real meaning, instead symbolizing an intangible goal. As Lizabeth Cohen has argued, being a good consumer was critical to claiming this identity and to being a good American citizen.[9] Yet racial minorities, especially African Americans, were excluded from much of this mass consumption, limited by economic restraints and racist policies, such as housing covenants.[10] Indeed, the dream of middle-class citizenship was primarily a white one. African American magazines like *Ebony* advertised suits to black men as a way they could share in the fantasy of middle-class respectability.[11] Whiteness was even depicted artistically as an ideal. "Norma" and "Normman," statues representative of ideal male and female bodies that were created in 1942 and displayed in the United States and abroad for many years afterward, were based on anthropomorphic measurements of thousands of white men and women. In addition, they were both labeled "Native White American," making their whiteness explicit.[12]

Children during this era were encouraged to conform to social and cultural standards, and the possibility that they might not frightened adults. In the 1940s and 1950s, widespread panic about the alleged wave of juvenile delinquency engulfed educators, mass media, and even the U.S. Congress, which put comic books on trial as a potential contributor to the problem.[13] Mental hygiene films shown to schoolchildren encouraged boys to act manly and girls to be feminine and virtuous and warned both not to attract any undue attention for "strange" behavior like being a loner.[14] Residential treatment for emotionally disturbed children was tightly embedded in these larger concerns, and RTC professionals strove to help their troubled, deviant youngsters fit in with their peers, their families, and their larger communities. In the process, they articulated and enacted a "normal" childhood for these children. Making disturbed children into normal ones was the main goal of RTC professionals, who saw normal and abnormal children as two sides of the same coin. As Angela Baird of the Cincinnati Child Guidance Home explained, "The disturbed child has rendered an invaluable service for the normal child as the normal child has for the disturbed. The difficulties of the one have given insight into the difficulties of the other."[15] Studying and treating disturbed children, they hoped, would give them greater insight into healthy ones.

Catchall or Catchphrase?

Although the milieu was central to residential treatment, RTC professionals were uncertain about how it should be defined. Some described the milieu vaguely, referring to the "total environmental setting within which [the child] lives," or "the child's daily life and his contacts with adults."[16] Others listed its elements: "food, clothing, and the housemother's care; play activities, toys, school, jobs to be done, and the companionship of other children and of staff."[17] All emphasized that it was not just the existence of the environment that created a milieu but its planned use as part of a child's treatment.[18] Every activity that happened in the milieu, explained a 1959 Southard manual titled *Handbook for Parents*, had meaning and therapeutic potential, whether it was a child's performance in school or the way she spent her weekly allowance.[19] At the 1957 American Psychiatric Association conference on residential therapy, RTC professionals engaged in heated debate about the term's meaning and connotations, particularly its vagueness.[20] The conference participants ultimately concluded that this new concept of milieu, despite debates over its nuances, needed a label and was central to residential treatment.[21] The idea that every activity and relationship in a child's daily life could be made therapeutic played a central role at almost every RTC in the mid-twentieth century.

Origins of the Milieu

The roots of the therapeutic milieu concept lay in several disparate attempts to understand and reimagine the role of the environment in psychiatric treatment. In nineteenth-century asylums in Europe and the United States, severely mentally ill individuals received variations on moral treatment, which was based on the premise that treating patients like rational beings would encourage them to behave normally. On the rolling grounds of enormous asylums situated far away from bustling cities, patients lived in carefully designed buildings intended to maximize the circulation of fresh air, participated in outdoor work programs intended to nurture their souls, and played the role of children in large institutional families. Of course, intention and reality were quite different, and there were very few physicians for hundreds of patients who were sometimes chemically or physically restrained as alternate means of behavioral control. But asylum treatment during this period represented an attempt to engineer the patient's environment to serve a therapeutic role.[22]

A century later, British psychiatrists during World War II developed the therapeutic community as another means of using the environment as a mode of treatment. In what are now called the Northfield experiments, a group of psychiatrists at the Northfield Military Hospital in Birmingham fostered a quasi-democratic institutional community in which soldiers had a say in their own care and participated in activities intended to reintegrate them into society. In London, psychiatrist Maxwell Jones attempted a similar approach at Mill Hill Hospital.[23] In 1945, Karl Menninger led a group of American psychiatrists on a tour of Northfield, and by the 1950s and 1960s, the therapeutic community concept had become integrated into American psychiatry as part of larger efforts to make psychiatric patients active participants in their own treatment.[24]

While these two instances certainly made critical contributions to the concept of the therapeutic milieu, RTC professionals in particular pointed to the work of Austrian psychoanalytic educator August Aichhorn in the 1910s and 1920s as having originated the idea.[25] Of course, the idea of the therapeutic environment had a much longer history, and this tidy line of succession also belied a messier reality in that RTCs all over the country were simultaneously developing and enacting their own ideas about milieu therapy. Their work, part of a longer tradition of adjusting a patient's environment to serve a therapeutic purpose, played a critical role in establishing an American tradition of milieu therapy that still exists today.[26]

Making Sense of Milieu

The therapeutic milieu operated in a multitude of ways, and RTC professionals developed several overlapping theories to explain and justify its use. The first focused on the potential of the milieu to nurture a child and foster positive relationships with others. For children who had been deprived of parental love, staff members believed open love and affection would replenish their supply.[27] In particular, they believed that physical affection in the form of hugging, kissing, rocking, and carrying children made them feel safe and loved.[28] As one patient at the Cincinnati Child Guidance Home explained, the job of a psychiatrist was easy: "You just have to love your patients and let them know it."[29] When children came to accept this proffered love, they would learn to trust the adults around them and see "that it is a safe, honest, and good world."[30] Although this approach departed from the caricature of orthodox psychoanalysis, in which the therapist was physically and emotionally aloof from his patient, psychoanalysis in the United States had always been a heterogeneous practice. By the 1950s, a number of new psychotherapies were emerging. In humanistic therapy, for example, a nonjudgmental therapist promoted loving oneself and "self-actualization."[31] So although hugging and loving children in residential treatment did not represent an orthodox analytic approach, it reflected the heterogeneity of American therapeutic practices at the time.

Staff members were cautioned not to suffocate a child with love but simply to offer support without expectation of reciprocation, an approach they learned could be quite effective. When thirteen-year-old Billy, a completely withdrawn boy who frequently had outbursts of violence toward others, arrived at Hawthorne Cedar Knolls in 1948, his experienced cottage parents did not shower him with love and affection. Instead, they respected the distance he placed between himself and other people and offered kindness and support, but nothing more. Billy gradually approached his cottage parents more and more, carrying on conversations and letting his cottage mother write thank you notes for him when he received presents from home. By the time he had to switch to a cottage of older boys three years later, he was very upset because he had come to rely on the couple for emotional support.[32] Their cautious approach, brought about "by respecting his fears and avoiding any direct overtures toward greater intimacy," had encouraged Billy to develop some of the first meaningful relationships in his life, according to Hawthorne administrators who later reflected on his case.[33]

The fact that this development had taken place in the cottage, a small building intended to approximate a home and run by two staff members called cottage parents, was significant. Constructing a homelike atmosphere was essential to RTC professionals and their goal of providing normalizing experiences to their children. "The intent and purpose of a small unit cottage plan," explained a Hawthorne social work student, "is to give to each child as far as possible the care he would receive in a normal family setting."[34] Only by living in a setting approximating "normal" family life could an emotionally disturbed child be loved, love others, and grow.[35] RTC professionals referred to these experiences and others in the milieu as "corrective," a term that implied that they were making up for pathological experiences in the child's past.[36] Corrective experiences were, by necessity, different for different children. A child who had lived in an overly strict household might need more leeway, whereas a child whose parents had let him act on every impulse might need more structure and discipline.[37] But in general, most RTC professionals felt that corrective experiences could best occur in an environment that provided at least some structure. Structure could help disturbed children interact with one another, calm down symptoms like hyperactivity, and force children occupied by fantasy worlds to engage with reality.[38]

Corrective experiences were not intended to be harsh. In fact, RTC professionals hoped they could help their children achieve mastery over the world around them. In the therapeutic milieu, children would be presented with a watered-down reality, "a reality which is strained down to a consistency which [a child] can absorb somewhat like a prepared baby food."[39] When disturbed children took behavioral baby steps in an encouraging, simplified environment, they would learn the self-confidence and pride that came with success.[40] In the long run, they would ideally be prepared to deal with the requirements of life outside the RTC, having learned to operate in the constraints of a structured environment with rules and limits.[41] In reality, administrators struggled to determine just how watered-down to make the milieu. On the one hand, it was important for children to experience success and mastery over their environment. On the other, they worried that children would not be adequately prepared for the real world when they left the safe confines of the RTC.[42] Residential life, however idyllic, was only temporary.

The final rationale for using milieu therapy was more practical than theoretical. Simply put, RTC professionals wanted kids to be kids. Fun and games were essential to mental health, and it would not be right to let children miss out on the normal activities of childhood just because they were in treatment. Instead, they should keep playing just as they would (or should) have at home as part of their natural growth and development.[43] Most of the children they saw had not experienced much fun in their home lives, and RTC professionals hoped they might give the children "positive memories and images of what it means to enjoy" that might eventually "become something that they look forward to and something which may urge them to continue to grow."[44] Play, they were arguing, was the right of all children, even disturbed ones.[45]

A Kinder Institution

In order to develop and play like normal children, RTC patients needed an environment distinctly different from the punitive or custodial training school or state mental hospital where they might have otherwise ended up. On arriving at Hawthorne Cedar Knolls in 1950, one journalist noticed a palpable difference from the tenor of other institutions: "Over the whole community was an amazing atmosphere of normalcy. I found no guards, no locked doors, no fences, no prohibiting signs. I did find, both in environment and spirit, a great sense of openness and freedom."[46] If this account was a bit dramatic, it encapsulated the atmosphere that RTC professionals aimed to create.[47] Unlike training schools, RTCs were typically not closed institutions; that is, they did not lock children in.[48] Even those that did, which were typically hospital units, instructed nurses to wear street clothes instead of uniforms and to stop using techniques like sedation and restraints to control the children.[49] The result, one nurse explained, was "a much more friendly and homelike ward atmosphere."[50] No locked unit, no matter how warm, could ever approximate a home. Still, staff members worked hard to make them as physically and emotionally dissimilar from hospital wards as possible.

Painting their centers as noninstitutional institutions was an especially important task for RTC professionals in light of growing public and professional distrust of psychiatric institutions. Overcrowding in large state mental hospitals had become unsustainable by the mid-twentieth century. Hospitals were packed to the brim with chronically ill patients (almost all adults), and a miniscule number of psychiatrists faced the impossible task of caring for hundreds or even thousands of patients at a time. Treatment was largely custodial, and patients remained for years, even decades.[51] Starting in the mid-1940s, journalists and photographers documented the often-horrid conditions in which these patients resided and sounded the call for reform in a series of widely read exposés, the most famous of which was Albert Deutsch's collection *Shame of the States*.[52] These anxieties were also reflected in films like *The Snake Pit*, which documented a seemingly normal housewife's descent into insanity and admission into an overcrowded, prisonlike mental hospital.[53] It is thus particularly ironic that RTCs should flourish just as most psychiatric institutions were under attack. Much of their success was due to their administrators' successful rebranding of their work as noninstitutional in nature.

The terms "permissive" and "permissiveness," both used frequently to describe the general tone of RTCs,[54] invoked an approach to child rearing that was emerging in the late 1930s.[55] In permissive child rearing, a parent not only gave a son or daughter increased freedom but also adopted a more child-centered point of view.[56] In an RTC, permissiveness meant many things. It might mean not adhering to a strict schedule. At Southard, children typically woke up at 7 A.M., with breakfast served until 8:30, but children who missed breakfast entirely were still fed regardless.[57] Permissiveness might also mean ignoring irritating, hurtful, or frustrating behavior. Ten-year-old Hattie's arrival was marked by "irritable, demanding, noisy behavior," but the director reported that staff members "accepted [her behavior] without comment" instead of scolding or punishing her.[58]

Children had often come from homes where breaking rules meant getting punished, and they were anxious to test the limits of staff members' permissive attitudes. At the Orthogenic School, one child took a single bite out of eight different sandwiches to see how the staff would retaliate. When he saw that they would not, he stopped.[59] Not only was it acceptable to break rules that might exist at home, it was also normal to speak honestly about the consequences (or lack thereof) for doing so. Hank, a newcomer who worried how the staff would react if he didn't brush his teeth every night, was told that it didn't really matter, and that it was perfectly normal to forget to brush.[60] Another student at the school, Mary, saw paint in the playroom and told her counselor that she had gotten "a bad licking" at home for getting paint on herself. When she inquired how the staff would respond if this happened again, her counselor told her that they would just wipe the paint off. Distrusting this simple explanation, Mary proceeded to place paint all over her own arm, but found that even then, she was not scolded.[61]

Working with disturbed children in a setting like this demanded tremendous patience. A nurse at the New York State Psychiatric Institute's children's unit needed "a sense of humor, enthusiasm, [and] a tremendous amount of patience," according to the unit's director.[62] At the NIH child psychiatry unit, it was completely normal to have fights and runaway attempts daily, yet staff attempted to stay open-minded.[63] "This requires that the adults in the environment be nonjudgmental persons, tolerant and understanding of child behavior which would not be socially acceptable in other settings," explained NIH child psychiatrist Donald Bloch.[64] Only by putting up with a wider range of behaviors, RTC professionals believed, could staff help children develop independence and self-control.[65] Even in the most extreme situations, staff members struggled to remain calm, focus on helping the child, and not retaliate.[66] Fighting back, they believed, would only demonstrate to a child that the staff member was unable to handle or understand his behavior and would preclude any therapeutic gains.[67] Taking this stance could be extremely difficult and took a personal toll on staff members. "It is usually very hard to show a relaxed attitude towards a child who starves himself," reflected a psychiatrist at the Illinois Neuropsychiatric Institute.[68] Even more difficult was working with a hyperactive, violent child. In one case, the psychiatrist remembered, a psychotic boy's "extremely dirty, obscene, and aggressive behavior" was so disturbing that the staff members had to take turns working with him one hour at a time so they didn't get too overwhelmed.[69]

Permissiveness was not infinite and had to be balanced by a healthy dose of limit setting. Destructive behavior toward oneself or other people was universally unacceptable, for example.[70] While setting boundaries was a realistic necessity of the permissive approach, it could also be interpreted as therapeutic in its own right. In particular, RTC professionals believed that children experienced comfort and security when adults established limits.[71] In one extreme scenario, a group of children at the Cincinnati Child Guidance Home declared mutiny on the staff in August 1949 when their ringleader announced that "the children were tired of taking all this stuff from the adults and were now going to take over." For several hours, they destroyed property, threw food, set fires, and physically attacked staff members. The staff was able to regain control only when they decided to divide and conquer, with each staff member physically holding down a child. The children's reaction was not one of frustration and rising anger. Instead, they "seemed relieved and one commented, 'We sure had you scared, didn't we?'"[72] When a local policeman stopped by after dinner to let the children know he was there to protect them, they again seemed relieved and the home director noted that "they responded readily to the setting of further limits on attempted destructive behavior."[73] Examples like these, including many far less extreme, convinced staff members that circumscribing children's behavior and balancing permissiveness with limit setting was not only necessary but also therapeutic. While child-centered permissiveness was theoretically the goal, as with everything in an RTC it had to be balanced with the practical demands of caring for a varied and challenging group of children.

The Landscape of Care

The physical aspects of the milieu were just as deliberate as its emotional tenor. The purposeful process of constructing the physical milieu is especially visible in the few instances when RTCs were able to build entirely new campuses. In the mid-1950s, the Menninger Clinic built a larger, more modern child psychiatry campus to replace the dilapidated mansions then in use at the Southard School. In planning documents and communications, administrators discussed building visiting rooms for parents and special therapeutic spaces, like playrooms with one-way mirrors for observation.[74]

At the University of Michigan in the mid-1950s, a brand new children's hospital with both general pediatric and child psychiatry wards was built to provide a specialized space that could accommodate more patients. In early planning meetings, administrators discussed constructing seclusion rooms and group therapy rooms.[75] They also made detailed plans for recreational facilities, including a gymnasium, a swimming pool, an auditorium "for movies, plays and other entertainment in which they themselves will participate," and a three-level outdoor playground "with facilities for baseball, volley ball, slides, swings, built-in sand piles, a wading pool and other resources that we have found that children most enjoy."[76] The wards would promote children's autonomy, with snack bars where children could prepare popcorn and hot cocoa for themselves at night.[77] The two chief planners, Neuropsychiatric Institute director Raymond Waggoner and Children's Psychiatric Hospital Ralph Rabinovitch, went so far as to theorize the ways in which the new building's spaces would serve different purposes. Classrooms would provide a quiet refuge, the recreation floor with gym and swimming pool would promote "noise and free fun," and the living area would support activities that fell in the middle.[78]

On a more pragmatic level, these administrators knew they would be housing some extremely destructive children and took special care to use materials and building techniques that would accommodate rough behavior. The new Menninger Children's Division buildings, for example, used sheet vinyl on the floors and a Portland cement plaster finish on the walls to "resist hard use."[79] At the University of Michigan, administrators publicized the measures they had taken to keep the unit intact in a *Time* magazine feature and a pamphlet advertising the unit. Seven-foot tile walls resisted damage, as did "rugged" oak furniture (compared to the previous beds, which had been steel and "only lasted a few months"). Hinges were "slam-proof" and could not be taken apart, light switches were controlled by keys, and electrical outlets were controlled inside a centralized nurses' office. Radiators, which the children had destroyed in the old unit, were exchanged for an innovative ceiling-based heating system.[80] Still, the planning committee hoped to avoid a harsh, "prisonlike" atmosphere, so they suggested that the wall tiles be colorful.[81] This approach was not universal. Staff members at Bellefaire, Southard, and the Camarillo State Hospital believed that providing comfortable, new furniture was essential, because it encouraged the children to take care of their surroundings. When the children damaged institutional property, it was replaced quickly to demonstrate the staff's respect for the children and their belief that living with damaged furnishings would negatively influence their self-esteem.[82]

A New Home

Despite the need for durable furniture, RTC professionals tried hard to approximate the physical environment of a home. In one image from the University of Michigan, a boy sits at his desk, wearing dark slacks and a checked button-down shirt. In front of him is a radio, a small shelf with books and other personal effects, and a lamp with a square base and a design (perhaps cherries?) on the lampshade (fig. 5.1). On his right is a large window, half-covered by a curtain with a colorful, modern print. On his left, a neatly made bed with striped bed sheets and two of his own drawings, tacked to the wall. This is not a typical hospital room, and it is certainly not a typical psychiatric hospital room. While there are screens on the insides of the windows to prevent children from jumping out (not visible in the picture) and tiled walls, in many respects this looks like a typical boy's bedroom.

In another photograph from the Southard School, a boy of similar age sits in his bedroom (fig. 5.2). Flowered curtains cover the windows and a

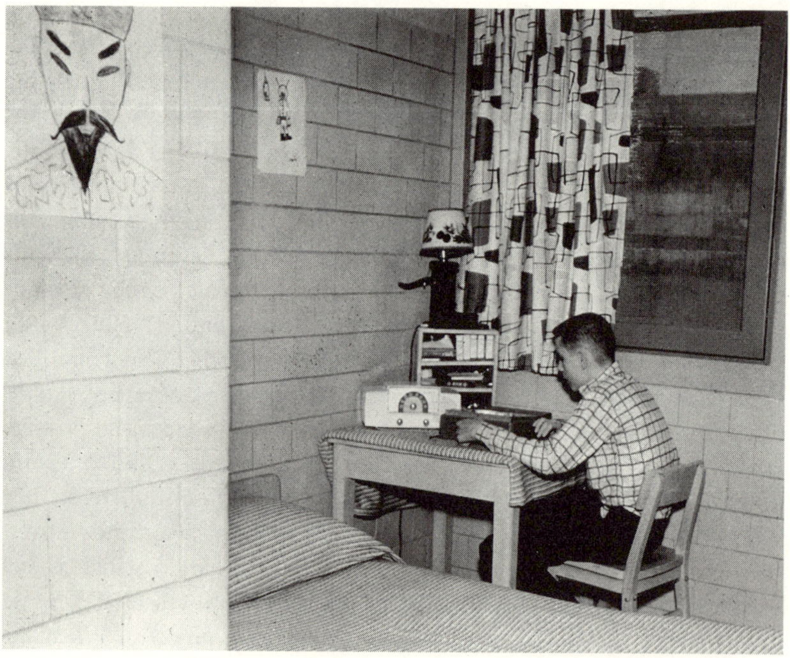

5.1. Boy's bedroom at the University of Michigan Children's Psychiatric Hospital, 1950s. (Untitled photograph, Box 15, Children's Psychiatric Hospital, ca. 1950s, Raymond Waggoner papers.)

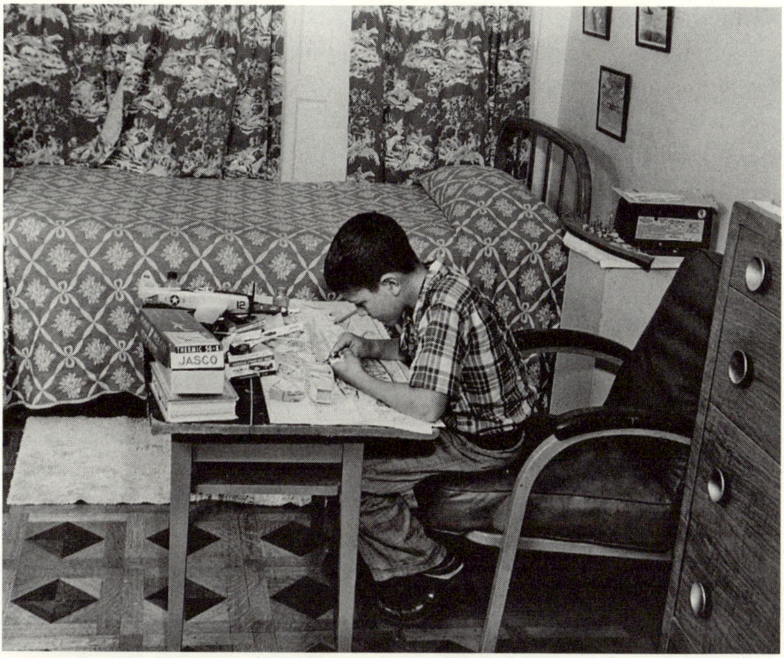

5.2. Boy's bedroom at Southard School, February 1955. (Untitled photograph, *Look* Magazine 1955 #86, Box 118-4-3-6, KSHS.)

fleur-de-lis bedspread covers his twin bed. Nearby, the boy sits at a desk putting together a model airplane. Without a caption, one would assume that he was at home in his own bedroom. This resemblance was very intentional. Re-creating the atmosphere of a white, middle-class, suburban family home, physically and emotionally, was an essential part of imparting corrective, normalizing experiences in the therapeutic milieu.

In the postwar era, the suburban, middle-class ranch home became an American ideal.[83] The neighborhoods and buildings in which RTCs were situated reflected this mission. For example, CWLA researchers Helen Hagan and Joseph Reid noted that the Cincinnati Child Guidance Home was located in a "middle class, residential" neighborhood, and described the setting of the Evanston Receiving Home of the Illinois Children's Home and Aid Society as "an upper middle class [neighborhood] in a typical community suburban to a large metropolitan city."[84] Many RTCs were physically situated in old houses, from the private Southard School, which until 1961 was housed in a set of old Topeka mansions, to the Arthur Brisbane Child Treatment Center, run by the state of New Jersey, which occupied an old private estate.[85] Social work student Bernice Crumpacker described the Cincinnati Child Guidance Home as "a small, attractive brick dwelling not unlike an old English cottage in design."[86] The idyllic forty-acre wooded grounds of the Bradley Hospital, a former private estate, were the epitome of comfortable living. A pond was used for swimming, fishing, and ice skating, large fields were perfect for sports, flying kites, and planting small gardens, and many of the trees were "well suited for climbing and tree house building"—all aspects of the grounds that staff members and observers were eager to mention. At RTCs that were too large to occupy houses, administrators divided children into cottages that offered "experience in family living" for approximately ten to twenty children.[87] This would theoretically provide them with the same homelike experience as much smaller institutions that were situated in actual houses, like Southard.

When one teenage boy first walked into a receiving area at Hawthorne Cedar Knolls, he was surprised at what he found: "First, a big room. With homey touches. Plants and curtains and matched blonde wood furniture. A big console TV stands across the wall. . . . A hinged ping-pong table on wheels stands folded in two against the wall."[88] None of this was an accident, reflecting the great lengths to which RTC professionals went to ensure that the interiors of their institutions would approximate "a modern family home."[89] At Bellefaire, radio-victrolas and pianos were installed in individual cottages, and at Bradley, Mother Goose illustrations covered the walls.[90] At Southard, "warm soft colors" and "colorful drapes, curtains, and paintings of the children themselves" covered walls and windows.[91] A 1946 photograph of the Southard living room is in many ways the picture of an upper middle-class home, with a dark wood side table topped with a vase of flowers, a large upholstered chair, drapes covering tall windows, and wall-to-wall carpeting (fig. 5.3).

The deliberate quality of RTC interior decoration was particularly evident at the National Institutes of Health, where a $100,000 "rambling, modern piece of upper-class suburbia" was built in 1957 to replace the small existing child psychiatry unit in the campus hospital.[92] Administrators specifically intended the building to serve a normalizing function in the lives of the children who lived there. According to NIH child psychiatrist Joseph Noshpitz, the purpose of the new home was "to re-teach many of the details of normal home living to this group of very disturbed children," a task that required a "middle-class typical" environment.[93] Although he did not specify what he meant by this, the house featured air conditioning, a twenty-one-inch television, a living room and fireplace,

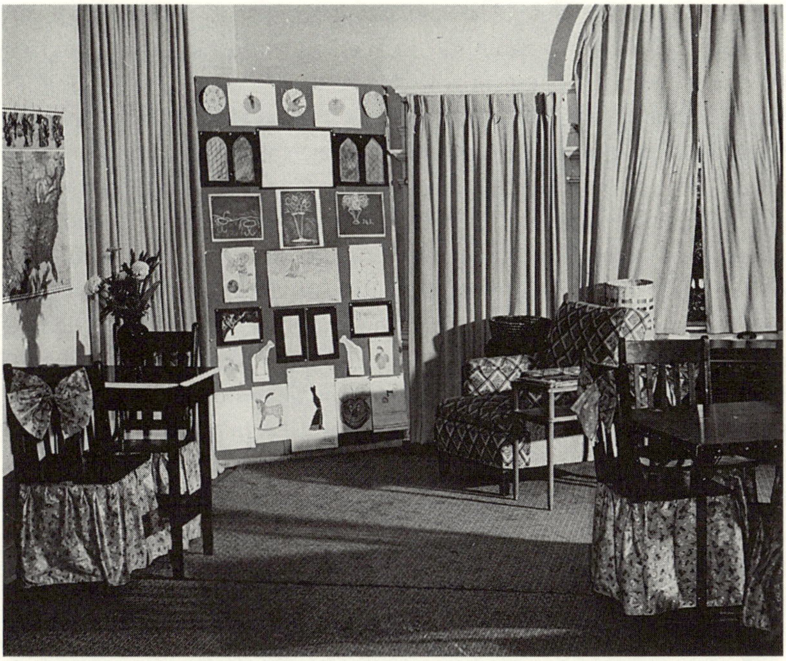

5.3. Remodeled living room at the Southard School featuring patients' artwork tacked to a wall, 1946. (Untitled photograph, Box 118-4-3-6, Children's Division cont. Misc. A-B Photos Box 4, KSHS.)

three bedrooms, a playroom, and a kitchen, "where the refrigerator can be raided for Cokes and snacks," among many comforts.[94] This composite description was put forth not by Noshpitz or any other NIH employee but by journalists, who conveyed to their readers that RTCs were quite different from the harsh mental hospitals increasingly in the public's imagination and that the children who lived there, though extremely disturbed, were still kids who raided Cokes from the refrigerator. Perhaps, they were suggesting, disturbed children could be helped. Perhaps they were just like other children, different only as victims of pathological homes.

At Wiltwyck, which housed primarily African American and Latino boys, administrators went to great expense to create this middle-class environment. A 1954 furniture order for the school included sixteen Eames chairs, denim for thirty bedspreads and for living room curtains, and three televisions, one of which had a twenty-one-inch screen.[95] A record player donated by Columbia Television and a phonograph rounded out the center's 1954 acquisitions.[96] These new items took on added significance at Wiltwyck. The middle-class domestic consumer ideal in postwar America was undoubtedly a white ideal, and the great efforts of a perpetually cash-strapped institution to create this ideal speak to the racially normalizing aspect of residential treatment as well.

In RTCs located inside larger hospitals, it was understandably more difficult to create a homelike atmosphere. Most child psychiatry units were located inside preexisting hospitals; in the case of psychiatric hospitals, the atmosphere was especially uninviting. Windows might be covered with screens and doors locked to prevent children from escaping or hurting themselves.[97] Within these constraints, RTC directors did their best to make their units as welcoming as possible. The University of Michigan Child Psychiatric Hospital, which had gone to great lengths to make the new building virtually indestructible, divided the complex into "living units" with individual dining rooms, kitchens, and play areas that would "provide an atmosphere closer to a family grouping rather than a large institutional design."[98] At the Illinois Neuropsychiatric Institute, staff members acknowledged that they were working on a traditional hospital ward with concrete floors, but tried to dress it up with colorful walls, bedspreads, a piano, plants, and plenty of toys.[99]

Most of the time, a child lived in a room with one or two other children. Still, RTCs strove to give children their own space. The Lakeside Children's Center in Milwaukee had rooms for one, two, three, or four children that featured bulletin boards so children could hang up their own drawings or posters. They were also encouraged to decorate their rooms as they wished; one baseball fan kept his bat and ball out for display, and another boy featured cars and planes on his wall.[100] At Bellefaire, wrote a boy named Bobby, children were three or four to a room, but each child had his own drawers and locker for personal possessions and was allowed to decorate his areas as he wished with "pictures of baseball stars, pin-ups, and so forth."[101] Children at the University of Michigan were avid arts and crafts students, designing curtains and building bookshelves and fish tanks.[102]

Having a private or semiprivate space was also important because it would give children the opportunity to be alone. The few single bedrooms at Lakeside, director Burmeister believed, "satisfy a need each one of us has. This is the enjoyment of being by oneself at times, to read undisturbed, to listen to music, to study or write, to putter about—in other words, to gratify one's own needs in one's own ways."[103] Burmeister's observation is particularly important in light of the socializing, group-oriented nature of the milieu. Although promoting effective group interaction was one of the milieu's main purposes, it was just as important that children at Lakeside had time and space to themselves. This balance between the group and the individual reaffirmed the notion that the normal child was also the *moderate* child: not alone all the time, but not without alone time, either.

Part of the Family

Physical objects and decorations were one major part of making the RTC like a middle-class home. The other was providing the children with a new nuclear family with whom they could build new memories. At the head of the family were the parents, who in an RTC might be played by nurses or nonprofessional residential workers. By experiencing life with a substitute set of parents, RTC professionals believed, a child could learn to manage his relationships with his own parents in a safe, nonthreatening environment.[104] In RTCs based on the cottage system, a married couple called the cottage parents or a single cottage mother was in charge of an individual cottage and the children who lived there. She or they were responsible for guiding the children through the day's activities from morning until night and maintaining order in the cottage, setting out rules and meting out punishments like extra chores or having to stay home from a fun activity. Cottage parents were also responsible for their children's emotional well-being.[105] The director of the Lakeside Children's Center noted that the cottage mother "is with [a child] twenty-four hours a day, through thick and thin. She takes care of him when he is ill, mends his socks, sews on his buttons. He hears her talk of, and stick up for '*my* boys' or '*my* girls.'"[106] In some instances, cottage parents spent more time with a child than his real mother or father likely would have, especially if that parent worked outside the home.

Cottage parents were not new to the landscape of children's institutions; they had been and were still working at most training schools for delinquent children. But at RTCs, their emphasis was more on the child's emotional health than on running a tight ship. At Hawthorne, which had previously been a training school, some cottage parents who maintained the "old" approach had initially stayed on. They saw themselves as "custodians" and their cottages "were places where children slept and dressed" but nothing more. Whether of their own volition, these couples left quickly, remnants of an antiquated system that had paid little attention to a child's psychological needs.[107]

In RTCs that did not operate on the cottage system, other staff members assumed parental roles. Nurses and attendants on hospital units, most of whom were unmarried women, functioned as replacement mothers, going far beyond their professional training to assume new roles.[108] "One female attendant seemed to be the fountainhead of motherly love," described a nurse at the Illinois Neuropsychiatric Institute.[109] In one instance at Hawthorne Cedar Knolls, a plumber served as "father surrogate."[110] Because these staff members, rather than physicians, were with children from dawn till dusk, it seemed natural to administrators that these bonds might form. At times, it seemed they were the only staff members who could reach a child.[111] Popular press stories tended to focus on and glorify staff members' roles as replacement parents. In a *Chicago Tribune* feature on the University of Michigan Children's Psychiatric Hospital, the author described nurses who "often curl up on the patients' beds for a night time story and a bit of mothering."[112] A similar feature on Ryther in *Time* magazine described a nurse to whom troubled Butch opened up, "finding in her some replacement for his mother," and a male caseworker who "was assigned to . . . take the place of a father in Butch's mind."[113] In some ways, publicizing these relationships was a way of dealing with the distasteful fact that children were being kept away from their own homes and families.

These relationships often played a tremendously important role in the daily lives of the children. For an eight-year-old boy named Sam who had tics and frequent temper tantrums, his close relationship with his cottage father (who was also the campus gardener at Hawthorne) helped him learn responsibility and self-confidence. According to Hawthorne's director, this had occurred because Sam now had a strong father figure in his life, presumably correcting the damage his biological father had wrought.[114] Some pseudo-parental relationships were so strong that when they were threatened the effects were devastating. In his memoir of his childhood at the Orthogenic School, Stephen Eliot described his counselor Diana as "the center of [his] world," who made him feel "truly loved for who [he] was inside."[115] When Diana left the school to get married, he reflected that "losing her felt like losing a parent."[116] For Eliot, Diana had essentially become his mother, someone who spent almost every day with him, knew him inside out, and actually liked him despite his (self-described) annoying, competitive personality.[117]

Whether one or more cottage parents, nurses, or other staff members were serving in loco parentis, these staff members were expected to model appropriately gendered behavior for their charges. At Hawthorne, married couples were chosen to run cottages because they could aid children who themselves were confused about their gender roles or who had seen only troubled marital relationships. "The experience of living with a happily married couple in which man and woman play their respective roles in a normal fashion can be most helpful" for these children, explained two

Hawthorne social workers.[118] Cottage parents could also instruct boys and girls in gender-appropriate activities. A cottage father might teach his boys fishing or carpentry, while his wife might teach girls how to cook, sew, and care for their appearances.[119] For the child with a weak, effeminate father or a smothering or manly mother, these experiences would teach them what a "real" man or woman looked and acted like.

From these staff members, children also learned what was expected of them as girls or boys who would one day be women and men. One particularly revealing conversation between a residential worker and several girls at the Cincinnati Child Guidance Home covered the possible roles they could pursue as adult women:

AQUA [*DESPAIRINGLY*]: I sometimes think it is much better to be a boy. They have everything.

WRITER: That is because you have not found out how much fun it is to be a little girl and grow up to do all the things a woman can do. Sure thing we don't think you have to be a boy to do things and be happy. Do we Susan and Maude?

SUSAN: I use to [*sic*], but I don't now.

MAUDE: Women can do a lot of things and have babies.

WRITER: Yes, girls grow up and can do many things. They fall in love and get married; keep house and learn to make their houses pretty; have babies and fun taking care of their babies.

SUSAN: And clean up and wait for him to come home and he sends roses to the house.

MAUDE: I am going to get married and have three babies.

SUSAN: I am too.

AQUA [*INTERESTED BUT NOT CONVINCED!*]: That's nothing men have all the jobs and can do anything they want to.

WRITER: You can have a job in an office, or be a teacher, or a nurse. Many women have jobs, but most women think keeping house is more fun.[120]

Despite Aqua's reluctance to buy into this line of thinking, the worker was clearly trying to convince the girls that homemaking and mothering was an aspirational ideal. Yes, some women worked outside the home—but didn't homemaking sound "more fun?" Interactions like this provided opportunities to ensure that disturbed children learned how to behave according to socially appropriate gender roles.

Residential treatment center "families" involved brothers and sisters too. One director called his RTC a "substitute sibling setting," arguing that the relationships formed among children could be therapeutically significant. Bellefaire formed other pseudo-sibling relationships through its volunteer Big Brother and Big Sister programs, which matched up Jewish adult volunteers from the community with boys and girls to give them role models and an opportunity to form a meaningful personal relationship.[121] These relationships were also opportunities to reinforce gendered behavior; Big Brother relationships gave boys an opportunity for "constructive male identification" and Big Sisters took teenage Little Sisters shopping in the community and ran a six-week charm school to teach girls how to manage a budget and groom themselves.[122] For quiet, suspicious Sandy, having a Big Brother was transformative. He learned independence when his Big Brother suggested he earn money to buy the bike he wanted so badly and formed his first close relationship with another person, which led to new friendships with other children.[123]

Pets rounded out the RTC family. The children at the Cincinnati Child Guidance Home took in stray cats and dogs, and a dog was included with the brand new house built on the NIH grounds for its disturbed children.[124] At Southard, pets were limited to fish and turtles because several children had mistreated some larger pets.[125] Pets could serve a therapeutic purpose. In particular, withdrawn children were often attracted to pets, who were "soft and warm to the touch" and made "no demands for response from the child."[126] Pets were also excellent public relations tools; visitors to the Lakeside Children's Center "usually anticipate finding the traditional old institutional picture. . . . The pets help to dispel any feeling of formality. . . . One can almost see the idea come over the visitors—'If they have all these pets for the children, they can't be so bad.'"[127] Creating the "RTC family" was important therapeutically, but it was similarly critical to presenting a friendly, nonthreatening image to the public.

Despite the prevalence of the home model in residential treatment, a minority of RTC professionals vehemently opposed it. The 1957 American Psychiatric Association conference report concluded that the popular tendency to re-create a homelike environment was misdirected and was more for the benefit of staff members than children. It was confusing to both parties, the report explained, but sometimes a fireplace was just a fireplace: "Fireplaces . . . are desirable because they make life more enjoyable for the child, not because they simulate what is found in a home."[128] Several RTC administrators specifically took issue with making staff members into replacement parents. While transference—the phenomenon in which a patient displaced feelings for others onto his or her therapist—was generally seen as an important element of successful psychotherapy, critics of the home model worried that transferring a child's parental feelings and needs onto staff members was a risky endeavor. Parent-child relationships, they argued, took years to form; how could they expect new ones to form almost immediately?[129] Other children might not need a substitute parent, and still others might not be emotionally ready for it.[130] One child psychiatrist believed that imbuing staff members with parental qualities would directly challenge the authority and responsibility of a child's real parents, who ideally would continue to parent the child even throughout his or her hospitalization.[131] In this sense, the "substitute family" plan directly competed with the therapeutic goal of treating parents and child concurrently. If a child's parents were being replaced, albeit temporarily, how could his or her family be treated as a whole? At Lakeside, children placed family photographs on their dressers to remind them of their real families waiting for them when they went home.[132] Despite this rhetoric, many RTCs still engaged in practices that upheld the home model. At the Children's Service Center of Wyoming Valley, where director Franklin Robinson wrote frequently of his opposition to the home model, cottage directors (they were purposefully not called cottage parents) attended their patients' PTA meetings "and may see the teachers when in doubt about why a child has been kept in after school." In this case, these "cottage directors" were enacting the roles of parents even when they had intended to do the opposite.

In and of the Community

In addition to constructing the milieu within their own walls, RTC administrators worked very hard to ensure that their institutions had reciprocal interactions with the institutions and members of their local communities. These interactions were in some ways in direct opposition to the therapeutic milieu ideal, which attempted to create intact local worlds with their own rules and actors in which the children would live. However, community integration, like milieu therapy, had the ultimate aim of reintroducing children into their communities as successful citizens. And good community relations could help bolster the image of RTCs as noninstitutional institutions.

Since the mid-twentieth century, institutions like training schools had served to keep the community safe from abnormal or dangerous youngsters. They were located far from cities and surrounded by fences with locked gates that not only kept the children in but also kept the community out.[133] The same had been true for institutions that only later became RTCs. When it was a training school, Hawthorne Cedar Knolls had been a closed institution, with locked doors and gates keeping the children segregated from the surrounding community.[134] At the Bradley Hospital in Providence, which had focused on treating children with neurological disorders in the 1930s, former director Maurice Laufer remembered that "we were sort of isolated conceptually . . . so that we did not do as much as we should have with the community."[135] The Southard School, which treated mostly intellectually disabled children in the 1930s, focused on "segregation and isolation from the community," believing that "the less the public knew about our children, the better."[136] Part of this was likely due to the stigma associated with intellectual disability at the time—such children were believed best hidden away from the prying eyes of unsympathetic neighbors.

As these institutions remade their identities and became RTCs in the 1940s and 1950s, their attitudes toward their surrounding communities changed as well. Hawthorne staff took all the locks off their doors, making the institution physically accessible to the outside community and vice versa.[137] Bradley started sending its children to public schools, and Southard staff members vowed to integrate their children into "the normal atmosphere of community activities."[138] By the late 1950s, a consensus emerged that RTCs should be well integrated into their communities.[139] The reverse was also true, the authors argued: the community should be a part of the RTC so that "the citizens and other agencies of the community . . . see the hospital service as a part of the health and welfare program for all its children."[140] If neighbors knew more about what happened inside RTCs, professionals reasoned, they would feel less frightened of the children and perhaps even become invested in their success. Integration also reinforced the image of RTCs as wholly different from custodial institutions that sought to remove themselves entirely from mainstream society.

Administrators at RTCs actively sought to expose lay and professional members of local community agencies to the public health demand for treatment of emotionally disturbed children and illustrate the work they were doing to meet this need. In just the first year of its operation, the director of the Arthur Brisbane Child Treatment Center in New Jersey spoke at the local Kiwanis Club, Rotary Club, Exchange Club, Lions Club, a local high school, four women's clubs, two churches, and two government social agencies.[141] These events not only spread information and awareness, they also helped RTCs raise money from these organizations. Residential treatment centers also offered educational programs to teach child welfare professionals, parents, and other lay members of the community about mental hygiene and emotional disturbance.[142] Southard School was particularly involved in community outreach, sending psychiatrists and psychiatry residents to work at nearby training schools, public schools, child guidance centers, and the local hospital.[143] The result of this exposure, reflected former director Edward Greenwood, was that they were "very much identified as a part of the city, and I think this has been a great contribution to Topeka."[144] Although RTCs were small institutions and their numbers few, this extensive education and outreach meant that their approach to helping troubled children was disseminated widely.

For the more general public who were not necessarily aware of or interested in visiting an institute or attending a talk, television programs and movies offered an easier means of disseminating information about emotional disturbance and residential treatment. At least two films about Bellefaire were produced and disseminated in the 1950s. While the films themselves no longer exist, pamphlets and stories about them describe their plots and modes of distribution. The first, a twenty-five-minute film titled *More Than Half a Chance*, told the story of Rocky, who had started associating with a gang. "Rocky didn't actually heave the brick that shattered the store window," the brochure about the movie declared. "Yet, why was he with the gang that did it? Where had his family failed him to make him the tough little fellow he was?"[145] The movie promised to explain how "the misfortune of broken homes" made children like Rocky so troubled, and how Bellefaire offered children like them a "chance for a happy childhood and opportunity for a happy future."[146] Between 1952 and 1953, the movie was shown thirty-eight times to community groups.[147] Another Bellefaire film, the twenty-eight-minute *Boy in the Doorway*, was reportedly shown to ten thousand people, ranging from members of Jewish groups like B'nai B'rith and the Jewish Federation to attendees at professional meetings like the National Conference of Social Workers and regional meetings of the Children's Welfare League Association. In November 1957, it was even aired on a local television channel.[148]

Television viewers in the Los Angeles area could learn about residential treatment from their local broadcast stations. In 1957, KNXT (which became Los Angeles's CBS affiliate) broadcast a series called *Focus on Sanity*, which explored the world of California state psychiatric hospitals.[149] The approach was both sympathetic and scientific; the narrator declared in the series' introductory segment that "mental illness is not a disgrace. It's a disease."[150] On the August 7 episode, viewers visited the Camarillo State Hospital children's unit. The narrator described his experience of entering the foreign world of the unit, from his initial surprise at the seemingly normal children running around outside on a playground, to his quick realization that "there was something different about this play yard. . . . Each of these children was in his own little world."[151] His description told viewers that these disturbed children were not completely foreign or even scary but emphasized their differentness as well.

Charitable groups and clubs offered structured ways for community members to contribute to RTCs. At the Cincinnati Child Guidance Center, volunteers from the Red Cross, Junior League, and women's groups, among others, participated in activities like "dancing and music classes [and] special outings and trips."[152] At Brisbane in New Jersey, community groups funded birthday parties for each child with cake and ice cream for all.[153] Some RTCs even had volunteer groups founded for the express purpose of supporting the institution. In Seattle, more than thirty Four and Twenty women's clubs (named for the number of women who could fit into the living room at the first meeting) raised money for the Ryther Child Center and promoted the center's programs to community members.[154] In Los Angeles, a women's group named Las Candelas visited the children at Camarillo State Hospital on a regular basis, playing with them on hospital grounds or taking them on outings to the beach for picnics.[155]

While formal community outreach programs raised awareness of emotional disturbance and residential treatment, RTCs most forcefully demonstrated their commitment to community integration by sending their children into the outside world. As a matter of policy, many administrators encouraged children to form friendships outside the center and participate in activities like scouting, team sports, and going to the YMCA.[156] Administrators were careful about when and how they placed children in these situations, however. Martin Gula, the director of the Evanston Receiving Home outside Chicago, pointed out that if the home was going to send its children to local public schools, they had to be more selective in their admissions standards "for the residence can treat only as much disturbed behavior as the neighborhood will tolerate."[157] Administrators at RTCs had to be thoughtful about running institutions that were both in and of the community, as not all neighbors were welcoming.

Many RTCs faced formidable resistance from community members who did not want any emotionally disturbed children living nearby. When child psychiatrist Frank Curran was recruited from Bellevue to open an inpatient child psychiatry unit at the University of Virginia, he recalled the opposition of community members who "stated that the kind of children that we would be treating would psychologically contaminate their children who might be riding on the same bus with them to and from that area."[158] Typically these issues were cyclical, flaring up when a particular child had done something visibly aberrant in the community and tapering down after concerted efforts at community engagement and education.[159]

Conflict with the neighbors was a regular occurrence at Wiltwyck in upstate New York. Runaways, common in the 1940s and 1950s, strained relations with the local community. Frustration with the institution came to a head in September of 1951, when four boys ran away from Wiltwyck and broke into a house where they played with a gun. One of the four boys was accidentally shot and killed, a tragedy that was "deeply upsetting to every member of [the] school."[160] After this event, the director recalled, "we were attacked as a 'non-punitive' institution," criticized for their permissive policies. But as the school recovered from the incident and the number of runaways decreased dramatically, Wiltwyck's relationship with the community improved.[161] By 1955, Wiltwyck boys were playing Little League baseball on American Legion teams and singing Christmas carols at a nearby air base.[162] Twelve years later, community relations again soured with numerous runaways who broke into and robbed nearby homes. The boys acted so poorly when they were arrested that "they left a bad impression with the police officers."[163] A few months after this report, a new campus had provided a fresh start and a local volunteer group, the Westchester Friends of Wiltwyck, seemed to be smoothing over community relations. Volunteers were planning birthday parties for the children, teaching arts and crafts, and helping run a local Boy Scout troop.[164]

Moments of transgression could be opportunities for community education. When Butchie, a boy staying at Bellefaire, started throwing trash over a wall into a neighbor's backyard, she asked him to stop. Instead, he began cursing at her, to which social worker Morris Mayer encouraged him to "Say it again!" This seemingly bizarre event—a young boy being encouraged to curse instead of being punished for antisocial behavior—would have been difficult for any outsider to comprehend. But Mayer later visited the neighbor, explaining "that she had been witness to a minor miracle and that this was the first time in his life Butchie had ever spoken any word." In fact, Mayer told the neighbor that Butchie's swearing was likely an expression of his pent-up anger, which had been repressed until then. As a result of this conversation, the *Bellefaire Voice and Views* article explained, the neighbor was able to make sense of Mayer's unusual tactic and better appreciate the needs of the troubled children living next door.[165]

Fostering good relationships with local community members and organizations was critical for RTCs, many of whom were dependent on local philanthropy. At the Child Guidance Home of Cincinnati, for example, 30 percent of the home's operating budget came from the city community chest and 8 percent from the Junior League of Cincinnati.[166] At the Evanston Receiving Home, the Community Fund of Chicago provided 50 percent of the money needed to keep the home running.[167] Not all RTCs were as dependent on philanthropy; the Arthur Brisbane Child Treatment Center in New Jersey and University of Michigan child psychiatry unit were almost fully supported by the state, while wealthier RTCs like the Children's Service Center of Wyoming Valley and Southard School were primarily funded by parents who paid high fees for their children's treatment.[168] It was common for RTCs to receive funding from public sources and philanthropy.[169] At Wiltwyck, the bulk of the budget was provided by New York City monies, with another large sum provided by the philanthropic Greater New York Fund.[170] While each RTC depended on a slightly different set of people and organizations to fund their operation, few could afford to burn bridges with their neighbors.

For children at RTCs around the country, treatment was not limited to hour-long sessions with a psychiatrist or social worker. Instead, the environment in which they lived—the therapeutic milieu—had been engineered to make every activity and every interpersonal interaction therapeutic. Campuses that resembled white, middle-class homes and staff members who played the roles of temporary parents would help the children become "normal" by creating a physical and emotional environment that embodied contemporary American ideals about the "good life." Fostering strong community relationships was critical to educating neighbors about emotional disturbance and its treatment while portraying children treated at RTCs as regular neighborhood kids.

Place became a marker of normality, from the neighborhood in which an RTC was located to its wallpapered living room. Just as Americans in the postwar period sought to attain a new middle-class ideal by buying houses, cars, and television sets, RTCs used these same markers to build environments that could "correct" abnormal children. In these carefully engineered settings, staff members would play the part of master puppeteers as they orchestrated activities and interactions that made "normal" children out of disturbed ones.

SIX

Building the Normal Child

If we can help the boys and girls to become normal and happy children, we have experienced a fine return on the investment we are making.

—Leon Richman, *executive director, Bellefaire, 1951*[1]

After she had reluctantly settled into life at Hawthorne Cedar Knolls and resigned herself to engaging in therapy sessions, fourteen-year-old Vivian told her caseworker, "I want to be a calm, happy, normal human being. I want to understand myself. I want to control myself and be able to accept 'no' without getting excited. I want to be able to work, save, and not be wild."[2] To Vivian, being normal meant developing insight into her own behavior, achieving self-control, adhering to basic social rules, and learning practical skills that would help her be a useful member of society. Normal meant well, not only to Vivian but also to her caretakers at Hawthorne and their counterparts at other RTCs, who candidly discussed what made a child normal and their hopes of moving their charges as close to this ideal as possible. Normal children, believed RTC professionals, were active participants in their schools and communities, maintained meaningful relationships with peers and adults, were able to express themselves as individuals, and could operate both in groups and alone.[3]

As we have seen, one of the ways in which staff members hoped to guide children toward normality was by fashioning a welcoming, permissive atmosphere that resembled a middle-class family home. Within that environment, RTC professionals believed every activity and every interaction in the milieu, no matter how minor, was meaningful and had potential therapeutic value. In many cases, reality did not reflect this ideal: children could be cruel to each other, and surely not every activity fulfilled its intended purpose. Moreover, not every child *wanted* to be normal. Still, staff members tried to foster an environment in which children could simultaneously take control of their own lives and be gently guided by adults who would help them learn how to function successfully in a social world.

The normality that RTC professionals hoped to foster was characterized by moderation and a balance between conformity and individuality. On a daily basis, they hoped, children would learn how to relate to others and obey basic social norms. But fitting in did not mean being a mindless automaton. Instead, children were encouraged to form meaningful relationships with one another and with adult staff members so they could learn to understand and be responsive to the needs of others. During activities like art therapy and school, they were taught to express themselves as independent thinkers and artists, whose often-unorthodox thoughts or goals were welcomed as special and unique. The milieu served as a complex framework for imparting social norms as treatment, as RTC professionals strove to balance togetherness with aloneness and social conformity with independence, creativity, and self-expression.

This balance reflected the tension in postwar America between "normality" as cultural ideal and individuality as a bulwark against Communism. After the upheavals of World War II, which resulted in the physical relocation of families and their destabilization as fathers went to war and mothers went to work, the cultural ethos became a reactionary one. As American families attempted to "get back to normal," they found themselves confronted with new anxieties. Polio seemed to threaten families across lines of race and class. Americans found themselves wondering how they had gotten so behind in science and math when the Russians launched Sputnik. And mothers found themselves the targets of critics who blamed them for their children's deficiencies and, at times, for a perceived national epidemic of juvenile delinquency. As a result, families turned inward, hoping to raise children who would quietly fit in and get along well with others. Parents enrolled their children in activities like scouting and Sunday school to help inculcate common values.[4] At school, children watched mental hygiene films that taught them that social conformity, from what they wore to how they behaved, would lead to popularity and happiness.[5] For all Americans, normality was not just a statistical average. It was an ideal they strove for.[6]

Yet normality did not always mean conformity. In fact, many liberal social scientists cautioned that too much conformity was dangerous and would produce rigid, closed-minded citizens who dangerously approximated the Communist mindset.[7] Rather, the ideal American had an open, creative mind.[8] This creative mind, as Jamie Cohen-Cole has demonstrated, "would inoculate America against the dangers of mass society," which cultural critics believed had the potential to threaten individuality and turn Americans into an unthinking conglomeration of consensus.[9] The structure of therapeutic milieus at RTCs reflected a desire to balance these two approaches, suggesting that the tension between these ideals extended beyond academic discourse into clinical practice. Furthermore, this approach was apparent at RTCs in the late 1930s and early 1940s as well, suggesting that some of the cultural norms we label postwar or typical of Cold War culture were actually present much earlier.

Exploring the therapeutic milieu at the "ground level" allows us to get a better sense of daily experience and especially of the children's own experiences. Although children's voices appear here filtered through the recollections of the adults who cared for them, it is still possible to grasp aspects of their experiences at RTCs—experiences that were at times pleasant and comforting but could also be frightening and disturbing.[10]

Every Little Thing

In the carefully planned milieu of RTCs, every moment mattered. When nine-year-old Kenny arrived at Pioneer House on November 29, 1946, the staff members recorded their detailed recollections and impressions of the boy's first day. That evening, two counselors had joined Kenny in playing with a model train. While they played, the female counselor later recorded, Kenny repeated the phrase, "Ain't I smart," about fifteen times, "several times when it seemed out of context," and told her that "girls can't work this sort of thing," ordering the counselor around and demanding that they construct the train tracks his way.[11] At the end of the day, Pioneer House director Fritz Redl concluded that Kenny liked to get his own way, boast about his (nonexistent) skills, and tell others that he was superior to them.[12]

The detailed records staff members kept of activities in the milieu are notable because they included minute detail about the activities as well as staff reflections on their significance. In the milieu, every interaction had meaning, and it was up to staff members to discern it, a process that was essential to diagnosis and treatment.[13] In Kenny's case, observing his behavior helped staff members understand his personality and characterize his interactions with others. Seemingly insignificant events could also be harnessed as opportunities for therapeutic intervention. Redl was the originator of the term "life-space interview," which referred to on-the-spot discussions with a child immediately after a significant event had occurred in the milieu.[14] The life-space interview, espoused by most RTCs (even if not by name), was seen as a more organic alternative or complement to traditional psychotherapy.[15] For example, Bruno Bettelheim explained that, since children at the Orthogenic School tended to have difficulties with routine practices like bathing or eating, it was only natural to deal with these issues as they arose: "Anxieties that center around cleanliness or elimination are handled more directly and more easily with these children while they wash, or resent taking a bath, than by discussing their feelings in play sessions where the real experience can only be re-enacted with play dolls or toys."[16] This model enabled discussions that might have been limited to the artificial environment of the office to happen more organically.

One seemingly pedestrian area of great professional interest was food. Food could have a multiplicity of strong meanings for a child, and staff members worked to ensure that interactions around food would be positive and even therapeutic. A handbook for residential workers at Southard advised that interactions around food could reinforce anxieties, such as a fear of deprivation based on a child's past experiences. To counteract this possibility, staff were told that "the philosophy regarding food is basically that there is always enough. . . . It is never to be used by the worker as a means of depriving, punishing, or controlling, but is to be given freely and warmly."[17] Lauretta Bender likened the giving of food to the giving of a mother's love, and Bruno Bettelheim argued that disturbed children needed to learn that adults could meet their needs fully and without strings attached.[18] To show children that there was always enough food to meet their needs, these centers adopted special eating practices. At Southard, children had access around the clock to a special refrigerator that was stocked with candy bars at night.[19] At the Orthogenic School, an unlocked candy closet was available to the children, who could take as much as they wanted.[20] Mealtimes were relaxed, and picky eaters were not criticized. At Bellevue, meals were prepared in the central kitchen, but "modifications [could] be made in our own kitchen where milk, juices, cocoa, bread and jam, etc. are always available."[21] If a child at Southard disliked milk, "maybe a little choclate [*sic*] syrup in it will help. If not, there may be tea or punch or just plain ice water."[22] Staff at the University of Michigan offered plenty of seconds on dessert and did not worry much about enforcing good table manners.[23] If food represented love, RTC professionals made sure it was never in short supply.

In addition to establishing a generally positive environment around food, staff members recognized that mealtimes had particular therapeutic potential for certain children. For example, knowing that adults would never deny them food, even after bad behavior, could be helpful for children who tended not to trust adults.[24] Frank, a boy at the Orthogenic School with a long history of theft, told his counselor over a meal that he no longer felt the urge to steal because "at School you get everything you want. I don't have to steal."[25] Paranoid children might see that others were not trying to harm them. At Hawthorne, one social work student found that children with schizophrenia felt comforted when they saw staff members eating the same food as them, a sign that dinner was probably not poisonous.[26] For withdrawn Emily, the situation was quite the opposite. She was constantly scared that others were trying to kill her, but for some reason had no trouble eating food prepared in the Orthogenic School kitchen. Yet when she thought a cookie had come from her mother, she "screamed at the top of her lungs that the counselor was killing her" and was comforted only when the staff showed her that the cookie had come from the school kitchen.[27] Staff members' detailed recording of these events and reflection on their significance demonstrated their belief that every event in the milieu, no matter how small, had important diagnostic and therapeutic meaning.[28]

Friends and Enemies

Even with all the candy bars in the world, the milieu could be a chaotic place. A journalist visiting Southard in 1947 reported in *Collier's*: "At first you think it is bedlam. A teen-age girl kicks out a window in an upstairs bedroom. Two boys spill a bucket of varnish down the front staircase. Several children display flaxen streaks in their hair, where they have doused it with peroxide. A small boy dashes off the veranda and sets fire to dry grass in the yard. A girl hurls a teacup across the dining room."[29] A residential workers' logbook from Southard suggests that such havoc occurred on a daily basis. At the end of their shifts, workers left brief notes for colleagues taking over for them to update them on any major events. On February 24, 1960, Sam was angry when he was told it was time to go to bed at 9:30. To retaliate, he plugged the bathroom sinks and turned on all the faucets, flooding the entire room.[30] In November, childcare worker Beth wrote at 11 P.M., "There was a fire in the wastebasket in bathroom downstairs. General destruction of property continues. Masses of wet toilet tissue flung on bathroom wall. All is a mystery."[31] Living and working with these youngsters was no doubt extremely trying for residential workers.

Children could be cruel to one another. Ellen and Bonnie were constantly at each other's throats. On March 14, 1960, Bonnie hit Ellen in the face, leaving her with a swollen cheek. "This is why Bonnie and Ellen are not to be left alone at any time," reported childcare worker Phyl Fry.[32] Children also insulted each other about their emotional problems and family backgrounds. In April, Anita and Bonnie got into a physical fight after Bonnie called Anita sick.[33] Lee Stringer recalled an episode when a child named Pee Wee made fun of his race (Stringer was black) and poor family. Stringer retorted: "At least my mother shows up [to visit]," and the two began to punch each other wildly.[34] The milieu could be a dangerous place.

Staff members kept a keen eye on how children interacted with each other, hoping to gain insight into their personalities. In their prolonged work with a small group of boys at Hawthorne Cedar Knolls, two social work students observed that eleven-year-old Jimmy took on a "tough guy" role, threatening other children constantly but never following through and engaging in physical fights.[35] Walter, also eleven, was withdrawn, "distant from his peers and rarely relates to anyone," speaking "in a whinning [*sic*] voice."[36] Twelve-year-old Donald also failed to interact with others, but he was so "manipulative and exploitative" of the other children that none of them wanted to deal with him anyway.[37] Staff members also took note of children interacting well with other children. On the evening of March 22, 1960, Southard childcare workers Suzy and Roy found Brian "quiet + relaxed." He didn't fight bedtime, and calmly informed the workers that he had forgotten to brush his teeth. When he was done brushing, "instead of the usual jumping on beds + yelling at little boys to wake them up," Brian patted two boys and calmly went to bed. "I'm real proud of him," the worker reflected.[38] Staff observations and analyses of how children interacted with one another reflected their beliefs about what comprised "good" or "bad" behavior. Obviously physically attacking another child was bad behavior, but so were Donald's manipulation, Jimmy's threats, and Walter's whiny withdrawal, which the social workers identified as inappropriate group behaviors. Good behavior meant following the rules, of course, but staff members believed it was even more important that children knew how to relate well to one another. When Brian went to bed without argument, Suzy and Roy were pleased, but when he patted two boys on the head on the way, they were proud.

Despite the serious disturbances and varied backgrounds of RTC children, they lived closely and cooperated in surprising, powerful ways. David, a boy at Southard, frequently smeared his own feces all over himself, his shared bedroom, and his shared bathroom. The boys on his floor, disgusted by this behavior, set up a meeting with a staff member to ask if David might be moved down to the second floor and away from them. The staff member was sympathetic but explained that it might not be possible because the children on the second floor had a different bedtime. In response, a boy named Gary "stated quite thoughtfully and with rather deep sincerity, 'Your reasons are good but you are not taking into account our feelings about the matter,'" explaining that the area smelled and that David's feces were everywhere. Together the boys came up with a number of suggestions. One proposed placing deodorant sprays and a can of liquid deodorant for David's underwear in the bathroom, and another boy offered to switch bedrooms so David could be alone.[39] Though it was not a perfect solution, the boys had worked it out together, with the support of a staff member who was sympathetic to their expressed needs. In the process, they had delineated their own needs and expressed sympathy and understanding to a severely troubled boy, demonstrating to staff members that they had successfully taught these boys how to interact meaningfully with their peers.

The Power of Peer Pressure

RTC professionals believed that all interactions among children had the potential to be therapeutic, because children would help each other learn to behave according to designated norms. Lauretta Bender called this phenomenon the "socializing effect," or "a means of aiding the child in becoming a more successful social personality."[40] Not everyone saw this effect as beneficial. By the early 1950s, social psychologists like Solomon Asch warned that what they called "group pressure" could squelch individual opinion and produce a false consensus as individuals sought to conform to a group norm.[41] But at RTCs, staff members felt that group influence, or peer pressure as they often called it, was a positive force that children would naturally use to keep one another in line. During both informal and formal work with groups of children, RTC professionals attempted to engineer children's interactions with each other as deliberate therapeutic tools. In the process, they refined their concept of what it meant to have a "successful social personality" and, consequently, what it meant to be a normal child.

Organized groups like student councils gave children a voice in their daily lives while encouraging productive peer interactions. Bellefaire's Campus Council met every week and made suggestions to the board on topics like "allowances, dating, bedtime hours, sports equipment, [and] programming."[42] A student recreation council at Hawthorne played a similar role.[43] At Southard in the late 1930s, the Children's Court featured a child "judge" in black gown and white wig who made rulings on children who had misbehaved or had other complaints about the institution.[44] While a teacher was present, the final verdict was delivered by the judge, who also meted out "the fine or other penalty for misdemeanors."[45] These groups were usually monitored by adults. But at the Illinois Neuropsychiatric Institute, the children's desire to organize was so great in the late 1940s that they spontaneously formed a "highly organized military organization" on the ward with ranks, drills, and insignia.[46] While this system imposed a great deal of pressure on children whose behavior was deemed "abnormal" by their peers (bedwetters, for example), it also resulted in increased privileges and responsibilities. "The children were encouraged to feel that they were acutally [*sic*] working as ward staff members, and their job assignments went up on the bulletin board along with nurses' assignments."[47] Organized groups and councils, whether overseen by adults or not, gave children spaces to interact meaningfully and shape the milieu to their liking.

Groups of children could police children whose behavior was seen as disruptive or annoying. Bruno Bettelheim told the story of Jack, a delusional boy who interrupted a group bedtime story when he began yelling about a dead man hiding under a table. In response, the other children shouted "quite forcefully and almost in unison . . . 'There is not and shut up; we want to hear the story.'"[48] This order, along with several other similar reassurances, quieted Jack, who went to bed peacefully. Bettelheim believed that this worked so effectively because, unlike the other people in Jack's life, the children were not afraid of Jack's strange beliefs and were a cohesive enough group to stand up to his bizarre statement with certainty. While examples like these were described by staff as helpful to the "odd child out," in reality they were likely also hurtful or threatening at times.

At a few RTCs, staff members created formal programs to harness these therapeutic interactions, gathering children in carefully engineered groups to participate in activities with an adult supervisor.[49] Throughout, the supervisor would serve as both teacher and therapist, handling conflicts as they arose and helping a small group of children learn how to interact with one another. At Langley Porter in the mid-1940s, a psychiatrist and social worker formed an experimental therapeutic group as a response to wartime staffing shortages, which had left the children without a teacher and with tensions rising in the absence of structured daytime activities. The setup was flexible and unorthodox: for one and a half hours twice a week, a group of between five and eight children met with a leader and an assistant. The composition of the group changed over the five months of the experiment with some new children put in and others taken out for behavioral reasons (such as children being dangerously aggressive toward one another) or practical limitations (if a child was discharged, for example). Sessions involved unstructured play among children with very different personalities, supervised to ensure that things did not get too out of hand. The staff members noted each child's progress in a daily chart, using open and shaded circles of different sizes to describe the children (fig. 6.1).

Although there were many bumps along the way—three children were simply too aggressive to be around the others, for example—the psychiatrist and social worker found that the children improved much more quickly than they would have expected. In particular, there seemed to be a direct benefit for different kinds of children to be around one another. Eight-year-old Judith was initially extremely aggressive and led the group in two games of strip poker, but being part of the group helped her calm down, although she remained a ringleader. Her black dot fluctuated in size, but had become quite small, approaching "normal," by the end of the five months. Eight-year-old Tony was aggressive at home, threatening to kill his mother, but on the ward, he had been very withdrawn and anxious. Staff members were encouraged to see Tony begin to express his aggression in group therapy, as his large open circle housed a larger and larger black

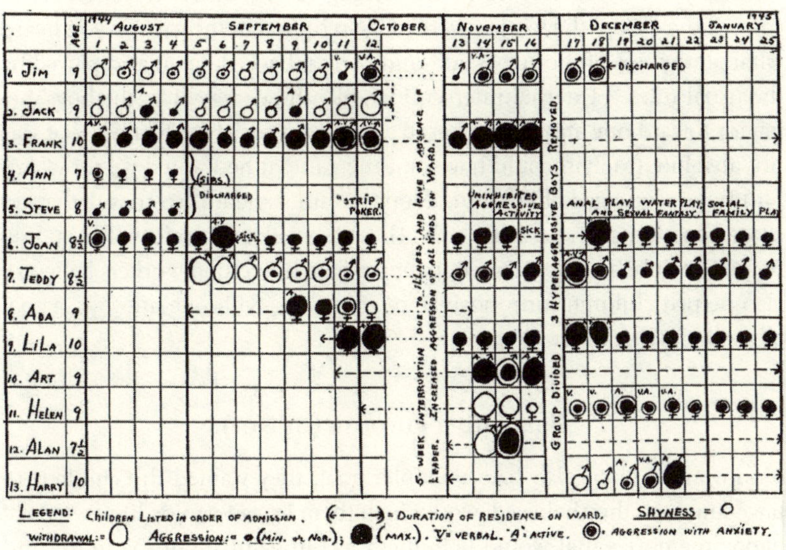

6.1. Tracking group therapy progress at Langley Porter, 1947. Withdrawn = *large open circle*, shy = *small open circle*, minimally aggressive or normal = *small dark circle*, aggressive = *large dark circle*, and aggressive and anxious = *dark dot surrounded by a circle*. (Kathleen K. Stewart and Pearl L. Axelrod, "Group Therapy on a Children's Psychiatric Ward," *American Journal of Orthopsychiatry* 17, no. 2 [1947]: 315.)

dot (withdrawn to anxious/aggressive) and finally became a small, healthy black dot.[50] Although the experiment ended when the staff members involved in group therapy had to assume administrative roles, it seemed to demonstrate that when different kinds of disturbed children played together, the result could be therapeutic. Notably, group leaders described children as improved the closer their behavior inched toward normal—not too shy or too aggressive, but somewhere in between. "Normal" meant moderate, neither one extreme nor the other.

Group workers, who either were lay workers or had social work degrees, played an important role in identifying unproductive behaviors and encouraging children to abide by group standards. Hawthorne group workers Marvin Bloom and Adrian Cabral referred to this process as helping "them to become more socialized by playing more in accordance with group accepted rules."[51] This process was integrated into group play in the tiniest of moments, like when Melvin tried to make up a new rule just as a game of hide and seek was about to start. None of the other boys wanted to use this rule, and the group worker told Melvin they would not use it, to which Melvin announced, "I quit." The worker refused to accede to Melvin's pushiness and replied, "So quit," to which Melvin attempted to introduce yet another new rule. Continuing to resist Melvin's attempts to control the group, the worker warned, "No hiding in the game—you heard what all the rest of the guys said," and Melvin backed down and played by the usual rules.[52] External interventions like these, as well as the boys' behavior toward one another, enforced a degree of social conformity that was not absolute (Melvin could have quit the game if he wanted to, for example) but encouraged children to adopt certain standards so that the group could function as a successful unit. These "socializing" endeavors not only helped limit behaviors deemed inappropriate but, group workers believed, also helped children form positive relationships with one another, a goal of residential treatment in general.

Fun with a Purpose (or Not)

Bloom and Cabral also had a simpler goal: they wanted the children to have fun. Fun, they believed, would help them learn to enjoy life and make happy memories that would help them feel hopeful about the future and "urge them to continue to grow."[53] There was no shortage of opportunities for fun at RTCs. The first annual report of the Arthur Brisbane Child Treatment Center reported that "the children engaged in boxing, roller skating, swimming, fishing, baseball, walks," picnics, sledding, television and movie watching, and a visit from a magician.[54] Bellefaire was notable for its abundance of extracurricular activities, from arts and crafts, woodshop, the student newspaper *Blue and Gold*, drama, fishing, scouting, baseball and basketball in the local Jewish sports league, Stamp Club, and music lessons to special events like the soapbox derby and county fair, where the children sold items they made to the public at their individual cottages' booths.[55] Children typically were allowed to choose their own recreational activities. "All the activities are voluntary," explained Arnold in the introductory pamphlet written by Bellefaire children. "You can go to any groups you want and drop out any time you want."[56] Sometimes spontaneous activities were the most memorable. Harry Wade, Southard head childcare worker from 1949 to 1952, remembered "bike rides, swimming at the old Gage Park pool, endless games of kick the can, the annual camping trip . . . and individual shopping trips with various children," a mix of planned activities and "in-between" moments.[57] On one evening during Reid and Hagan's visit to the University of Michigan's child psychiatry unit for their CWLA study, the boys put on girls' clothing and were primped by the nurses while another group of children made fudge and another group worked on their photography.[58]

All this was not to say that fun had no purpose. In the eyes of staff members, "The youngsters' recreational diet was as carefully planned as a medical prescription would be for physical disturbances."[59] The idea that play should have an educational function was common among American parents, who by the 1950s were starting to dictate the terms of their children's play with planned activities.[60] The rationales for play at RTCs were as numerous as the adults dictating them. Strenuous activities like boxing could help children get rid of excess energy or negative emotions, some argued.[61] Other RTC professionals focused on the potential for play to build self-confidence and independence as a child learned new skills, including how "to hold his own with his peers."[62]

Above all, they hoped children would learn how to play with each other. The road to successful group play required the individual child to move away from his or her behavioral extreme: "The withdrawn child is encouraged to be more competitive; the demanding child to share; and the aggressive child to utilize his energies constructively," explained a social work student at the Illinois Neuropsychiatric Institute. The process could be extremely trying. At Southard in the mid-1940s, the children preferred more individual activities like swimming or horseback riding as opposed to more cooperative ones like volleyball, much to the frustration of the staff, who hoped to use team sports to reinforce appropriate social behaviors.[63]

Recalled former Bradley director Maurice Laufer, "We had to teach them how to play, literally how to play . . . but also how to be a team player."[64] By learning how to play as a team, staff members like Laufer hoped they would also learn to behave according to basic societal standards.

Another important purpose of recreation was teaching girls how to be girls and boys how to be boys. Many activities were divided by sex: at Brisbane, boys learned how to take care of the grounds and worked with the carpenter and painter, while the girls worked in the dining room and learned grooming and sewing.[65] At Hawthorne, boys were involved in scouting, while girls did "cooking, cleaning and sewing," which the staff deemed "therapeutic."[66] At Michigan, staff felt that teaching girls how to groom themselves was "part of the therapy."[67] Staff members of the appropriate gender were encouraged to take an active role in these efforts in tangible ways, teaching them to sew, cook, or style their hair and providing positive feedback to girls who embraced these activities.[68] The goal of these interventions was to encourage children to behave according to traditional gendered expectations.[69] Staff members also helped by modeling appropriately gendered behavior. In the case of Wilma, a teenager at Michigan who only wore boys' clothes and always looked "unkempt," a close relationship with a "young blonde nurse" and work in occupational therapy sessions making jewelry and learning interior decorating helped her "accept her feminine role."[70] These efforts were in line with expectations for teenagers in general, which were rigid and gender-specific.[71]

Recreational activities could also be designed to deal with an individual child's specific emotional needs. Billy was a withdrawn thirteen-year-old boy at Hawthorne who was subject to violent outbursts toward others, stealing, running away, and fire setting.[72] When he arrived at Hawthorne, the staff described him as "withdrawn, moody and depressed, except for his periodic rages, repulsing all friendly advances, unable to endure physical contact . . . almost like a hunted young animal."[73] The staff found Billy very suspicious of everyone around him and sent him to the community farm, hoping time there would foster emotional growth. Soon after, he began to bathe, wear clean clothes, and interact with the other boys in his cottage, encouraging signs that farm work was helping Billy grow as a person.[74]

Initially, farm work went to Billy's head. He started selling the chickens' eggs and made a good deal of money. At school, he would read only about farming and arrogantly lecture the other boys about how to properly take care of the cows.[75] But by his third year at Hawthorne, Billy's progress accelerated. He formed authentic friendships with other boys and started putting more effort into his schoolwork so he could learn to run a farm one day.[76] In therapy, he demonstrated new insight as he spoke of his tendency to distrust others. Farm animals, he told his therapist, would listen to what you say but not talk back or try to manipulate you.[77] After four years at Hawthorne, staff members helped Billy get a job on a nearby farm. Eventually, he moved back to his hometown, completed high school, and went to an agricultural college to work toward his dream of owning his own farm.[78]

Reflecting on Billy's stay at Hawthorne, former school director Herschel Alt commented that his time alone at the farm had helped calm him down and diminish his violent thoughts and impulses. Only then could he learn to form trusting relationships with the children and adults around him and gain insight into his own character.[79] Spending time on a farm was not a traditional "fun" activity like baseball or swimming, but it was a meaningful activity that staff members specifically chose for Billy based on his interpersonal difficulties. In situations like these, RTCs were literally adapting the milieu to the child to achieve the greatest therapeutic benefit.

Art and the Creative Mind

Traditionally lowbrow activities like farming or sports were paired with explorations into the fine arts, which were felt to offer children additional means of self-expression. At most RTCs, visual art and other creative activities like drama and music were considered pillars of milieu therapy. The products of these activities were largely not intended for the public eye. Instead, these forms of creative expression served as alternative modes of communication between children and adults and provided opportunities for a child to explore his or her own feelings without any judgments or repercussions. Here, it was the act of creating art, music, or drama and sharing it with others that mattered most. Each creative activity offered a multiplicity of purposes and meanings for children and staff, and their sum was intended to foster creativity and self-expression.

To help children explore their creative sides, RTC administrators constructed specialized, on-site arts and crafts facilities. At the University of Michigan, the planning committee instructed the architects to build three different shops, one of which would specifically be used for woodworking.[80] They also requested a kiln, two sewing machines, and a lathe, along with other supplies. Classrooms were to have painted Masonite walls "so the children can paint designs on them."[81] At the Menninger's new Children's Division building, special walls would let the children hang up their artwork or even express themselves freely in chalk and paint.[82] Even on Southard's old campus, the specially built crafts shop provided a dazzling array of equipment and materials, including "equipment for finger painting, potter's wheel, an electric kiln, loom for weaving, easels, tools for leather work, jewelry, linoleum block printing," "materials for photography, carpentry, model boat building, metal etching, [and] wood burning."[83] This equipment was no doubt very expensive, reflecting the importance staff members placed on artistic activities.

For the child, time to paint, sew, or build was time alone with little adult intervention.[84] The goal was not to make children good artists but to foster freedom of expression, which RTC professionals believed was inherently therapeutic.[85] Children could communicate thoughts that they otherwise perceived as too dangerous to talk about, release physical jitters, or even express aggression or rage.[86] A 1938 Southard pamphlet described the impressive craft shop, where activities ranging from pottery to finger painting "encourage many a timid child to dream, to dare and to create." In the same room, "the destructive child finds an ideal place to vent his rage by pounding mightily on nails, by rending boards with whirring saws, by thumping clay with doubled fist."[87] Art might even serve a socializing function as children worked together in a craft shop or art room, watching one another create.[88] Even though children were not receiving formal training or being judged on the quality of their work, the variety and depth of their creations is stunning.

For the therapists and other adults taking care of them, art offered a way to connect to children who were hesitant to participate in therapy or other activities. Ruth Faison Shaw, the founder of modern American finger painting, was an extremely popular visitor and guest instructor at Southard because she was able to talk to children at their own level and make them feel comfortable.[89] At home in New York, Shaw taught finger painting at the Dalton School, where art was promoted as a form of creative self-expression. It was this same ideal that she and her counterparts sought to introduce into the residential treatment setting.[90] Nancy, a five-year-old girl at the Lakeside Children's Center, was prone to losing her temper and arguing that things were never fair. But it was in art that the staff learned the most about her. Every time she created something, she would immediately destroy it, "diagnosing each piece as a failure, denouncing herself and her shortcomings." This behavior convinced the staff that Nancy felt that she was herself a failure, that "she felt inferior and inadequate."[91]

The real prize for the therapist or staff member was gaining access to thoughts and feelings that even the child herself might not be aware of. Used in this way, art could be "'a language of the unconscious' for the child."[92] At Southard, Ruth Faison Shaw and staff member Jeanetta Lyle asserted that fingerpainting was similar to playing with mud and amounted to adults letting children express thoughts that were otherwise forbidden. While a child made multiple drawings on the same piece of wet, painted paper, Shaw would record how he or she described her work (fig. 6.2).[93] These descriptions would be analyzed later to gain insight into the child's unconscious thoughts and feelings.[94]

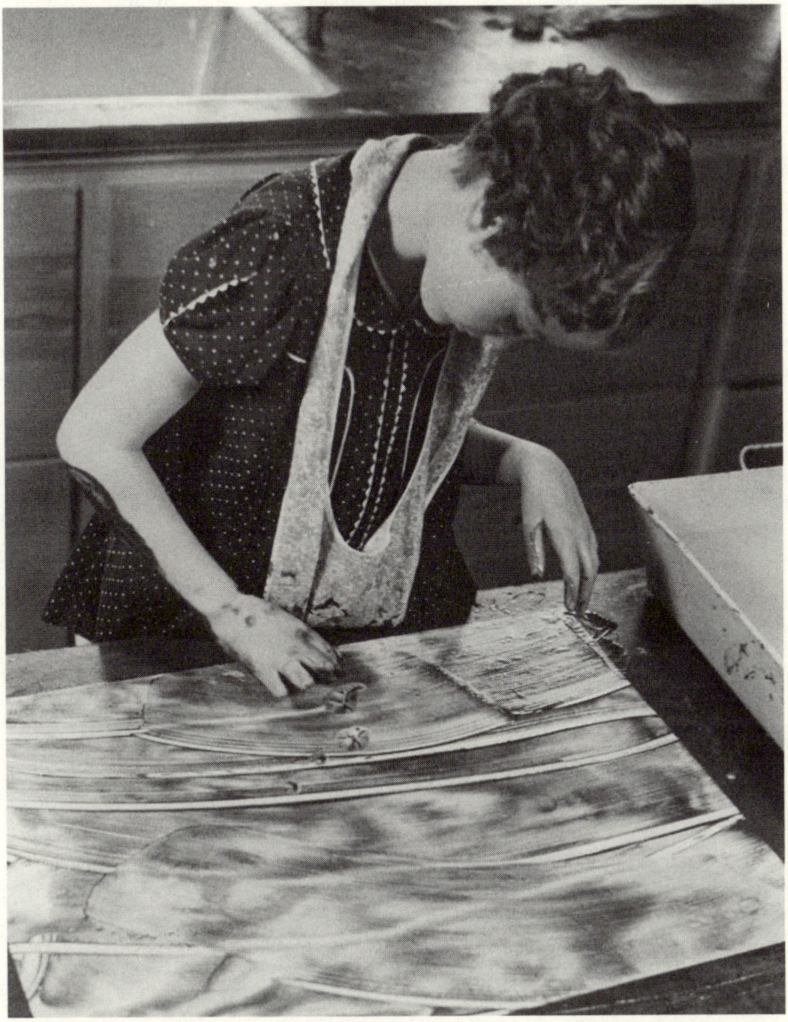

6.2. Finger painting at Southard School, 1940s. (Jeanetta Lyle and Ruth Faison Shaw, "Encouraging Fantasy Expression in Children," *Bulletin of the Menninger Clinic* 1, no. 3 (1937): 78–79.)

Drama and puppet therapy, though used less widely, played a similar role in promoting self-expression and providing material that staff members could analyze for conscious and unconscious content. At Wiltwyck in upstate New York, children wrote and performed their own plays, which staff believed would help them practice interacting with other children and give them "an opportunity to talk about [their] own feelings in a disguised and nonthreatening way."[95] A similar psychodrama program existed at Michigan but was done in small groups of three or fewer children who met with a psychologist.[96] Perhaps the most elaborate program existed at Bellevue in the 1930s, when Works Progress Administration funds supported an elaborate puppet therapy program. Led by puppeteer (and later, psychoanalyst) Adolf Woltmann, hand puppets like protagonist Casper played out common trials and tribulations of childhood and family life, such as sibling rivalry, jealousy of a new baby, and deprivation of parental love (fig. 6.3).

At certain points in the show, Casper would ask the children in the audience what he should do next, and the children would shout out their

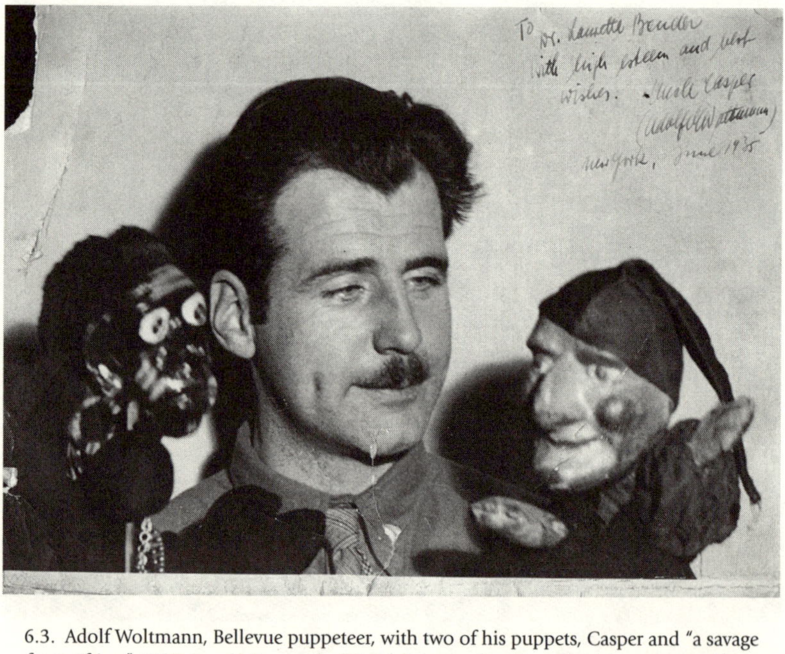

6.3. Adolf Woltmann, Bellevue puppeteer, with two of his puppets, Casper and "a savage from Africa," 1935. Inscription reads: "To Dr. Lauretta Bender with high esteem and best wishes. Uncle Casper (Adolf Woltmann) New York, June 1935." (Untitled photograph, Box 17, File 10, File #10 Photographs 1930–40 [From Scrapbook on Puppet Shows], LB.)

preferences. In theory, the children were unconsciously projecting their own problems onto Casper in front of other staff members, expressing feelings that they might not have felt comfortable communicating directly to an adult. In the puppet show audience, a child was surrounded by other children shouting out their suggestions for Casper and ideally would feel free to express herself without fear of judgment or punishment.[97] At one show, Casper's mother explained to him that she was going to have a new baby. Casper then turned to the audience and asked, "Would you want a little baby brother or sister, children?" Reported one observing journalist in the *New York World-Telegram*, "There is a tumult of voices. There are forty decided opinions, no reluctance in shouting them. Cries of 'No, no!' ring out; cries of 'Yes, yes!' resound."[98] In front of Casper, the children were free to express their opinions, socially desirable or not.

Casper could bring out the darker side of children as well. In the same puppet show, Casper found his new baby sibling sleeping and was trying to wake him up. One boy encouraged him to shout louder at the baby and another suggested shooting it. When Casper asked the audience if he should kill the baby, "Some children cry out he should. Others shout to stop him."[99] One visitor from the Brooklyn State Hospital was "chilled by the vicious responses of the audiences" when she saw one of the puppet plays at Bellevue.[100] But according to Bender and Woltmann, instances like these helped children learn that their peers had similar concerns and that it was all right to express them openly.[101]

Also at Bellevue, Works Progress Administration workers from the Federal Music Project ran a program in music therapy on the unit that similarly sought to promote self-expression. The group did a variety of activities, including group singing, freeze (when the music stopped), and rhythm band, in which children could beat as loudly as they wanted to on drums and other percussion instruments. The effects were so calming, especially for children deemed hyperkinetic, that one staff member commented, "'Music hath charms to sooth the savage beast' was written in Queen Elizabeth's day but today we might add and the 'problem child.'"[102] Music seemed to bring children together. For even the most sullen child, hiding in the corner, one staff member observed that the allure of the group was too great to ignore for long. Ultimately, she commented, "the music socializes him in spite of himself."[103]

During a second era of music therapy at Bellevue in 1946, the activity was completely different, focused almost entirely on the children's integration into and subjugation to the needs of a larger group. Led by a man who can only be identified as "R. Dreschler" by his signature at the bottom of his final handwritten note, the five-month experiment began with the goal of "getting children who were withdrawn or asocial to integrate with a group through the non-verbal medium of music."[104] Each day, the children would come into the room and choose an instrument out of a box. They would request songs from a small, familiar roster, and Dreschler would play them on the piano while the children "accompanied" him. The notes he wrote pay particular attention to children who deviated from the group in any way and describe how he tried to help them reintegrate into it. Charlotte, for example, had difficulty playing along with the group and kept banging her cymbals after a song had ended, making it difficult for the others to talk in between.[105] The goal was not to produce lovely music but, rather, to engage all of the children in the same atonal feast of noise without physical or emotional violence.

In his final comments on the five-month experiment, Dreschler reflected that "this music group has not been very therapeutic, but in the cases of some children it has served an integrative purpose quite well, drawing withdrawn children into a group, and giving aggressive children a non-destructive outlet for their energies."[106] While Dreschler never explained what would have made the group more "therapeutic," his comments reflect the therapeutic goal, prevalent in most RTCs, of bringing "extreme" children back to a behavioral middle ground. His detailed summaries of each child's performance also reflect the premium he placed on an individual child's ability to function in a group of peers. Elmer was a leader, choosing the group's songs, but also insisted on occupying the teacher's attention as much as possible. Bruce always wanted his way and cried when he didn't get it, but "his ability to get along with the other children improved" when the teacher "adopted a stern attitude toward him." Wilbur initially spent sessions "attacking other children for real or imagined wrongs which were constantly being done him" but adopted the role of "policeman" for the group, integrating himself into activities by monitoring the participation of other children.[107] It was these tendencies, rather than the boys' musical talents, that were the subject of music therapy.

Just like other activities in the therapeutic milieu, art, puppet, and music therapies were intended to foster normality in RTC children. Art and puppet therapy relied more heavily on self-expression and creativity, while Dreschler's music therapy was intended mainly to foster group interactions. Still, each activity had elements of both: music therapy let children bang out their frustrations, and Bellevue staff believed that children felt more comfortable yelling at the puppets because they were doing so together.

More than any other aspect of the milieu, though, these activities fostered the belief that the normal mind was individualized, open, and creative.

In the Classroom

While activities like painting or puppet shows happened only once in a while, RTC professionals tried to make daily life resemble life outside institutional walls as much as possible. The major way in which they did so was by requiring children to participate in educational activities on a regular basis. The task was not an easy one; most of these children had a long history of difficulties in the classroom. They were typically behind their grade level, and many RTC professionals observed a high prevalence of reading disabilities.[108] More commonly, they hated academic work and associated it with emotions like "feelings of failure and unworthiness" or disinterest.[109] When it came to school, it was often impossible to separate learning problems from emotional ones.[110]

Special education in the mid-twentieth century was a well-developed idea that was often executed suboptimally. From the 1930s to the 1950s, many states mandated that special classrooms be available to meet the needs of so-called exceptional children. In almost all cases, these children were educated in separate classrooms or schools; by 1948, more than 439,000 children were involved in a special education program.[111] Yet the education of children with emotional or intellectual disabilities—a varied group often artificially grouped together in policy and practice—lagged behind.[112] In the 1950s, most intellectually disabled children were still being institutionalized by their parents, an option recommended by most experts. However, new groups of middle-class parents organized to provide support and build opportunities for their children, believing that all children should be given a chance to learn. They agitated for expanded special education, working with state officials to increase funding and sometimes even forming their own schools.[113] RTC professionals similarly felt that all children deserved an education, although they often found it extremely challenging to reach their population.

Although the push to integrate children into "typical" classrooms would not mature until the 1960s, RTCs were constantly experimenting with the most effective way of educating their charges.[114] A few RTCs sent their children to local public schools.[115] It was far more common, though, to keep children on the grounds at an on-campus school or set of classrooms.[116] At Bellevue and Hawthorne Cedar Knolls, on-site schools were officially part of the local public school system.[117] Children at Bellefaire attended a local public school in the area until the late 1940s, but when teachers complained that some children were too difficult to manage, administrators divided up the children and scattered them among some twenty local public schools in 1950. Though better communication between the institution and teachers improved community relations, Bellefaire increasingly was admitting more disturbed children, some of whom were not capable of attending public school. The same year, administrators founded a small on-campus school for the most troubled, disruptive children, a solution that met the changing needs of the center so well that by 1956, 65 percent of Bellefaire's children were attending the on-campus school.[118]

On-campus schools often bore little resemblance to public schools. A few centers aimed to keep their children on par with their peers in public schools. Brisbane accomplished this goal by holding classes year round, and Bradley teachers focused on teaching the three R's (reading, 'riting, and 'rithmetic) and expecting children to behave just as they would in a mainstream school.[119] More commonly, administrators and teachers hoped their students would learn to enjoy school and succeed there.[120] Reflected Charles Bradley, "Our purpose is to show children that school can be fun and that teachers are human beings."[121] According to Bradley and his contemporaries, a successful educational experience at an RTC would be emotionally fulfilling and foster creativity and independence.[122] These goals were reflected in the nontraditional content of residential schooling. Teachers at the Illinois Neuropsychiatric Institute based their lessons on the curriculum of Chicago public schools but made sure that "assignments [were] usually short, easy, and quite varied" so students could experience success "and avoid frustrating and failure situations."[123] Classrooms had pianos and painting materials, and student writing and artwork was on display. Assignments might include putting on a play with a group of students or taking care of a goldfish, which would encourage productive group interactions and teach responsibility, respectively.[124] At Hawthorne Cedar Knolls, "school" might include group activities like the Explorer's Club and creating a school magazine or vocational training in gardening, plumbing, or homemaking to prepare students for life on the outside.[125] Each activity had a purpose, aimed at shaping a child's development as an expressive individual and a functional member of a group or society at large.

The classroom atmosphere reflected the rest of the milieu: it was permissive, but not without limits. In a 1958 booklet celebrating Bellefaire's ninetieth anniversary, photographs of two classrooms illustrate this relaxed approach (figs. 6.4 and 6.5). In the first, six young students sit in individual

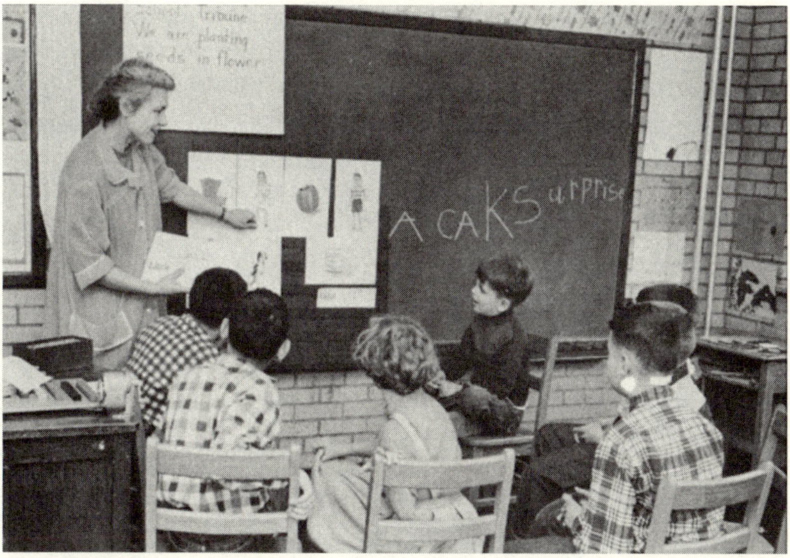

6.4. Bellefaire children in the classroom, late 1950s. (Untitled photograph, "Bellefaire 90th Anniversary 1868–1958," Container 19, Folder 7, BA.)

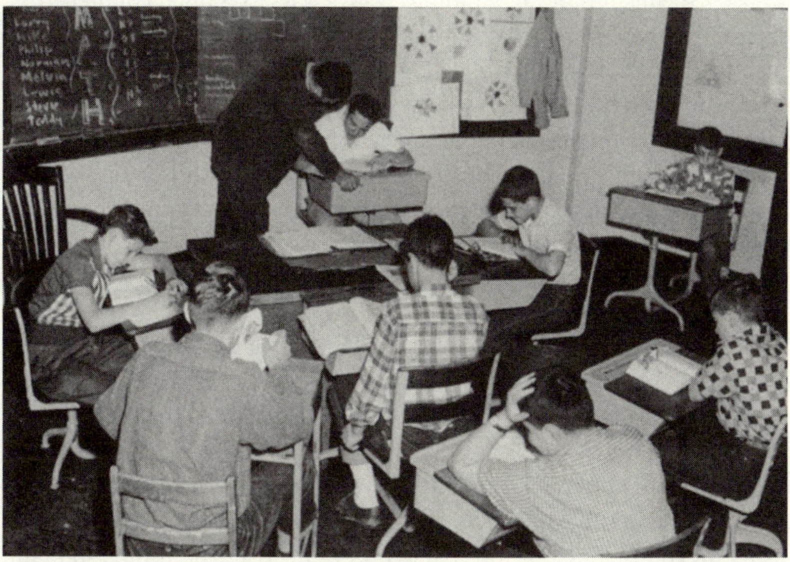

6.5. Bellefaire children in the classroom, late 1950s. (Untitled photograph, "Bellefaire 90th Anniversary 1868–1958," Container 19, Folder 7, BA.)

chairs, huddled a few feet away from the chalkboard as the teacher points to images she has taped there. In the second, a slightly older group of eight boys sit at their desks, which are strewn about the classroom. One boy at the front is being helped by the teacher, and nearby is a clump of four boys near the teacher's desk and two others farther back; a single boy sits away from the others near the wall. Freedom to move around the classroom contributed to its permissive, unorthodox atmosphere. One boy at the Orthogenic School was so distrustful of this policy that one day he announced to the class that he was leaving, ran out of the classroom, and immediately returned to repeat the cycle again. Meanwhile, the teacher ignored his strange behavior and told him he was free to move about as he wished. When the boy saw that he was really not going to get in trouble, "he finally came in, took his seat, and with no further acting out took up his assignment."[126] This laissez-faire approach had limits, though. At Hawthorne Cedar Knolls, the line was drawn at smoking, fighting, and walking out.[127]

Motivating children who mostly had terrible memories of school was difficult, and teachers had to adopt unorthodox methods of persuasion. Leonard Kornberg, a teacher at Hawthorne, adopted a wide repertoire for handling and encouraging his students, including using humor, staying patient during outbursts, standing physically close to his students, nipping new disruptions in the bud, and encouraging positive behavior and good work.[128] Staying nimble and finding creative ways to counter children's disinterest in work was key. When one boy told Kornberg, "You ain't gonna make me work today," he replied, "I never make you work—you're the guy who wants to be an electrician." The boy replied, "Aw, cheap psychology," and started to work.[129] Instead of ordering him to work, Kornberg used his knowledge of the boy's personality and life goals to motivate him to take the work on himself. His approach was typical of RTC staff members, who wanted to help children help themselves rather than telling them what to do. In some cases, the process cut to the core of a child's emotional disturbance.

George was an eight-year-old boy who arrived at the Orthogenic School in the late 1940s. At the age of three, he had begun running away from home on a regular basis, and at six, he tried to drown another child to get his fishing tackle. By the age of eight, he was known for "violent attacks on children, plus strong delusions of persecution."[130] At the school, he continued to run away (though he always came back), but on one occasion he let his counselor come too. When they came to a good fishing spot, the counselor pointed out a sign that said fishing wasn't allowed there and suggested they move. George protested, "I can't read so that doesn't apply to me."[131] But the counselor did not let the comment go and told him that not being able to read the sign didn't mean you didn't have to follow the rules. Reading might actually help a person know what was and wasn't legal, she explained. After the failed fishing trip, George learned to read, a sign staff members interpreted as his recognition that ignorance was not a sufficient excuse for bad behavior and that reading might be a valuable skill. Soon after, George confided to his teacher that he was worried he might again try to drown someone and "be sent to the [electric] chair."[132] If that happened and he could read and write, he explained, he wouldn't be able to claim ignorance. Here, the teacher intervened and reaffirmed that ignorance was never an excuse for breaking the rules.[133] In this complex example, learning (reading) provided a point of intervention into George's academic and emotional troubles, and his teacher served as both confidant and counselor in the process. The end result was not only an educational victory, but a social one as well: the counselor and teacher had helped George to see that he had to behave in accordance with basic societal expectations.

Discipline and Punish

Had George been at a training school for delinquent boys, the story we just heard would likely not have played out as it did. George would probably have received some physical punishment for his repeated runaway attempts and might have been sent to an especially difficult work detail or isolation cottage.[134] Just as they did with every other aspect of care, RTC professionals constantly compared disciplinary methods at their institutions to those at the worst of their training school counterparts. In particular, they boasted about having moved past the "old" methods of corporal punishment and isolation and toward more enlightened approaches, like trying to understand why a child had acted out, limiting physical interventions to holding a child tightly, and reinventing isolation as a voluntary, temporary solution. The result was an inconsistent hodgepodge of policies that aimed to contain a child's behavior within certain boundaries while addressing his individual emotional needs. Ideally, they aimed to hold a child to basic social standards without impinging on his right to be angry or upset.

Though some of these attempts were more effective than others, RTC professionals were anxious to demonstrate to their colleagues, charges, and the popular press that their approach to bad behavior exemplified their great distance from the training school approach. When Ernst Papanek became the director of Wiltwyck in the early 1950s, he called a large assembly to tell the boys that life would be different from now on, and "boys were not to be beaten or even slapped by counselors any more," as Claude Brown recalled.[135] Popular magazine stories about Wiltwyck specifically noted the absence of corporal punishment and the advent of a new, more thoughtful approach to discipline. A 1949 *Newsweek* story noted that "Wiltwyck deals with its boys through kindness rather than discipline. . . . If boys are negativistic or skip out of the schoolrooms during classes, the counselors will not force them but try to find out the reason in consultation with a psychiatrist."[136] Nine years later, a *Readers' Digest* piece explained that the school emphasized the consequences of bad behavior instead of handing down blanket punishments. For example, a boy who had broken a window would be required to pay for it out of his own allowance "until he understands that society will not countenance destruction of property."[137] Just because harsh punishments were forbidden did not mean punishment was not used as a teaching tool.

For staff members dealing with a very challenging population of children, this approach was formidable. At Hawthorne Cedar Knolls, which had previously been a training school for delinquent children, many of the cottage parents were holdovers from the previous era and believed that corporal punishment was an appropriate response for "bad" behavior. The new administrators were extremely opposed to it and held a number of meetings with the cottage parents to encourage them to use alternative methods of discipline. If they formed close relationships with the children, administrators explained, outbursts that demanded disciplinary responses would diminish. Although the incidence of corporal punishment decreased after this intervention, it never entirely vanished, much to the chagrin of administrators.[138] Elsewhere, corporal punishment either did not exist at all or was used sparingly. At Bellefaire, administrators "recognized that cottage parents will lose their tempers with children and administer an occasional slap," but this slap had to be reported to their superiors.[139] Bradley Hospital reserved corporal punishment as an absolute last resort that had to be approved by administrators.[140]

In reality, disciplinary measures at RTCs comprised a patchwork of policies. Ideally, staff members would identify undesirable behaviors as manifestations of a child's feelings and seek to understand them through talking. This scenario was borne out in the case of Gary, a boy who ran away from Southard. When a staff member found him a few blocks away, he did not scold or slap the boy but instead took him into a drugstore for a soda where they discussed why Gary was unhappy and how the staff could help him deal with his anxiety and lack of self-control. The approach seemed effective; "later throughout that evening Gary seemed relaxed, calm, and relieved," reported the staff member.[141] But talking didn't always work with children who were completely out of control. In these cases, staff members at many RTCs resorted to holding children tightly to keep them from hurting themselves or others.[142] When ten-year-old Brenda began to boss the other children around intolerably, having slapped and kicked staff members just a few hours earlier, her childcare worker encouraged her to go to her room but was forced to escort the girl physically after she refused. The worker then tried to speak with her about her actions for two hours while Brenda "screamed foul language for fully a half hour" and threw things. Finally, the worker simply sat on her while she kicked and spat. In Brenda's case, talking it out was not an option despite the worker's best efforts and physical force provided a means of exerting authority and protecting Brenda and the other children. Whether or not we choose to view this approach as "social control," it is important to note that staff members were careful to avoid striking the children, believing that their role was simply to prevent the child from injuring himself or other people. In addition, this method seemed to calm children down. When Stephen Eliot was threatening to kill himself, his counselor Diana Kahn wrote in her daily note that "I just hold him firmly and tell him that I certainly will stop him. That seems to [do it], not the talking, but the holding on to him. I think it's because I'm bigger and it seems as if I could stop him is reassurance."[143] Talking was not always enough to stop a child's self-destructive behavior.

Even in moments of crisis, staff members still tried to communicate with children and express their desire to help. When a fifteen-year-old boy at Southard abruptly jumped up at lunchtime and hit the director over the head with a bottle of ketchup, the staff immediately formed a calm plan of action. In order to keep the other children from getting too excited, they removed the boy from the lunchroom and told them that the director was fine.[144] Then, a team of staff members told the boy that they were there to protect him and apologized for not noticing that he was becoming "restless and anxious."[145] They encouraged him to simply use words in the future to tell others why he was so upset. In the process of a few minutes, the crisis had been resolved, and staff members had assumed some of the blame for the boy's actions. All was not idyllic about this interaction; they also warned the boy that if he could not control his behavior in the future, he could not stay at Southard and would have to be sent to a psychiatric hospital. Moments like these illustrate how in many ways RTCs were extremely progressive institutions, but staff members were still faced with the reality of extremely troubled children and used threats to establish their authority and keep these children under control. Southard may have been a relatively progressive, permissive environment, but this interaction demonstrates that the staff's tolerance only extended so far.

From its careful construction as an instrument of normality to its apparent resistance to close evaluation, the therapeutic milieu remained an elusive creature. Dynamic and experimental, RTC professionals believed it offered the best chance of restoring abnormal children to productive lives in their communities. However idyllic the idea might have seemed at times, the milieu still had to withstand the physical and emotional strain of extremely disturbed children who did not necessarily want to play by the rules adults set out for them. But as new social and cultural pressures began to threaten the vitality of residential treatment in the late 1960s, defending the fragile milieu as a unique form of treatment would become RTC professionals' last line of defense.

INTERLUDE

Homeward Bound

After several months or even a few years, it was finally time for a child to leave the RTC. Staff members decided that a child was ready for discharge for several different reasons. Some were sudden and without clear indication: a child's therapist left the institution or a parent decided treatment should end because the family was going on vacation. Other times, staff members decided a child was too disturbed to benefit from the RTC and needed to go to a different, usually custodial institution.[1] For children who were getting better, discharge ideally came when a child could independently manage in the "real world." Ryther Child Center staff looked for a child's ability to "meet the demands of a more normal and less understanding group" of peers, and staff members at the Evanston Receiving Home anticipated discharge when a child "no longer [required] the special protection . . . of a total treatment environment."[2] Southard administrators' standard for discharge was a child's ability to attend public school, form relationships with others, and "work and live within a group."[3] Just as inability to function within social environments had led many children to RTCs in the first place, it was an acquired ability to operate in these environments that made them ready to leave.

In other cases, it was simply time for a child to leave the RTC when staff members felt they had done all they could do.[4] In the case of one ten-year-old girl who had come to Bellefaire "withdrawn, unhappy, [and] unable to relate to others" after her parents' divorce, treatment had been beneficial. Three and a half years later, she "became more mature, made friends, and was happier." At that time, staff members decided she would benefit more from individual attention in a foster home than from continuing to live at Bellefaire.[5] Another girl at Bellefaire, who had arrived at age sixteen after a suicide attempt, went on vacation with her father one year into treatment and never returned. The staff did not encourage her to return, though, "as [they] felt she had achieved as much as she was able to from her placement."[6]

When children left residential treatment, where did they go? Although statistics varied widely from center to center, approximately half of them went back to the home they had originally come from.[7] As one Bellefaire annual report explained, this solution was in everybody's best interest: "We have not yet met a child who ultimately did not want to return to his own home," the report explained.[8] The fate of the other half was dependent on the RTC from which they were discharged. At Bellevue and Bradley, both of which treated many severely ill psychotic children, a group went to other institutions like state mental hospitals or institutions for so-called feebleminded children.[9] Foster homes were likely destinations for children at the University of Michigan or Bellefaire, and Langley Porter and Hawthorne sent almost all of their children back to their original homes.[10]

For some children, therapeutic work with RTC staff members ended after discharge. At Bradley and Southard, where children typically came from out of state, outpatient follow-up treatment and contact was left to local referring agencies to administer.[11] At Bellefaire and the Children's Service Center of Wyoming Valley, which had similar patient populations, the centers did their best to stay in touch with recently discharged children, especially at first, and the Children's Service Center had children who had been discharged return for a six-month follow-up visit.[12] At Langley Porter, the Cincinnati Child Guidance Home, and the University of Michigan's Child Psychiatric Hospital, where patients tended to come from the surrounding region, discharged children (and parents, in many cases) who lived nearby returned regularly for outpatient psychotherapy.[13] Hawthorne Cedar Knolls operated on this basic framework as well, trying to ensure that discharged children could continue to see their regular therapist on an outpatient basis.[14] Their methods of continuing care were partially shaped by the needs of the children they had discharged, who tended to return to Hawthorne during particularly rough moments or to spend vacations or weekends in an environment where they felt completely comfortable.[15] Return visits were not just a Hawthorne phenomenon; some children who had completed treatment at the Illinois Neuropsychiatric Institute came back and "expressed pleasant reminiscences" of their time there, as one social work student recalled.[16]

Given their stays of several months or even several years within a veritable "bubble" created by the therapeutic milieu, it is no wonder that children would come back to visit well after discharge. According to a current

Ryther administrator, one former patient, now in his eighties, still visited the center regularly as of 2010.[17] A looming discharge could bring mixed feelings. Lee Stringer remembered that when his caseworker at Hawthorne told him he would be going home at the end of the school year, "I [told] her it would be just great. At the same time, I [felt] a tug. For camping in the woods. For trips to Coney Island. For winning ribbons in the Maccabeah. For all the fun things of the summer here. And more than anything, a tug for all the kids here to do them with."[18] Once a child returned home, all of the planned activities and outings he or she had come to expect were replaced with a daily life that might seem drab in comparison. For Claude Brown, returning to Harlem from Wiltwyck was a disorienting experience: "The Harlem that I had dreamed of and wanted to get back to seemed gone," he recalled. "I didn't know this place. . . . I was like a stranger. I longed to get back into Wiltwyck."[19] Brown's solution was to pay regular visits to Wiltwyck director Ernst Papanek in his Harlem office, where the two chatted sometimes about Brown's life and sometimes about nothing at all.[20] Maintaining a connection to Wiltwyck was crucial as Brown sought to reintegrate himself into his old life.

How to Succeed

Claude Brown's return to Harlem was rocky, even with Papanek's help. After he once again became involved in a neighborhood gang, Brown was sent to Warwick, a training school with steel bars on its windows. Although the juvenile judge had suggested Wiltwyck, the RTC was unable to take him back, and Brown was sent to a custodial institution, branded a failure.[21] Was Brown a failure? He ultimately graduated from Howard University and became a highly respected novelist, essayist, and lecturer. But before that, he spent most of his childhood moving between gang life on the streets of Harlem and custodial care at Warwick. How did RTC professionals judge whether a child's treatment was successful, and how did they deal with children who did not seem to benefit from residential treatment?

Some RTC professionals believed that efficacy should be measured with respect to an absolute standard, which they referred to as "adjustment." "Adjustment" was a vague but popular psychodynamic term that referred to an individual's successful functioning in the larger world, and RTC professionals took advantage of its malleability.[22] "Adjustment" for a child discharged from residential treatment could alternately refer to his or her successful functioning in the community, ability to form relationships, diminishing symptoms, or successful emotional self-regulation. It was not uncommon for RTC professionals to summon all of these definitions in describing a child whose treatment had been effective. For example, psychiatrists Anne Benjamin and Howard Weatherly of the Illinois Neuropsychiatric Institute described "adjusted" children as those who "have no symptoms of emotional disturbance or insecurity, who adjust without difficulty to the routine of home and school, have satisfying relationships, and both enjoy and are working up to their mental capacity in school."[23] In 1946, social work student Bruno Herbert evaluated the adjustment of nineteen girls discharged from Hawthorne Cedar Knolls using different meanings of "adjustment" to assess different girls. Polly, whom he judged to be "markedly improved" (qualitative assessments of improvement were standard for measuring efficacy in psychiatry at the time), was "well liked" by staff members and peers and had a "mature" relationship with her caseworker.[24] Kathleen, who was "somewhat improved," was "more accessible emotionally" and "more self-controlled" but still had "cravings for dangerous excitement."[25] Anita, whom Herbert declared was "unimproved," had difficulties at school, had "never really been accepted by the other girls," and was unable to form a good relationship with her caseworker. Polly's adjustment was based on her ability to form relationships, Kathleen's on her emotional status, and Anita's on her functioning at school and ability to form relationships, yet all three were being evaluated on their "adjustment."

One especially popular measure of adjustment was a child's ability to assume traditional gender roles on discharge. In a 1947 study of the effectiveness of residential treatment at Ryther Child Center, Lillian Johnson and Joseph Reid described three young adults leading perfectly "normal" lives. One boy graduated high school "a good student, a leader in his class, a football player, a buoyant and apparently well adjusted individual."[26] Another, they noted, "served in the Army during the war and has since married and established a home. He is independent and responsible."[27] A teenage girl who had arrived at Ryther after attacking her foster mother was "now the wife of a young professional, looking forward to having her own child."[28] These young people were presented as stereotypical postwar ideals: the leader and football player, the hardworking father and veteran, and the young wife and soon-to-be mother. When former patients achieved these universal cultural benchmarks of success, they were considered to be as good as cured.

Although it had a multitude of meanings, adjustment was still "an arbitrarily established absolute norm," as two proponents of the concept explained.[29] Other RTC professionals rejected this model and urged their colleagues to consider a child's improvement relative to how they had presented on admission. Only this approach, they argued, could effectively measure how residential treatment had changed them.[30] Social work student Shirley Camper illustrated the mismatch between absolute and relative evaluations of efficacy in her master's thesis on children discharged from the Illinois Neuropsychiatric Institute in 1944 and 1945. Evaluating children with respect to an absolute standard, Camper found, often underestimated the progress they had made in residential treatment.[31] For example, one ten-year-old boy had been admitted due to failing in school, hyperactivity, frequent tantrums, enuresis, and masturbating, among many other problems. Although he still had difficulty in school after discharge, he had stopped wetting himself and masturbating, treated his sister with more respect, and no longer spoke in a "high-pitched, unpleasant voice." Camper explained that if the boy were evaluated according to an absolute standard of adjustment, he would be considered "fair" within a range of good, fair, and poor adjustment. But if one considered the significant progress he had made during residential treatment, he was actually greatly improved.[32] Absolute standards of efficacy, she argued, would have undermined his substantial improvement and the role residential treatment had played in it.

When it came to determining just what proportion of children had been helped by their stays at RTCs, statistics were confusing, unstandardized, and at times, misleading. In general, estimates of success rates were quite high. In 1947, Ryther administrators concluded that 74.1 percent of children cared for there were successfully treated and "were able to return to the community and lead normal lives."[33] In 1958, Othilda Krug estimated that 75 percent of the children treated at the Cincinnati Child Guidance home had "a significant improvement toward a healthier and happier life."[34] Not only did RTCs' assessments rely on different standards of successful treatment, but on further examination, they also often revealed less than ideal rates of improvement. For example, Hawthorne Cedar Knolls administrators calculated that more than 75 percent of the children treated there in the early 1950s were "improved" or "partially improved," but only 22 percent of all children were "improved."[35] Success rates could also change over the course of only a few years. In 1944, the Southard School annual report announced that eight of nineteen children there were "improved" compared to their initial presentation.[36] In 1945, this figure changed to twenty of thirty-two, and in 1946, sixteen of thirty-three children.[37]

Qualitatively, there was enthusiasm among children and administrators who felt that treatment was generally effective. After University of Michigan administrators widely advertised their recently renovated child psychiatry unit in 1948, the superintendent of one child welfare agency wrote the hospital director to express his enthusiasm for the renovations "and the offer of service that has been so beneficial to the children whom we have sent you for treatment."[38] For the superintendent and his colleagues at the Michigan Children's Institute, the University of Michigan's child psychiatry unit offered hope for children the agency was not able to treat in the community. Children also spoke about the benefits they had gained from residential treatment. In July of 1948, four teenagers who had recently been discharged from Bellefaire spoke to the board of trustees about their experiences there. "There were some differences of opinion as to whom helped them most—the social worker or the cottage mother or some one else," the meeting minutes stated, "but they were all very positive about the fact that they had been helped."[39] Another Bellefaire success story, a boy named Jacob, wrote in the *Bellefaire Bulletin,* "I am glad that I am going home. I think that Bellefaire has helped me a great deal . . . The main thing is that I know I will get along as I will try to be kind to people, and do the things my mother tells me."[40] No doubt, statements like these helped attract donors and promote camaraderie among staff members who believed they were doing real good. Concluding that treatment was effective—and believing this to be true—gave RTC professionals encouragement to continue on in their difficult work and gave parents and children hope that their treatment had been or would be worth the expenses, time, and hassle incurred. It promoted an environment of optimism amid the harsh reality of the children served by RTCs, which was disproportionately reflected in media coverage of residential treatment.

Although sunny images like these were common, RTC professionals were also open to discussing their failures. As Wiltwyck director Ernst Papanek told the *New York World-Telegram,* "If we have our victories, we have our failures, too . . . when you set out to salvage the bruised and twisted young minds of a city's slums, every victory is a miracle and every half-victory a triumph."[41] Being the "last stop" for otherwise hopeless children gave RTC professionals permission to admit failure, for they had tried when everyone else had given up.[42] At times, they even took the blame for a child's lack of progress. In their evaluation of Ryther's first ten years of service, director Lillian Johnson and social worker Joseph Reid told the story of a boy who had failed treatment by continuing to steal bicycles and cars until he was sent to a reformatory. Several years later, the boy returned for a visit and learned of Johnson and Reid's study, asking a staff member whether "he had been classified as a failure." The staff member replied instead "that it was not that he had been classified as a failure but that the agency's work with him was considered a failure."[43] The staff member's willingness to take responsibility for the boy's poor outcome and Johnson and Reid's publication of the story in a report that was likely distributed to community members and donors suggests that open admission of failure was not something RTC professionals felt they should be ashamed of.

At the same time, failures were sad and frustrating. Stephen Eliot recalled the day when Bruno Bettelheim called all the children at the Orthogenic School together to let them know that Paul, another child at the school, would be going home. Remembered Eliot, Paul's parents "had had a frank discussion with Dr. B., who told him that Paul had gone as far as he could at the School and it was unlikely the staff could get him ready even for high school."[44] The news made Eliot "terribly sad," and two residential workers told the children how difficult Paul's loss had been for them as well.[45] Bettelheim's detailed discussion of one child's problems with the other children was probably unusual, but Paul's story suggests that failures at the Orthogenic School were mourned collectively.

Failures cut deep among staff members who often felt *they* were the ones who had failed their charges. At Southard School in 1965, a girl attempted to hang herself when most of the staff members were at a meeting out of town. When they returned and learned of the girl's suicide attempt, they were angry and confused. "We spend our staff meeting in a miasma of denial," said child psychiatrist William Easson to three psychiatrist colleagues. "No one talks about things in case you say too much or in case some unpleasant reality comes out into the open . . . reality may catch up with us and we cannot deny it much longer."[46] No matter how impossible the situation, Easson was arguing that open discussion was the only way to resolve the emotional chaos that already existed. RTC professionals like Easson, accustomed to working with children on whom others had given up, freely admitted their naïveté when they were faced with children who failed to improve or even got worse on their watch. But as new cultural and financial pressures threatened the existence of RTCs in the 1960s and 1970s, events like these did not help improve the impression that residential treatment lacked evidence of efficacy. Failures became yet another piece of public evidence that RTCs were not equipped to handle the wave of children with which they would soon be confronted.

SEVEN

The Breakdown of Emotional Disturbance

In the late 1960s and in the 1970s, RTCs were faced with a number of new challenges that threatened their very existence and, by extension, the existence of emotional disturbance as an organizing concept for providing services to this vulnerable population of children. When a major federal government report announced that the United States was suffering from a crisis in its ability to provide care for troubled children, it quickly became clear that RTCs could not meet the needs of thousands of recently identified disturbed children. Moreover, residential treatment was becoming an undesirable option as a result of larger cultural anti-institutional sentiment and enthusiasm for community-based care. As a means of responding to these critiques and in an attempt to stay afloat financially in the midst of rising costs, many RTCs adopted "continuum of care models," offering services that bridged institution and community. Yet experts continued to question whether there was a role for residential treatment and, indeed, whether it was even effective.

Even as RTCs struggled to justify their value, other forces relabeled groups of children and contributed to the fracturing "emotional disturbance" as an organizing political and therapeutic concept. With the rise of new special education legislation and debates over mainstreaming, emotionally disturbed children were reimagined as "emotionally handicapped." Autism proved another fracturing force. Studied by researchers for several decades, its power as an organizing disease model solidified in the late 1960s and early 1970s with help from experts and parent advocates. Children who might formerly have been called withdrawn or psychotic were given a new label and became part of a new movement, as parents and advocates fought to keep them—and treat them—at home. Finally, it became clear that many troubled children never made it to an RTC or even an outpatient clinic.

Even in the heyday of residential treatment, many children labeled delinquent remained in detention centers and training schools. Even while advocates fought to improve or dismantle these institutions and new laws gave children the legal right to due process, a large group of primarily poor, minority children remained under the purview of a juvenile justice system that became more like the adult criminal courts and less like the rehabilitative agencies once imagined by their progressive founders. By the end of the decade, a group of children who had once been identified and targeted using the concept of emotionally disturbed were spread haphazardly within a broken network of agencies, professionals, and institutions.

A "Crisis" in Child Mental Health

One senator called the findings "shocking." Indeed, the 1969 final report of the Joint Commission on the Mental Health of Children had demonstrated that "only a third of the children who need care receive it. Nearly one million receive no care at all."[1] The commission's million-dollar study, conducted between 1966 and 1969, had been commissioned by Congress and funded by the National Institute of Mental Health (NIMH) after a number of child welfare organizations demanded increased attention to children's mental health needs.[2] The final product represented the findings of over five hundred experts in the field of child mental health and welfare and provided a damning critique of the state of children's mental health in the United States. Although the NIMH estimated that 1.4 million children under eighteen needed some kind of psychiatric care in 1966, the commission reported that almost one million of these children received no treatment of any kind.[3] These numbers represented a "crisis in child mental health," as the commission titled its report. Notably, the report referred to "mental health" rather than "emotional disturbance," signaling not only a change in terminology but also a shift in how troubled children would be understood and treated in the future. Although "mental health" and "mental illness" had been used to describe adults for decades, these terms were new to the field of child welfare, which had previously used the language of mental hygiene and emotional disturbance. In the 1960s and 1970s, the term "mental health" did not yet represent the biomedical model of emotional distress that would arise in the 1980s and 1990s. Still, it signified a turn toward understanding child and adult emotional distress as part of the same public health problem.

According to the commission, there was an enormous number of previously unrecognized emotionally disturbed children in the United States who were ill enough to require some psychiatric care. However, resources needed to treat all of these children properly did not exist. Instead, the report explained, many children ended up warehoused in large state institutions for the adult mentally ill. Others slipped through the cracks, "bounced around from training schools to reformatories to jails and whipped through all kinds of understaffed welfare agencies."[4] All of these disturbed children had not materialized out of thin air. In fact, child welfare and child mental health experts had long warned the public about the growing specter of childhood emotional disturbance. In 1953, the Child Welfare League of America had estimated that there were five hundred thousand emotionally disturbed youth in the United States, and a 1954 study by Columbia University's Department of Psychiatry had concluded that 10 percent of all American schoolchildren were disturbed.[5] But neither of these findings had provoked a congressionally mandated study, and five hundred thousand disturbed children were a fraction of the 1.4 million disturbed children estimated by the NIMH in 1969.

Two major factors contributed to the identification of so many disturbed children and the declaration of a crisis in child mental health. The first derived from the events of November 22, 1963. The Warren Commission, tasked with investigating the assassination of President John F. Kennedy, found in its 1964 final report that Kennedy's assassin, Lee Harvey Oswald, had been an emotionally disturbed child. As a three year old, Oswald had spent thirteen months in an orphan asylum because his widowed mother was unable to take care of him and his two brothers.[6] In elementary school, one neighbor noticed that Oswald "kept to himself" and did not "want to be with any other children."[7] Another called him a "bad kid" and noticed he was "quick to anger."[8] At the age of twelve, he threatened his brother's wife with a knife.[9] Oswald skipped school on a regular basis. This finally captured the notice of the juvenile court, which sent him to a detention home for twenty-two days of psychiatric observation.[10] There, psychiatrist Renatus Hartogs determined that he was an "emotionally, quite disturbed youngster who suffers under the impact of really existing emotional isolation and deprivation, lack of affection, absence of family life and rejection by a self-involved and conflicted mother."[11] He diagnosed the boy as having a "personality pattern disturbance with schizoid features and passive-aggressive tendencies" and recommended he be treated in an outpatient child guidance clinic.[12]

On discharge, Oswald had never received any further treatment, which journalists interpreted as evidence that the boy's murderous tendencies had never been checked.[13] Hartogs told newspapers immediately after the assassination that his initial exam had found the boy to be "dangerous," a charge that the commission later determined to be inaccurate after it examined Hartogs's original records.[14] Quickly, mental health experts and journalists seized on Oswald's story as a means of fomenting fear about the epidemic of childhood mental illness sweeping the nation and raising awareness about the importance of early intervention. One psychiatrist declared that "the world is full of potential Oswalds," and another warned readers that "it is impossible to estimate how many boys like Lee Oswald are still being shoved through their classroom years, never receiving the attention which could avert future tragedies."[15] Oswald's probation officer reminded Americans about the shortage of residential treatment facilities, remembering that he had tried to place the boy in two different RTCs but both had rejected him, citing a lack of available beds.[16] Oswald's history of emotional disturbance was even used by Connecticut senator Abraham Ribicoff to justify an ultimately unsuccessful 1965 amendment to the Social Security Act that would have provided $5 million in federal funds to support treatment of emotionally disturbed children.[17] In short, Lee Harvey Oswald was evidence that America was experiencing a dramatic swell of childhood emotional disturbance that was going untreated.

The second factor contributing to the perceived crisis in childhood mental health was the determination that the African American "culture of poverty" was causing a groundswell of emotional disturbance among young black Americans. One sociologist found in 1969 that African American youth in New York City were twice as likely to be emotionally disturbed as white children.[18] Experts attributed this disproportionate number to both structural and cultural factors. According to Senator Daniel Patrick Moynihan in his 1965 report, *The Negro Family: The Case for National Action*, African American families were fundamentally pathological institutions, led by "matriarchs" who emasculated their husbands or led single-parent households. The result was a perpetuating cycle of poverty, a culture of low self-esteem, and a predominance of fractured families.[19] Living in these families, it was believed, was fundamentally psychologically damaging.

As Mical Raz has shown, the culture of poverty model utilized and often conflated the psychological concepts of maternal, sensory, and cultural deprivation to explain why African American families were unhealthy environments for children. Matriarchs, Moynihan's report argued, were unable to pay significant attention to their many children, causing maternal deprivation. Furthermore, their disorganized, messy homes were paradoxically sources of sensory deprivation as the children were considered to be deprived of the regulated stimuli that promoted healthy growth and development. The result was cultural deprivation, a concept that reinforced the idea that African American children were somehow robbed of a normal upbringing. We now recognize *The Negro Family* as implicitly racist and paternalistic, and a number of contemporary social scientists rejected Moynihan's argument. Still, the report and its associated, deeply entrenched concept of cultural deprivation provided the theoretical foundation for Johnson's War on Poverty.[20] Black families in the 1960s, according to many social scientists, were the perfect breeding grounds for emotional disturbance.

Other policy makers and mental health experts pointed instead to structural problems like poverty and racism as the root causes of emotional disturbance among black children. The Joint Commission on the Mental Health of Children assembled a separate, multiethnic Committee on Children of Minority Groups after members "recognized that the mental health problems of minority-group children [were] severe enough to warrant special consideration."[21] The committee found that poverty and racism were to blame for higher rates of emotional disturbance in this population.[22] Poverty, which they determined was inextricably linked to minority group status, resulted in unstable families, poor education, and an unhealthy environment. For example, the report explained that poor housing was linked to poor sleep, reduced attention span, exposure to violence, "irrational [parental] discipline," and fatigue.[23] Racism, the committee continued, contributed to emotional disturbance because minority children learned from an early age that society considered them to be inferior, causing widespread demoralization. Once psychological troubles emerged, mental health services were too limited to be of any help.[24] The psychologically damaging effects of poverty and racism were well-worn concepts, popularized most prominently by psychologists Kenneth and Mamie Clark, whose evidence that racism degraded how children thought of themselves had proven key to the 1954 *Brown v. Board* decision.[25] In presenting these structural issues as the cause of poor mental health among minority children, though, the committee rejected the theory of deprivation, calling it "a residue of a racist society."[26] But whether high rates of emotional disturbance were linked to a culture of poverty or the combined psychological effects of poverty and racism, the fact remained that they were contributing to what now appeared to be a "crisis" in child mental health.

A Question of Supply and Demand

In the 1970s, residential treatment increasingly seemed like an unsustainable solution to this perceived epidemic. Even though there were more than seven times as many RTCs in 1965 as there had been in 1952, the Joint Commission calculated that only eight thousand of 1.4 million "seriously ill children under eighteen," or 0.005 percent, were being treated in RTCs. Furthermore, many states had no RTCs, and western and southeastern states were particularly underserved.[27] Even if there had been enough RTCs to serve all of the disturbed children in the United States, residential treatment was extremely expensive; the Joint Commission estimated that one year of residential treatment for a child cost between $10,000 and $18,000 (or approximately $126,000 today).[28] As two social workers explained in a 1972 review of residential treatment, "It is obvious that residential treatment programs are serving only a small proportion of disturbed children."[29] There were simply too many children and the cost of providing residential care to them all was too high to make residential treatment a realistic solution to the perceived child mental health "crisis" of the late 1960s and 1970s.[30]

Despite these concerns, proponents of residential treatment argued that the high cost of treating a small number of children intensively was worth it. In particular, they contended that not treating these children would cost their communities more in the long run.[31] Bruno Bettelheim warned child mental health professionals that "it is high time we stopped being penny wise and dollar foolish. True, it may cost $50,000 to rehabilitate an Oswald, or the killer of Dr. Martin Luther King," he argued, but the cost was worth it.[32] He argued that the child who did get treated, even at a tremendous cost, would ultimately pay dividends as a tax-paying, responsible adult.[33] Bettelheim told the story of a boy referred to the school, whose community agencies decided they were unable to foot the $50,000 estimated cost of treatment. "While the letter was on its way to me saying that this was much too expensive," Bettelheim recalled, "the boy set fire to a building, killing three people and doing $350,000 damage. I guess this was something the community could well afford. . . . I can also predict that the boy will cost the community a lot more before he dies, during which time he will contribute no tax money whatsoever."[34] Others argued that money should not be the determining factor when a child's life was under consideration. Explained Bradley's president, "Cost is not the yard stick to use when care of children is being measured. There is that very important element called the quality of life."[35] But in the 1970s, even these noble considerations were dwarfed by concerns about money and the stark reality that RTCs could only accommodate a tiny fraction of children who would qualify for treatment.

A Changing Mental Health Ecosystem

Even if RTCs could have cared for America's estimated 1.4 million emotionally disturbed children, the infrastructure of the American mental health system was undergoing significant upheaval in ways that directly challenged the legitimacy and feasibility of residential treatment. The growing popularity of community mental health care, the inextricably linked yet independent movement toward deinstitutionalization, and fundamental changes in how psychiatric care was paid for created a fractured, hostile ecosystem in which RTCs had no clear role.

Community mental health as a concept and a movement had its roots in World War II, when treatment of neurotic soldiers on the front lines convinced a generation of psychiatrists that mental illness was influenced by larger social and environmental factors and could and should be treated in the community.[36] After the war, the federal government built demonstration community mental health centers funded by the 1946 National Mental Health Act.[37] Funds to expand the model increased in 1963, when the Mental Retardation Facilities and Community Mental Health Centers Construction Act provided significant federal assistance to build new community mental health centers across the country.[38] Young psychiatrists in particular looked to this model as a means of addressing deep-seated social issues like poverty and racism.[39]

At the same time, anti-institutional sentiment was growing, particularly with respect to the management of mentally ill adults. In the early 1960s, a diverse group of intellectuals was pointing to psychiatric hospitals as dehumanizing tools of social control.[40] By the end of the decade, the populations of large, state-run mental hospitals were declining significantly, albeit at widely varying rates across the country. Although it is tempting to explain deinstitutionalization by the rise of community mental health centers, imagining a direct flow of patients from hospital to community, Gerald Grob and Howard Goldman have argued that this oversimplified narrative is incorrect. Instead, they have demonstrated that changes in the financing of mental health care drove the emptying of mental hospitals. With the passage of Medicaid in 1965, populations of elderly mentally ill adults were simply moved to nursing homes, where the federal government paid for their care. As a result, a population of somewhat younger severely mentally ill adults were left with few resources. Community mental health centers, hailed as the answer to the country's psychiatric woes, were better suited to treat mildly troubled adults using psychotherapy. For those covered by private employer insurance or Medicare, mental health provisions were minimal and required high copays. Insurers preferred to pay for short stays at general hospitals, leading to a population of younger adults treated with a decentralized, "revolving door" approach.[41]

While these developments primarily addressed adults in need of mental health care, they all had major consequences for troubled children. Riding the wave of anti-institutional sentiment, advocates and journalists presented a series of often shocking depictions of institutions for intellectually disabled children. In 1966, Burton Blatt and his photographer friend Fred Kaplan documented the horrid conditions at five state institutions for such children in their photo-essay *Christmas in Purgatory*.[42] Another series of exposés focused on abuses at Willowbrook State School, an institutional for intellectually disabled children in Staten Island. In 1965, Senator Robert Kennedy declared after an unannounced visit that the facility was "less comfortable and cheerful than the cages in which we put animals in a zoo."[43] The most damning evidence was presented by television reporter Geraldo Rivera, whose 1972 footage of naked, neglected children at Willowbrook drew unprecedented attention to the institution and triggered even more media coverage.[44] Although these institutions had not housed emotionally disturbed children, these exposés established a link between institutions and mistreated children that contributed to anti-institutional sentiment in the child mental hygiene realm.[45]

As for residential treatment centers, the news was not good. While the Joint Commission affirmed that "there are a few superb [residential treatment] institutions in the country," it conceded that there were "many that are marginal . . . most are disgraceful and intolerable."[46] A few journalistic exposés appeared about the poor quality of care for children housed on adult wards of state mental hospitals and the terrible conditions at new for-profit RTCs that were "springing up across small-town and rural America."[47] But for the most part, concerns about residential treatment lacked the moral stridency that had accompanied attacks on state mental hospitals and institutions for the retarded. Critiques were softer and largely limited to the pages of professional journals, most likely because RTCs had established a reputation as a more humane alternative to traditional, custodial institutions. But as community-based programs flourished, critics wondered if it was still ethical to perform "parentectomies," a term they used to describe the act of separating children from their parents.[48] Would separation, they wondered, actually damage a child's chances of improvement by failing to address the problematic family relationships that had caused his or her troubles in the first place?[49]

Money Troubles

Apart from larger social critiques of institutions and the movement toward community-based care, money remained a limiting factor for RTCs and indeed for all providers of mental health care in the late 1960s and the 1970s. Residential treatment centers were used to relying on community and organizational philanthropy, endowment interest, and government funds to cover stays ranging from several months to several years. Since World War II, third-party insurers had increasingly assumed greater responsibility for health-care costs.[50] Short-term psychiatric care delivered in general hospitals was their preferred mode of treatment, with much better reimbursement than longer stays in dedicated mental hospitals or freestanding RTCs.[51] The result was an artificial split between freestanding RTCs and those situated inside larger hospitals.[52]

In this scenario, freestanding centers like the Emma Pendleton Bradley Hospital were the losers. In 1961, Bradley had provided $130,000 worth of free care to children whose families couldn't afford the hefty price tag of residential treatment. Reimbursements from the state and third-party insurers only covered half of this cost, and the tiny proportion of treatment costs covered by parents made little difference.[53] By the 1970s, Bradley's financial situation had worsened, and the hospital was forced to raise its rates to keep up with rampant inflation and the rising cost of providing free care to most of its patients. In April 1976, Blue Cross Blue Shield of Rhode Island decided it was no longer going to foot the bill for children treated at Bradley.[54] As a result, the hospital struggled with a $145,000 deficit and parents were reluctant to have their children admitted, worried that they would be asked to pay for their children's care. Fortunately, the two parties settled out of court. Blue Cross Blue Shield was required to cover eight months' worth of unpaid bills and least forty-five days of a child's intensive inpatient stay—still significantly less than the average stay of two years.[55]

Although the short-term fight had been won, larger struggles with insurers left their mark on the hospital and its ability to serve emotionally disturbed children. By the late 1970s, insurance companies like Blue Cross Blue Shield were covering a large proportion of children's stays at Bradley.[56] Not coincidentally, this corresponded with a gradual decrease in the length of hospital stays. In 1961 and 1963, average stays at Bradley were 2.69 and 1.94 years, respectively; by 1980, they were less than six months.[57] The hospital's 1980 annual report explained that third-party insurers, which included both private insurers and the public Rhode Island Department of Mental Health, Retardation and Hospitals "will not pay one more cent than is deemed necessary."[58] What insurers were happy to pay for were short stays in the hospital's new Intensive Treatment Unit, where children were admitted for brief stays averaging one month to provide "rapid intervention in an emotional crisis," such as the onset of suicidality. By the spring of 1977, only a few months after the unit had opened, all of its beds were full and more children were placed on a waiting list.[59] The appeal of ever shorter-term psychiatric care was growing and offered a cheaper solution for insurers who primarily reimbursed patients for inpatient stays.[60]

In Cleveland, Bellefaire was in a similar bind. Trustees argued about how they could best attract patients and, by proxy, funding. One trustee suggested outreach efforts to Cleveland and the surrounding region. "As of now we have only fifteen regional children . . . if that source should dry up, we would really be in a crises [*sic*]," he warned.[61] Another suggested courting wealthy families "like [the] Menninger" Clinic, which collected up to $50,000 from patients who could pay the entire fee.[62] Executive Director Samuel Kelman thought that abandoning the institution's Jewish identity (even though non-Jewish children were already freely admitted) would make it easier to obtain government funding.[63] By 1980, the institution was taking in more and more patients whose care was covered by third-party payers, but reduced coverage for residential treatment meant that the institution's financial troubles only escalated.[64]

In the 1970s, Americans were frightened by what they perceived as the rapidly spiraling cost of health care in general. In 1969, President Richard Nixon told Americans that they were currently facing a "massive crisis." "Unless action is taken," he warned, "we will have a breakdown in our medical care system which could have consequences affecting millions of people throughout this country."[65] This perceived crisis, he contended, was primarily due to skyrocketing health-care costs. As third-party payers like Medicare and Medicaid increasingly reimbursed patients for health-care costs, physicians and the hospitals they worked for were steadily asking for more and more money to cover their services, and insurers were complying. As the 1970s wore on and inflation came to dominate the economy, costs continued to increase, alarming policy makers, insurance companies, and the public. Insurers worried that they wouldn't be able to cover rising costs, and Americans worried that the crisis would create an environment of rationing and shortages. These concerns spurred presidents Nixon, Carter, and Reagan to promote prospective payment systems like health maintenance organizations (commonly known as HMOs) to limit the amount that medical providers and hospitals could charge patients and insurance providers for care.[66]

In the late 1960s and 1970s, efforts to reduce governmental spending on health care resulted in slashed funding for mental health care of all kinds, including residential treatment. In California, Governor Ronald Reagan cut $17.7 million from the state's mental health budget, laid off thirty-seven hundred mental health workers, and implemented a hiring freeze, all the while maintaining that California had the best mental health care system in the country. The maximum length of inpatient stays in state facilities was reduced from sixty to a mere eight days. Reagan did not hide his distaste for psychiatry. In response to one psychiatrist's criticism of the cuts he retorted that the man was "a headshrinker. . . . He can see me on a couch now. Well, I want to tell you, if I get on that couch it will be to take a nap."[67] At Camarillo State Hospital, the site of a nationally recognized RTC, parents and physicians were dismayed by the cuts and sought non-traditional means to maintain the quality of its services. Chief of children's services Norbert Rieger told the *Los Angeles Times* that Reagan's assertion that services would not be affected was "absolutely untrue."[68] Three student professional assistants faced layoffs and parents raised money in an effort to keep them at Camarillo. One pediatrician began buying medication for the children out of his own salary.[69]

Stretching the Institution

Faced with these financial pressures, RTCs adapted. Most became complex organizations that offered a spectrum of services linking institution and community, many of which were cheaper to operate than residential care. Even without concerns for the bottom line, larger cultural anti-institutional sentiment and enthusiasm for community-based care made change to a continuum of care model essential for survival.[70]

Bradley Hospital introduced new treatment elements that sought to link the institution and its surrounding community. Starting in 1961, a preschool program offered educational and milieu treatment for disturbed young children while respecting "the belief that very young children should live at home if at all possible."[71] In 1965, hospital administrators built the Samuel B. Swan House, a halfway home to help a small number of adolescent boys gradually return to community life after hospitalization by attending public school and participating in community activities like joining Boy Scout and Sea Cadet troops.[72] Explained house administrator Buell Barton, "We try to stretch the walls of the hospital to encompass the community and to establish links with community systems."[73] In 1971, the hospital established a day treatment program "for children too disturbed to attend public school, but not requiring full hospitalization."[74] Children attended for five hours a day on weekdays and spent evenings and weekends at home.[75] Day treatment held many advantages, both cultural and financial. By sending children home at night, the Day Hospital avoided the cultural stain of prolonged institutionalization. Treatment typically lasted about fourteen months, far less than inpatients, who remained for an average of two years.[76] It was also much cheaper; in 1977, Blue Cross agreed, committing to cover 50 percent of the cost of day treatment.[77] Eight years into Bradley's experiment with a day treatment program, the hospital newsletter stated that "day hospital is less expensive than inpatient treatment; it involves parents and other community influences without the pain of separation."[78] It was a win-win situation: children could be treated at Bradley for less money while avoiding separation from their families. By creating programs that extended the institution's reach into the community, RTCs were demonstrating their embrace of the community as an ideal locus for care while establishing a model of vertical integration. If community care was to be the goal, RTCs would guide a child's entire journey from institution to home and every step in between.

Similar changes were occurring at other pioneering RTCs. By 1969, Hawthorne Cedar Knolls offered group homes, a halfway house in New York City for twenty-seven young men, and a day treatment program for thirty children, which offered "a transitional phase between the institution and return to the community."[79] At Bellefaire, a day treatment program was introduced in September 1970 in addition to the foster homes and group homes affiliated with the center and its supervising organization, the Jewish Children's Bureau of Cleveland.[80] Administrators found that the program offered many advantages. Children remained a part of their families, which enabled their parents to stay more involved and engaged in the treatment process.[81] Staff morale was high, and an unexpected community formed among the parents and children, cemented by carpools, sleepovers, and birthday parties.[82]

Southard School tried an even more progressive approach. At the Carriage House, an abandoned two-story building on the old school campus, teenagers from the community and staff members came together to design a casual environment where young men and women could drop in to talk with a mental health professional about personal issues or participate in group rap sessions.[83] There, staff members wore no uniforms, the decor resembled "the shabbiness of a clubhouse or a teenager's room," and everything was free.[84] The Carriage House was an ideal link between the community and the prestige of the Menninger Clinic, providing a place for young adults who didn't fit anywhere else, financially or medically.

Other programs aimed at community-based care of emotionally disturbed children emerged independently. One movement gained particular notoriety for its integration into the community and economic feasibility. Project Re-ED (Re-ED stood for "reeducation of emotionally disturbed children), founded by Nicholas Hobbs in the early 1960s, offered a weekday residential program based at local community schools. Run by "teacher-counselors" with nine months of training, Re-ED schools saved money by using professionals like psychiatrists and social workers as consultants, enabling them to multiply "the effectiveness of scarce and expensive mental health personnel."[85] Even when they were at the schools, children were physically close to their homes, where they returned on weekends.[86] Project Re-ED did not seek to cure the children's troubles. Instead, teacher-counselors strove for limited ends, hoping to alleviate bad habits so a child could return to a community "where the probability of continued successful function somewhat outweighs the probability of failure."[87] As a result, stays were shorter, lowering costs.[88] The project was such a desirable alternative that the NIMH supported its development with a $2 million grant in 1961 and the Joint Commission on the Mental Health of Children specifically recommended the model in its 1969 report.[89] By 1981, there were twenty-three Re-ED programs in nine states, ranging from California to Connecticut and Kentucky.[90]

But Did It Work?

Even aside from a shrinking pot of money and critiques of institutional care, there was still the nagging question of efficacy. Did residential treatment work, and how well? The answer to this question—which remained uncertain for the child mental health professionals who continually posed it—had important consequences for RTC funding, the careers of these professionals, and most of all, children who were treated either at RTCs or in other settings. Not only did RTC professionals spend little time discussing efficacy, they also varied greatly in their definitions of effective treatment, using "adjustment" as a vague marker of success that could mean just about anything. When they did begin to systematically assess whether residential treatment worked, their findings were both limited and disappointing.

Since the 1940s, RTC professionals had stressed the importance of performing research to evaluate their outcomes, but decades later they had done very little.[91] The 1962 publication of social worker Howard Polsky's *Cottage Six*, a thinly veiled chronicle of life at Hawthorne Cedar Knolls, offered disconcerting evidence that there was a lot more to residential treatment than the structures put in place by the adults in charge. Polsky found that the boys in Cottage Six, who were deemed the most disturbed of all, created their own deviant subculture separate from that of the institution. For example, the cottage was divided into cliques, with the "higher-status" boys regularly scapegoating and physically punishing the "defenseless low-status boys—the sneaks, punks, and the sick."[92] Even worse, Polsky concluded that their cottage parents co-opted and reinforced this subculture. "The unwritten compact of cottage parents and toughs," he concluded, "make[s] it unbearable for the 'deviants' because they are blamed for everything." Essentially, he had found that the cottage parents were complicit in their charges' subversion of the system.[93] When Polsky presented his findings at the annual meeting of the American Association of Children's Residential Centers, recalled James Whittaker, "it was a very difficult message for people to receive. . . . Here was an agency that prided itself on the depth of its clinical expertise . . . and the central fact that a determinant factor within that setting was the peer culture [suggested] that you couldn't just define residential treatment in terms of these formal arrangements."[94] If teenagers at one of the most highly regarded RTCs were getting away with subversive behavior with the help of their cottage parents, the prospects for residential treatment as a successful intervention looked dim.

In the late 1960s and early 1970s, independent mental health professionals and the Joint Commission called for more long-term follow-up studies of residential treatment and fretted that there was no way to compare the efficacy of individual RTCs because they were so varied.[95] At the end of the 1970s, the issue of efficacy remained unresolved. Whittaker proclaimed to his colleagues that "the impetus for evaluation is not simply political," urging them to "learn more about what works and what doesn't . . . to build knowledge in an area of practice sorely in need of hard data."[96] Regardless of how progressive or humane residential treatment might be at its best, its value was limited if no one could show that it worked. Who would be willing to foot the bill for a treatment that was extremely expensive and limited to a small number of children, and whose efficacy remained unproven?

Justifying Their Existence

Even with the many challenges presented by the cultural and economic milieu of the 1970s, RTCs still had an ace in the hole: they often worked with children no other agency or group could handle. Not even the innovative, government-supported Project Re-ED could help the most disturbed children. Conceded Nicholas Hobbs, "Re-ED is not a substitute for a hospital. There are children too disturbed, too out of touch, too aggressive, too self-destructive to be worked with successfully in small groups in an open setting."[97] Other defenders of community-based treatment similarly admitted that their programs were part of a larger continuum of care that had to include residential and inpatient options. For example, the founders of the Treatment Alternative Project program in Massachusetts, whose main goal was to keep children out of residential treatment, conceded that "there are some children who cannot be maintained by any available alternative method outside residential placement."[98] RTC professionals seized on this line of argument to defend their work. Gisela Konopka, a social worker and expert on group work in RTCs, explained that, "even under the best circumstances, there are children who must be granted total relief from the pressures of relationships that harm them over and over again; and there are families who simply cannot tolerate" their child's behavior.[99] Albert Trieschman, an RTC director, echoed Konopka's sentiments, maintaining that, even as community treatment opportunities developed, "there will still be youngsters who need to be away from their families, both for their own sake and that of the family."[100] Despite the growth of community resources to help troubled children, RTC professionals defended their work by pointing to children who were simply too disturbed to be managed outside an institution.

RTC professionals further defended their work by pointing out that they offered one thing no community treatment program could lay claim to: a continuous therapeutic milieu. Argued Trieschman, "The residential treatment center is the only laboratory that has developed the kind of ideas that actively extend mental health ideas to the natural circumstances of a day, a week, and a year."[101] This expertise could ideally be transmitted to practitioners in the community, Trieschman argued, although he did not specify how. Even if child mental health care was moving away from the RTC, Trieschman maintained that the knowledge produced in them was still uniquely valuable. This focus on milieu was reflected in two seminal works published in 1969 and 1972. The first, *The Other 23 Hours*, began as a manual for childcare workers at the Walker School in Needham,

Massachusetts, written by Trieschman, Whittaker, and Larry Brendtro. In it, the authors focused on the central therapeutic role of the milieu and the staff who worked there.[102] The second, a 1972 compendium of classic articles on residential treatment, edited by Trieschman and Whittaker, focused almost entirely on the therapeutic milieu.[103] Essential to the development of residential treatment as a progressive solution for emotional disturbance, the milieu was now the one thing that RTC professionals believed separated their institutions from a multitude of alternative treatment options for troubled children.

From Emotionally Disturbed to Emotionally Handicapped

Despite strong arguments for moving care out of the institution, there was significant lag time between the emergence of these new ideas and their implementation. In the 1960s and early 1970s, both the number of RTCs in the United States and the number of children in residential treatment grew. It was only after 1974 that the number of children at RTCs began to fall (see fig. 7.1). The number of RTCs did not decline until 1978 (fig. 7.2), suggesting that decreasing institutional populations may have led some centers to close their doors. In fact, one study estimated that 15,791 children remained in RTCs at the end of 1983.[104]

Despite growing numbers of children in RTCs, emotional disturbance as a category that mobilized money, care, and even public opinion was falling apart. Part of this was due to the larger threats to residential care, as we have seen above. But several other developments resulted in the reclassification of children who might formerly have been deemed emotionally disturbed and appropriate for residential treatment. As federal special education law classified severe emotional disturbance as a "handicap," many children were reclassified as disabled and in need of high-quality education in the community. Other children were subsumed under the expanding category of autism, powered by activist parents who sought normalization for a group of children they identified as sharing key traits. Finally, many delinquent children who might have been labeled emotionally disturbed at an RTC never made it to one. Instead, this increasingly poor and nonwhite group occupied detention centers and training schools, despite efforts to close the worst of these institutions and ensure children basic legal rights. By the end of the 1970s, "emotionally disturbed" had ceased to be a meaningful political category.

Since the 1950s, parents of intellectually disabled children had banded together to fight for publicly provided education for their sons and daughters.[105] Parents of emotionally disturbed children had fewer organizational outlets but made some strides toward educational advocacy and activism. In 1953, a group of parents under the aegis of the New York–based League for Emotionally Disturbed Children founded a school that they hoped could educate their troubled children while keeping them at home.[106] Although the school was privately run, it received funding from the city, state, and NIMH, suggesting that the model of community schooling for disturbed children was already attracting attention as a desirable alternative to institutionalization.[107] Three years later, the Godmother's League Day Treatment Center and School opened in New York City with a similar mission.[108]

Still playing catch-up to the larger special education movement, efforts to secure education for disturbed children in the 1960s resulted in new

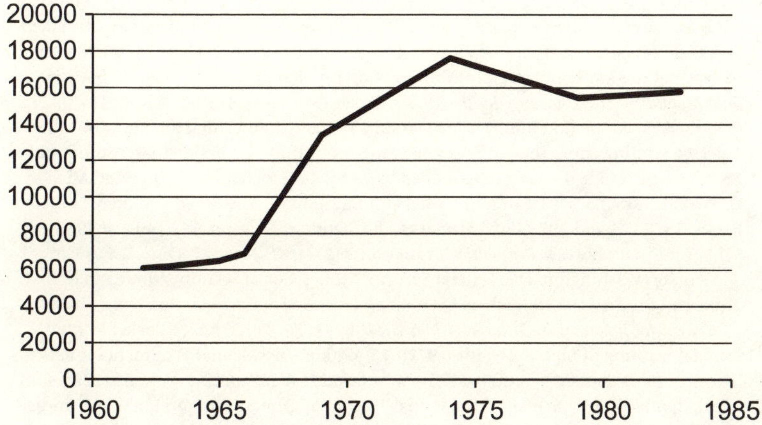

7.1. Number of children at RTCs, 1962–1983. (Sources: U.S. Children's Bureau, *Child Welfare Statistics, 1961* [Washington, DC: U.S. Dept. of Health, Education, and Welfare, Social Security Administration, Children's Bureau, 1962], 7, *Child Welfare Statistics, 1962* [Washington, DC: U.S. Dept. of Health, Education, and Welfare, Social Security Administration, Children's Bureau, 1963], 5, *Child Welfare Statistics, 1964* [Washington, DC: U.S. Dept. of Health, Education, and Welfare, Social Security Administration, Children's Bureau, 1965], 15, *Child Welfare Statistics, 1965* [Washington, DC: U.S. Dept. of Health, Education, and Welfare, Social Security Administration, Children's Bureau, 1966], 11; Michael J. Witkin and Mildred S. Cannon, *Residential Treatment Centers for Emotionally Disturbed Children, 1969–1970*, ser. A, no. 6 [Rockville, MD: National Institute of Mental Health, 1971], 22; Michael J. Witkin, "Residential Treatment Centers for Emotionally Disturbed Children 1973–74," *Mental Health Statistical Note*, no. 130 [April 1976], 1–23; Richard W. Redick and Michael J. Witkin, "Residential Treatment Centers for Emotionally Disturbed Children, United States, 1977–78 and 1979–80," *Mental Health Statistical Note*, no. 162 [August 1983], 3; Atlee L. Stroup et al., "Residential Treatment Centers for Emotionally Disturbed Children, United States, 1983," *Mental Health Statistical Note*, no. 188 [April 1988], 1010).

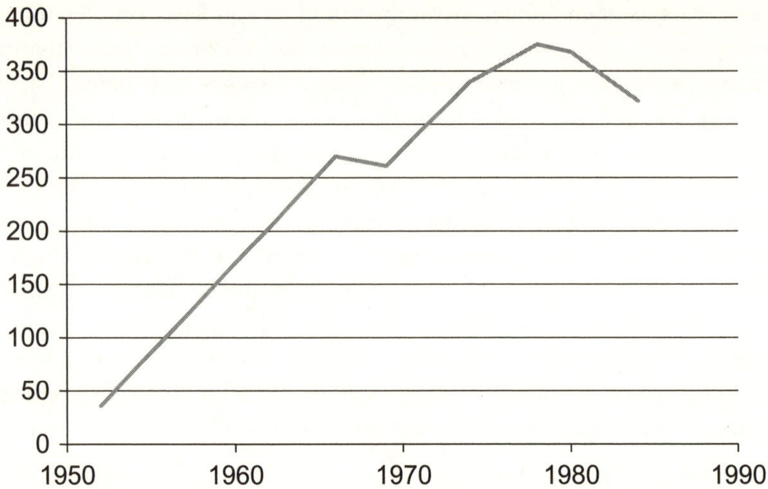

7.2. Number of RTCs, 1952–1984. It is important to keep in mind that each inventory of RTCs took its own liberties to define an RTC, and thus this information should be taken with the understanding that it represents a larger trend in the growth of RTCs rather than an exact tabulation.(Sources: Joint Commission on Mental Health of Children., *Crisis in Child Mental Health: Challenge for the 1970's: Report* [New York: Harper & Row, 1970], 272; Donnell M. Pappenfort and Dee Morgan Kilpatrick, "Child-Caring Institutions, 1966: Selected Findings from the First National Survey of Children's Residential Institutions," *Social Service Review* 43, no. 4 [December 1, 1969]: 447; Richard W. Redick and Michael J. Witkin, "Residential Treatment Centers for Emotionally Disturbed Children, United States, 1977–78 and 1979–80," *Mental Health Statistical Note,* no. 162 [August 1983], 2; U.S. Children's Bureau, *Residential Treatment Centers for Emotionally Disturbed Children: A Listing* (Washington, DC: Federal Security Agency, Social Security Administration, Children's Bureau, 1952); Michael J Witkin and Mildred S. Cannon, *Residential Treatment Centers for Emotionally Disturbed Children, 1969–1970,* ser. A, no. 6 [Rockville, MD: National Institute of Mental Health, 1971], 15; Witkin, "Residential Treatment Centers for Emotionally Disturbed Children 1973–74," *Mental Health Statistical Note,* no. 130 [April 1976], 2; Atlee L. Stroup et al., "Residential Treatment Centers for Emotionally Disturbed Children, United States, 1983," *Mental Health Statistical Note,* no. 188 [April 1988], 1.)

classes and schools founded across the country. In Baldwin Park, a Los Angeles suburb, two pilot classes of ten children with "cultural, emotional, or neurological handicaps" were founded in 1965 as part of the city's public school system.[109] In 1966, the Boston University School of Education and the city of Brookline, Massachusetts, sponsored a similar pilot program.[110] On Chicago's South Side, the School for the Treatment of Emotional Problems, or STEP, was founded to respond to the perceived crisis of emotional disturbance among poor African American children.[111] By 1966, almost half of states offered teacher certification programs for educating disturbed children and three-quarters offered at least some special classes for this growing population.[112] But this did not mean that there were enough classes to meet each state's needs, an issue that would elicit concern as new legislation mandated special education for all disabled children.[113]

The 1960s and 1970s were an era of dramatic growth in special education legislation. In 1965, the Elementary and Secondary Education Act Amendments included "seriously emotionally disturbed" children in its definition of "handicapped children."[114] The inclusion of emotionally disturbed children in the category of handicapped children was a remarkable change that would reverberate in policy making and shape the political identity of a group of children who would now be considered not just emotionally disturbed but disabled as well. In 1972, the Commonwealth of Massachusetts passed Chapter 766, a state law that affirmed the right of all handicapped children to state-sponsored education. Just as the federal government had a few years earlier, Chapter 766 included "emotional . . . factors" in its definition of "handicaps" eligible for special education.[115] It also included one other element that would influence future state and federal special education legislation: Chapter 766 encouraged mainstreaming, the act of educating disabled children alongside abled children in the same classrooms.[116] Drawing from this Massachusetts law and similar laws in twenty-seven other states, the watershed federal Education for All Handicapped Children Act in 1975 declared that "state and local educational agencies have a responsibility to provide education for all handicapped children."[117] The act employed a civil rights justification, referring to the "rights of handicapped children," a distinction that was likely not lost among the members of the growing disability rights movement.[118] Finally, the law incorporated a clause that had also been quietly used in a 1974 act extending federal grants to special education programs: "To the maximum extent appropriate, handicapped children . . . are educated with children who are not handicapped, and that special classes, separate schooling, or other removal of handicapped children from the regular educational environment occurs only when the nature or severity of the handicap is such that education in regular classes with the use of supplementary aids and services cannot be achieved satisfactorily."[119] Not only had the federal government mandated "free" and "appropriate" public education for disabled children, it had also suggested they be included in regular classes as much as possible.

The idea of integrating the education of differently abled children, termed "mainstreaming" by the early 1970s, had been controversial since the 1940s.[120] In the 1960s, the debate reached a fever pitch as experts debated the value of integration: Did disabled children perform better academically and socially in separate or integrated classrooms?[121] By the early

1970s, much of this controversy focused on the prevalence of minority children, especially African American children, in special education. Experts feared that minority children were being incorrectly identified as disabled and blatantly segregated from their peers.[122] But after the passage of the 1975 Education for All Handicapped Children Act, mainstreaming, as it was now known, became the new ideal.[123]

Although conflicting opinions about the mainstreaming of disabled children lingered, the situation was even more complicated for emotionally disturbed children.[124] As one education professor reflected, emotionally disturbed children were both similar to and different from other disabled children. Like other disabled children, "they have been identified, labeled, and thus singled out as needing special services." But disturbed children also offered practical challenges for mainstreaming. In addition to presenting new pedagogical challenges to underprepared teachers—a common concern about mainstreaming in general—emotionally disturbed children concerned teachers who worried they would be uncontrollable in the classroom or too draining on their time. Sometimes, basic classroom instruction was all the support a child could get. One fifth-grade teacher in Chicopee, Massachusetts, explained to the *New York Times* that her emotionally troubled student Joel was "supposed to receive counseling regularly, but he hasn't seen a counselor in some time. . . . They told me I should try to give him extra help here in the classroom. . . . But, you know, there isn't that much time, with all the other children, for me to help him."[125] If Joel's teacher didn't have enough time to teach her regular students, how was she supposed to make additional time for Joel?

Despite the legal and cultural pressures to mainstream disabled children, many emotionally disturbed children remained in special classes or schools. As late as 1978, a new school for emotionally disturbed children opened in Southern California to serve eligible children from twenty-three local public school districts.[126] Many of these segregated educational opportunities were suspiciously racially and ethnically segregated as well: a school for disturbed children in Springfield, Massachusetts, was largely composed of African American and Latino children whom an administrator commented had a very small chance of ever returning to a mainstream school. It was hard to find therapists who wanted to work with these difficult children, and without state resources to treat their families as well, many children stayed in behavioral holding patterns.[127] At the end of the 1970s, mainstreaming remained a contested concept, and emotionally disturbed children were educated in both standard and segregated settings. But more importantly, they had been legally and culturally assimilated into debates over special education, thereby co-opting them into larger debates about special education and disability and away from discussions of residential treatment and other predominantly psychiatric approaches to their troubles.

From Withdrawn to Autistic

A 1975 *Boston Globe* feature on the effects of Massachusetts Chapter 766 introduced readers to fifteen-year-old Christopher Johnson, who had been diagnosed as an "atypical autistic child" at the age of two and a half. Although a physician had recommended he be institutionalized, his mother had kept him at home ever since. "Instead of rocking in the corner at a state hospital ward," the article announced, "Christopher Johnson now spends most of his days in a bright, well-equipped public school classroom where has learned to read, to do simple arithmetic, to speak, to type and to knit."[128] Before Chapter 766, this scenario would have been unlikely. But how was Christopher's autism classified under the new law? Was he intellectually disabled or was he emotionally disturbed? In one sense, it didn't matter; the law guaranteed him a spot in his classroom alongside other children who required special education. But in another, Christopher's condition was somehow different from either intellectual disability or emotional disturbance.

Although autism had been defined in 1943 by Johns Hopkins child psychiatrist Leo Kanner, the condition had been discussed by a limited number of elite child psychiatrists without much popular awareness before the 1970s. No one could quite agree what it was. At times, autism was alternately blamed on bad mothering (a theory strongly propounded by Bruno Bettelheim), bad habits, and bad nerves.[129] Throughout this time, its identity as a discrete illness or disorder was fluid. In particular, it seemed to overlap with childhood schizophrenia, a disease entity with varying definitions.[130] To some experts, childhood schizophrenia was akin to adult schizophrenia, with delusions and hallucinations, while autism was broadly defined by a child's inability to relate to the world around him. To others, the two disorders were more similar than not.[131] Most child mental health professionals used the two terms interchangeably. One former Camarillo children's unit psychiatrist recalled that, during his time at the hospital in the late 1960s, the two entities were not differentiated, and "autism was [considered] really early onset schizophrenia," a theory Kanner also supported until the early 1970s.[132] When the *Journal of Autism and Childhood Schizophrenia* was founded in 1971, this diagnostic overlap was evident in its contents, which represented a multitude of theoretical backgrounds. By 1979, it was renamed the *Journal of Autism and Developmental Disorders*, reflecting the growing prominence of autism, its gradual integration within a larger set of developmental disabilities, and the disappearance of childhood schizophrenia.[133]

As we have seen, RTC professionals in the 1940s and 1950s had typically categorized emotionally disturbed children as either withdrawn and quiet or aggressive and acting out. When they applied diagnostic nomenclature to these groups, the former became "neurotic," "psychotic," or even "schizophrenic." However, they used the term "autistic" sparingly, typically as an adjective to describe a child's self-centered behavior; they almost never used "autism" as a separate category of emotional disturbance. In the 1970s, these words began to enter the RTC vocabulary. In 1975, Bradley Hospital psychologist Anthony Davids reported the institution had "established an 'autistic unit' composed entirely of psychotic youngsters, using a behavior modification approach to their treatment."[134] His language was noncommittal, recognizing the emergence of "autistic" as an organizing term but continuing to subjugate it to psychosis. The same year, Davids used a well-publicized diagnostic checklist in an attempt to differentiate among autistic and psychotic children at Bradley.[135] Academic texts on residential treatment began to mention autism and autistic children but did so fleetingly.[136] At least diagnostically, RTCs were behind the times.

While RTC professionals continued to speak of psychotic children, the number of children diagnosed with autism in the United States was growing rapidly. Sociologist Gil Eyal and his colleagues intriguingly suggest that this rise was attributable to the deinstitutionalization of intellectually disabled children in the 1960s and 1970s. In their schema, children who might have previously been institutionalized and labeled "mentally retarded" were occupying a new space between intellectual disability and mental illness, made possible by the growth of community treatment opportunities and a vocal parent advocacy movement.[137] Even if deinstitutionalization was not the driving cause of this phenomenon, broadening diagnostic criteria and increased public awareness were probable contributors.[138]

While a growing population of children were being labeled autistic, their activist parents, many of whom organized under the National Society for Autistic Children in 1965, were promoting autism as a neurological disorder rather than a psychological one. In the process, these parents rejected the blame placed on them by psychodynamic theories and included their children among those requiring special education services for their disabilities.[139] They also worked with experts (and became experts themselves) in the creation of behavioral therapies, which were given in the home with parents as primary caregivers.[140] In the 1950s and early 1960s, their children might have been diagnosed as withdrawn, schizophrenic, or psychotic and sent to RTCs. But by the 1970s, they had become a distinct clinical population whose optimal treatment was believed to be based in their own homes. As a result, autism "remade" many emotionally disturbed children into a different kind of person, contributing to the waning of emotional disturbance as a meaningful category of diagnosis and treatment.

Disturbed and Delinquent

While some emotionally disturbed children were being remade as disabled or autistic and were being cared for at home, many were placed in the custody of the juvenile justice system. Large, state-run training schools remained a popular option for many delinquent children and teenagers who were referred there by juvenile courts or sometimes even by parents who wanted their children to shape up. The 1960s were characterized by a significant increase in juvenile crime, due to a combination of factors including a larger population of teenagers born during the baby boom as well as structural changes, such as black urbanization, poverty, and racism, that contributed to the rise of delinquent behavior among African American youth.[141] Juvenile justice leaders and indeed the larger American public worried about the growing specter of delinquency, which seemed to be a tangible, ever-growing threat. Training school administrators were confronted with swelling populations and worried that their already large, unwieldy institutions would become dangerously overcrowded.[142]

As we have seen, RTCs housed many children who had been labeled delinquent and were often referred by juvenile courts. But most delinquent children had remained under the purview of the juvenile justice system. In the 1960s and 1970s, activism and legislation revealed a schism in how delinquency and even childhood were understood. Was delinquency merely crime committed by fundamentally "bad" children or was it a symptom of deeper emotional distress enacted by youngsters with undeveloped minds? Should it be treated punitively or should such children be rehabilitated according to a medical model? Just as they had in the early twentieth century, courts and children's rights activists struggled with these questions and sought to protect children's procedural rights and distinguish between minor and more serious offenders.

In the 1960s and 1970s, the children's rights movement arose from larger civil rights efforts, which sought to extend the same civil rights protections adults enjoyed to children but simultaneously ensure and protect their social and economic well-being.[143] To these advocates, children were vulnerable and in need of governmental protection.[144] Children's rights advocates pointed to what they deemed unacceptable conditions in institutions, schools, and courts. At many training schools, for example, advocates and sympathetic journalists uncovered inhumane practices such as prolonged isolation and physical and emotional abuse.[145] Detention centers, in which children were held while they awaited more permanent placement, provided a "penitentiary atmosphere" where "solitary confinement is readily employed for the slightest infraction."[146] Administrators and outside researchers alike acknowledged the prevalence of emotional disturbance in these facilities. One reform school clinical director reflected, "We have the most disturbed children in the juvenile correctional system. . . . Many have serious emotional disorders."[147] A University of Chicago study corroborated this statement, finding that, in March 1966, more than 80 percent of the children held in detention centers were emotionally disturbed.[148] Although many of these children would likely have been placed in these institutions even when RTCs were at the height of their popularity, their numbers were growing, as was public attention to their plight.

Jerome Miller, perhaps the most influential advocate for children in training schools, assumed this role almost by accident. When the Ohio State University social work professor was appointed commissioner of the Massachusetts Department of Youth Services in 1969, he was appalled by the conditions he observed in the state's training schools. At the Shirley Industrial School, he recalled a disciplinary cottage where children were beaten if they spoke at all, "strip cells [were used] . . . and no program [existed] except perhaps scrubbing floors in unison with brushes. . . . It was in sum, a horrific, brutal place."[149] After initially implementing reforms, Miller decided the system was beyond salvage and closed down all of Massachusetts's training schools in the space of two years. His work would serve as a model for the deinstitutionalization of training schools all over the United States.[150] Not all children had a Jerome Miller in their corner. In Texas, it took two decades of sustained legal and journalistic advocacy to shut down the two most egregiously punitive training schools for delinquents.[151]

In the 1960s and 1970s, the Supreme Court released several decisions that fundamentally shaped the juvenile court and the lives of American children. In *Kent v. United States* (1966) and *In re Gault* (1967), children were guaranteed the same due process applied to all adults charged with crimes.[152] *In re Winship* (1970) established that a child's delinquency had to be proven beyond a reasonable doubt—the same standard used for adults—rather than using the "preponderance of evidence," which had previously been the standard for juveniles. Although these decisions afforded children accused with crimes increased rights, they also had the effect of repudiating the rehabilitative basis on which the juvenile court had been founded and embracing a criminal justice approach.[153] Still, the court retained significant latitude. Juvenile judges could impose whatever sentence they felt was appropriate, and *McKeiver v. Pennsylvania* (1971) affirmed a judge's right to perform fact-finding and denied that children had a right to a jury. These decisions retained an element of paternalism, in which the court allegedly had the child's best interest in mind.[154]

In 1974, federal legislation removed a large population of children from the court's purview. The Juvenile Justice and Delinquency Prevention Act acknowledged that the juvenile justice system was overwhelmed, declaring that "understaffed, overcrowded juvenile courts, probation services, and correctional facilities are not able to provide individualized justice or effective help."[155] A new Office of Juvenile Justice and Delinquency Prevention would study the problem of juvenile delinquency, evaluate existing programs and formulate new approaches to prevention. Most importantly, the act redefined "juvenile delinquency" to exclude status offenders and stated that they could not be held in detention facilities of any kind.[156] In effect, runaway, truanting, or merely "difficult" children could no longer be placed in jails, detention centers, or training schools.

Although these changes seemed to be progressive responses to the broken juvenile justice system, many people were frustrated by their potential effects. Police chiefs in Virginia distributed a statement opposing the new law, maintaining they would no longer have any recourse to help status offenders like runaways and that the new rules would result in the extensive criminalization of these children in order to bring them into the system as delinquents.[157] Officials in Orange County, California, worried that they would "have virtually no sanctions to apply against incorrigible youths and chronic runaways."[158] If status offenders left a group home or counseling program, argued county chief probation officer Margaret Grier, she and her colleagues would be unable to intervene.[159] Officials from the Massachusetts Department of Youth Services charged that without training schools, children would no longer be threatened by the juvenile justice system and would become more dangerous and less controllable.[160]

The Juvenile Justice and Delinquency Prevention Act changed the fate of many children in unexpected ways. Many behaviors were reclassified as crimes rather than status offenses so children could be managed by the court. A heterogeneous collection of initiatives termed "diversion programs," often run by social service workers and alternately affiliated with or separate from the juvenile justice system, theoretically functioned to keep status offenders out of jail and on the right path by engaging them in therapy, community service, or other activities. This unexpectedly extended the reach of the juvenile justice system to many children merely deemed "at risk" who might not otherwise have become involved in the system. Finally, status offenders were in many cases diverted to private facilities, where their behavior was reclassified as mental illness or substance abuse. Many of these facilities were just as punitive and restrictive as the training schools from which these children had been excluded. Moreover, this group of children was predominantly white and middle-class. As Barry Feld has argued, this led to the division of juvenile justice into a two-tiered system segregated by race and class.[161] If poor, nonwhite delinquent children had been less likely to receive treatment in an RTC in the 1950s, by the 1970s their fate was almost always in the hands of a criminal justice system that saw their behavior not as a symptom of emotional distress but as simple lawbreaking.

Detention centers and training schools were often cruel, inhumane places into which a broad swath of children had been dumped. But they had also provided a concrete place for these children to go. Community care for emotionally disturbed children remained an underrealized hope, with insufficient facilities and professionals to treat the children who needed them. Residential treatment centers, straining under the demands of higher costs, decreased funding, a limited number of qualified professionals, and anti-institutional sentiment, were not a realistic solution to the growing child mental health "crisis." Moreover, the children they had treated were being claimed by other groups as broadly disabled or in some instances, autistic. By the mid-1970s, emotional disturbance, though still a prevalent concept in medical and popular literature, had ceased to exist as a politically meaningful category. This left RTCs without the cultural or political capital they needed to justify their existence in the 1980s, especially in the face of bipartisan advocacy for family preservation. Still, RTC professionals remained determined to participate in the national conversation about how Americans should treat their troubled children.

EIGHT

Discarded Children: The Last Thirty Years in Child Mental Health

The scenes depicted in the pamphlet advertising residential treatment look familiar. Photographs of children attending school and Cub Scout meetings are interspersed with photographs of puppet therapy, music therapy, parent counseling, and a bedroom with a floral bedspread, large leather armchair, and homemade art on the wall. The pamphlet advertises individual psychotherapy, a large interdisciplinary staff, and an emphasis on milieu therapy with a "family-like atmosphere." This could have been any RTC in the 1950s or 1960s except for a few key details: a photograph of a parent support group and another of "medication administered by licensed nursing staff." In fact, this brochure advertising the Children's Treatment Center at the Camarillo State Hospital was created in 1979.[1]

While materials from the Children's Treatment Center into the 1980s continued to describe trips to Disneyland, visits home every weekend, and Cub Scout meetings, the popular press detailed a constant series of threats to the institution's existence.[2] In 1982, the California State Health and Welfare Agency and Youth and Correctional Agency in a joint task force suggested that the hospital be transformed into a prison, its patients moved to other hospitals. As a consequence of the Wars on Crime and Drugs, prison space was in high demand; using the existing Camarillo structures would keep state operating costs down.[3] Although this proposal was defeated, staff continued to fear a prison transformation several years later, when state officials threatened to decrease the hospital population by 45 percent.[4] Hospital staff and volunteers protested that Camarillo was a progressive psychiatric facility that bore no resemblance to the "snake pit" portrayed in the 1948 movie of the same name that had been filmed on the Camarillo campus.[5] Nevertheless, Governor Pete Wilson closed the hospital in 1997, citing high costs and a declining number of patients.[6]

In the 1980s and 1990s, residential treatment centers faced a rising tide of opposition by independent and government child welfare experts who promoted "family-centered" mental health care for children in what they deemed the "least restrictive" environment possible. This approach was deeply embedded in late twentieth-century conservative family politics and child welfare legislation. The ideology of family-centered care fundamentally opposed residential treatment for troubled children as disrespecting the integrity of the family and cordoning children off from mainstream society. RTC professionals insisted that their centers had always involved families and protested that sometimes children had to be removed from pathological families to make progress. Faced with cultural pressures to keep children in the community and the strain of declining funding, RTCs responded with creative new solutions to treat a patient population that was poorer and seemed sicker than ever before. Outside RTCs, parents and child advocates focused attention on the experience of families with troubled children and used the language of the disability rights movement to agitate for services that could help keep their children at home. For desperate parents without the resources to act as advocates, the juvenile justice system offered an alternate solution. Some parents even relinquished custody to the state, hoping that their child could get better mental health care in a correctional facility. For other parents dealing with the declining number of inpatient and residential beds, for-profit RTCs and boot camp programs became another option in the late 1990s and early 2000s, despite evidence of physical and emotional abuse. As the "golden years" of optimism about child mental health receded in a fundamentally anti-institutional era, the child mental health system became ever more fractured and unable to serve its most vulnerable clients.

During this era of change, the phrase "emotionally disturbed" was still used to describe many troubled children. Indeed, the number of children in RTCs was still growing in the 1980s, despite the many challenges they faced.[7] Yet as residential treatment declined in professional and popular esteem, emotional disturbance became an empty descriptor. Without the cultural influence of RTCs, "emotionally disturbed" became a mere synonym for the more popular term "mentally ill," bereft of the rhetorical power that had once mobilized resources and symbolized hope for a vulnerable population.

Family-Centered Care and the Politics of Child Welfare

In his 1985 State of the Union address, President Ronald Reagan proclaimed that "as the family goes, so goes our civilization."[8] As the 1980s began, new federal legislation sought to emphasize the centrality of family in American life by providing funds to keep families together. A key goal of these efforts was to prevent or minimize the removal of children from their homes, which directly challenged the already strained budgets and cultural capital of RTCs. In 1975, the Education for All Handicapped Children Act had codified the phrase "least restrictive" to describe the optimal educational environment for a disabled child.[9] In 1980, the Adoption Assistance and Child Welfare Act, which sought to keep children in permanent homes and minimize out-of-home placements, such as foster homes, expanded the meaning of "least restrictive" to characterize the ideal setting for any child.[10] Although neither act focused on mental health care or institutional treatment, this phrase would come to dominate discussions about child mental health policy for the next several decades. For policy makers, "least restrictive" became a synonym for "noninstitutional."[11] Inspired by this legislation, the National Institute of Mental Health (NIMH) founded the Child and Adolescent Service System Program (CASSP), a program that promoted this goal by distributing federal funding to support community-based programs like regional Families as Allies meetings for parents of mentally ill children.[12]

In 1986, CASSP published a monograph suggesting how this new ideal might be incorporated into a coordinated "system of care" for emotionally disturbed children.[13] Such a system, the authors argued, would be characterized by two core values: it would be "child-centered" and "community-based."[14] Of course, neither idea was new; the idea that therapy should be unique to a child had characterized the early activities of both RTCs and child guidance centers, and cries for community-based psychiatric care had begun after World War II. However, child mental health experts were now incorporating the language of the least-restrictive environment in their writing. As the authors of the CASSP monograph argued, "Emotionally disturbed children should receive services within the least restrictive, most normative environment that is clinically appropriate."[15] The dominance of the "least restrictive" ideology built on the anti-institutional sentiment of the 1970s and created a hostile environment for RTCs, many of which had already been struggling for the last decade.

Not surprisingly, CASSP was opposed to residential treatment, which members felt was often used inappropriately for children who could have been taken care of elsewhere.[16] As the program's leaders explained, even foster or group homes would be preferable to larger institutions.[17] In a 1986 article, CASSP researchers described "state hospitals, training schools and other restrictive institutional facilities" as the traditional places where emotionally disturbed children could get care. These institutional options were compared to newer and more favorable treatment programs in the community "which provide less restrictive, more normative environments."[18] Thus, they defined an institution as the most restrictive placement, the worst of all the options for children who were living outside their original homes. In 1985, a large CASSP report on residential treatment declared that institutional care was now a synonym for custodial care.[19] This conception was only furthered by popular representations of institutions for troubled children. In the Oscar-nominated documentary *Children of Darkness*, mentally ill children were shown living in bleak custodial facilities, strapped to the bed to prevent self-injury, held down while they were given shots of antipsychotic drugs, and abandoned by staff who had no idea how to help them.[20]

Despite damning images and descriptions of institutional care, there was a bit of good news for independent RTCs: namely, that they were not hospitals. The authors of the 1986 CASSP report, for example, clustered them with group homes and therapeutic foster care—options they described as slightly better than traditional "institutions" like hospitals, training schools, and juvenile detention centers.[21] In their early years, freestanding centers and inpatient units had both self-identified as RTCs. By the 1980s, child psychiatry units in hospitals were considered one of the "most restrictive" options for children, second only to correctional facilities.[22]

As government experts and consultants developed a detailed program to support community-based care, mental health advocates also fought to keep troubled children at home. In 1982, the Children's Defense Fund published *Unclaimed Children*, the result of three years of research and interviews with public mental health and child welfare officials, mental health providers, and parents of troubled children.[23] In this landmark study, the authors concluded that, "of the three million seriously disturbed children in this country, two-thirds are not getting the services they need."[24] This was especially true for children from low socioeconomic or racially diverse backgrounds and for those raised in households affected by substance abuse.[25] It was no wonder that fourteen-year-old Joey, an intellectually disabled African American boy who had watched his mother get murdered, stopped making eye contact with others and refused to interact with adults. Psychiatric evaluations suggested intensive care, but he was rejected by numerous public and private facilities.[26] Peter, a "severely disturbed" eleven-year-old boy deserted by his alcoholic father and physically abused by his mother, was placed in jail for his own safety when his mother threatened suicide. Five days later, rejected by the state emergency shelter and without any nearby RTCs or therapeutic foster homes, he was simply returned home but kept in state custody.[27] When troubled children did get care, it was often in what advocates felt were unnecessarily restrictive settings. "Countless others get inappropriate care," the authors argued, estimating that 40 percent of hospital placements for this population were avoidable.[28] Six-year-old Jena, whom the authors presented as an example, had been placed in an adult psychiatric ward of a local hospital when she began setting fires at her third foster home. After one day, staff insisted she be transferred to a state psychiatric hospital for children, where she was placed in seclusion after screaming for her foster mother, who had not been allowed to visit.[29]

Not only were these admissions avoidable, advocates argued, they were also financially unsound. In 1989, the National Mental Health Association (known as the National Committee for Mental Hygiene in the early twentieth century) released the results of its national study on out-of-home placement, the *Invisible Children Project*.[30] The study involved a national survey focused on children placed in out-of-home settings (inpatient units or RTCs), emphasizing the high economic and emotional cost of this option. Whereas one year of treatment in a day program would cost $15,000–18,000, the study estimated, an average stay in a state hospital (4.2 months, based on the data the researchers collected) would cost $38,218; an average stay in an RTC (15.4 months) would top that at $52,300.[31] In comparison, the average cost of one year of tuition, room, and board at a private four-year university in the United States that year was $14,073.[32] Although these estimates compared different length stays, they emphasized the high cost of inpatient and residential care. In particular, the report lamented the placement of thousands of children in out-of-state RTCs and inpatient units, which was not only costly but made it extremely difficult for families to participate in their children's care.[33] Between 1986 and 1987, the authors found that 4,098 children had been placed in out-of-state facilities.[34] Most of these children, they believed, should have been treated in the community. Yet, as the report noted regretfully, there were not yet enough community resources to do so.[35]

If community-based treatment was so much cheaper, why were so many children being sent away from home? The authors of *Unclaimed Children* argued that a number of factors were at play. Intensive community-based programs were reimbursed poorly compared to residential or inpatient programs. For example, in Pennsylvania the Medicaid reimbursement rate for inpatient treatment was $300 per child per day, while the rate for day treatment at a child guidance center was $24. Moreover, community-based programs were often affiliated with schools, and education and mental health departments fought so much over who ought to be responsible for the cost of these programs that many never materialized.[36] While community-based care remained the gold standard, financial realities and bureaucratic struggles made it difficult to implement.

All in the Family

To mobilize support for community care in the least-restrictive environment, child mental health experts directed renewed attention to serving children "in the context of the family."[37] This meant that parents should be respected and involved in all decisions regarding their child and that mental health experts should "have a strong and explicit commitment to preserve the integrity of the family unit whenever possible," as two CASSP researchers explained.[38] Deputy Director Judith Katz-Leavy and several CASSP colleagues asserted that RTCs had failed to incorporate parents in their therapeutic plans.[39] "It was sometimes assumed," they argued, "that parents had no role to play once they had turned over their children's care to others. . . . When children had serious emotional disorders, it was often thought that parents' involvement would actually interfere with the child's treatment."[40] With outdated RTCs as their foil, the authors asserted that modern child mental health care ought to involve an array of services that would support parents as well as children, from home-based crisis services to assistance with housing and employment for parents. "A family with a 7-year-old boy whose problems include severe and unpredictable angry outbursts and difficulty sleeping," they argued, "may identify respite care, transportation to a day treatment program, information about behavior management techniques, and emotional support from other parents as their greatest needs."[41] To enforce this approach, CASSP stipulated that the grant money it provided to states be used to fund services and research supporting family-centered care.[42]

The idea that the best place for a child was at home was not new. In fact, it had been the centerpiece of the 1909 White House Conference on the Care of Dependent Children.[43] By midcentury, the Child Welfare League of America had promoted foster care as a temporary solution to help dependent and neglected children until they could ultimately be reunited with their families.[44] Although RTCs and child guidance centers had explicitly involved family members since their founding and RTCs had tried to re-create families within their walls, it had always been understood that a child's original family (or a foster or adoptive family, if need be) was preferred to placement in an institution. But in the 1980s, family politics gave rise to renewed rhetoric about the importance of "family-centered care" that explicitly discredited RTCs, which were seen as actively jeopardizing the American family.

Family politics as it applied to mental health care in the 1980s and 1990s drew from both conservative and liberal traditions. As Robert Self has demonstrated, backlash from the identity politics and liberal government programs of the 1960s resulted in a new alignment of parties in the 1980s dedicated to promoting what he calls "breadwinner conservatism," or the idea that families should be led by a male wage earner. This political position was closely tied to fiscal conservatism and attacks on big government, primarily by Republicans.[45] Although child mental health and welfare advocates employed the language of family politics in their pleas to keep children out of institutions, they also departed from this conservative model by promoting "big government" interventions. For example, CASSP, which was founded on the family preservation model, was funded by the federal government and dispersed congressionally appropriated funds to state and local child mental health programs. Ultimately, the work of CASSP led to significant federal spending in the form of the 1992 Children's and Community Mental Health Services Improvement Act (also called the Children's Mental Health Initiative), which distributed grants to states for building community-based "systems of care."[46]

In 1993, Congress officially made family-centered care a national policy when it passed the Family Preservation and Support Services Program Act, a subsection of the massive Omnibus Budget Reconciliation Act. The law allocated funds to states to fund programs, training, and research to help children stay in their homes and to help those living outside them to be reunited with their families or placed in other permanent settings with an adoptive family or other relative.[47] As a memo from the Children's Bureau explained, the law would enhance "parents' ability to create stable and nurturing home environments that promote healthy child development . . . and [avoid] unnecessary out-of-home placement of children."[48] Although many of these goals were vague, the memo did list crisis care, respite care, and follow-up services for adoptive families as examples of services that would be funded by the Act.[49]

Despite the basis of "family first" policy in conservative ideology, the law had broad liberal support from organizations like the Child Welfare League of America and the Children's Defense Fund.[50] In a 1992 editorial in the historically black *Atlanta Daily World*, Children's Defense Fund founder and president Marian Wright Edelman told the stories of several African American families in Detroit affected by drugs who had been helped by in-home counselors from an organization called Families First. "This is what we mean by family preservation—real life programs that strengthen family ties and empower communities," Edelman argued. She concluded by urging her readers to ask their senators and representatives to vote for the most generous version of the Family Preservation Act.[51] By the 1990s, family-centered care had become an attractive model to both conservatives, whose cultural views on the American family aligned with the spirit of this model, and liberal child welfare activists, who supported federal policies and programs that would help families stay together.

Under Pressure

Faced with advocates who promoted home-based care and family preservation, RTC professionals found themselves on the defensive in the 1980s and 1990s. Many chafed against the accusation that their work stood in opposition to family preservation. Nan Dale, the president and CEO of the Children's Village in New York, angrily told the *Atlantic Monthly*, "We're as pro-family a place as you can find. The fact that we serve a child who has been removed from a family does not make us anti-family. We involve parents."[52] Father Val Peter, the director of Boys Town in Omaha, Nebraska, dismissed family preservation as a fad. "What's in vogue right now is family preservation," he explained. "Just follow the trend. Watch the little lemmings dashing toward the sea. . . . It's as if they just discovered that it's a good idea to try to keep kids in families."[53] While family preservation and family reunification were always the goal, these professionals explained, sometimes one or both were not possible.[54] In fact, as another RTC director argued, most children in RTCs came from families or foster families that were inherently violent or unhealthy, making this ideal impractical at best.[55] Other RTC professionals felt that some children were so disturbed that it was unrealistic to expect that they could remain at home.[56]

Unresolved issues, like high costs and a lack of peer-reviewed evidence on the efficacy of residential treatment, continued to haunt RTC professionals in the 1980s and 1990s. Third-party payers remained reluctant to pay for long stays at an RTC and as a result, stays grew shorter and shorter.[57] At Bradley Hospital, for example, the average child remained in residential treatment for 201 days in 1981; this had shortened to fifty-seven days by 1987.[58] Similar trends existed for children in psychiatric hospitals. Mental health officials in Georgia reported that the average length of stay in 1986 was 77.5 days; two years later the average stay was 34.7 days.[59] The focus on providing least-restrictive care made it difficult to perform rigorous research on the efficacy of residential treatment, which in turn hampered the efforts of RTC professionals to advocate for themselves.[60] In a report on residential treatment, a Senate subcommittee determined that there was insufficient evidence to judge the efficacy of residential treatment or even to determine which children benefited from it most.[61] "In short," reflected three administrators from the Walker School, a prominent RTC in Massachusetts, "residential group care is a field under stress."[62] Without the luxury of longer stays, the administrators felt, it was impossible to build the strong relationships that children needed to get better. And because residential treatment was often used as a last resort, they believed that policy makers and mental health professionals held unfair expectations that RTCs would be able to "cure" this most recalcitrant population.[63] But without rigorous evidence that their interventions worked, RTC professionals were unable to make a convincing case for their value.

As debates about what child mental health care *should* look like continued, RTC professionals worked hard to adapt to these stresses. Much as they had started to do in the 1970s, individual RTCs continued to pursue a kind of vertical integration by creating as many elements of the continuum of care as possible. By 1985, the Children's Village in Westchester County, New York, not only housed three hundred boys in its flagship residential program but also ran four group homes, an adoption program, a set of foster homes, and a community-based program for families of troubled children.[64] RTC professionals also started using the same language as the advocates who wanted to shut them down. In the early 1990s, the Children's Division of the Menninger Clinic expanded its day treatment center, hoping it would serve as an alternate to residential care or as a transitional space between inpatient and community care. In a 1993 bulletin, the director embraced the language of family-centered politics, stating that the day treatment center "seeks to serve patients in the least restrictive therapeutically appropriate context with the goal of reintegrating children and adolescents back into their homes and communities as quickly as possible."[65] If the child mental health enterprise was going to emphasize least-restrictive care, RTC professionals were essentially demonstrating their willingness to alter their own programs to meet that need.

Residential treatment centers also had to pursue creative solutions to financial constraints. In the 1980s, they were heavily dependent on public funds from state departments of mental health and social services, county departments of mental health, and even local school districts.[66] Unfortunately, these funds were drying up quickly. In 1983, the Massachusetts Department of Social Services placed a temporary freeze on funding for all new RTC placements after projecting that its budget would run out three months before the end of the fiscal year. Proclaimed the mother of a fourteen-year-old suicidal girl who had been awaiting placement for two months, "I don't know if what they're doing is legal, but it is not moral."[67] As mental health funding dwindled across the country, centers struggled to pay for services that cost, by one 1985 estimate, between $21,000 and $69,000 per year (or between approximately $49,000 and $162,000 in 2018 dollars).[68] At Bellefaire, where children were accepted regardless of their ability to pay, staff noted that "the families we are currently serving are less able to pay even minimal fees than families who have previously been referred." As a result, the institution did its best to utilize funds from third-party payers like supplemental security income (or welfare for the elderly and disabled) but was still unable to recoup its costs.[69] The Children's Village, where one year of residential treatment cost $23,090, was funded by New York's Department of Social Services, Commission on Social Services, Department of Education, and Medicaid funds. Despite this, the center continued to suffer high staff turnover due to low salaries, and staff members themselves had to raise money to support the institution.[70] At the Bradley Hospital in Rhode Island, executives reclassified inpatient beds as "acute care" beds to improve insurance reimbursement and relieve financial strains in the 1980s. After two failed mergers—one in 1987 with what is now Hasbro Children's Hospital and one in 1993 with Butler Hospital, a psychiatric hospital in Providence—Bradley finally capitulated to its need for financial stability in 1996 by joining Lifespan, a not-for-profit organization with multiple academic member hospitals in Rhode Island.[71]

A Changing Patient Population

In the 1980s and 1990s, children being treated at RTCs were unlike their counterparts in the institutions' early days. Whereas most children treated in RTCs in the 1940s and 1950s had been white (with the exception of centers like Wiltwyck), those in residential treatment forty years later were far more diverse. As one 1985 study of eleven residential and day programs in the United States found, the demographics of an RTC tended to reflect its surrounding community. One of the largest and most prominent RTCs, the Children's Village outside New York City, had a patient population of 50 percent African American and 30 percent Latino children.[72] Another study of American RTCs in 1988 found that 25 percent of children in residential treatment were African American and 8 percent were Latino.[73] In comparison, the 1980 U.S. Census recorded that 11 percent of Americans surveys identified as black and 5.3 percent identified as being of "Spanish origin," suggesting that these populations were overrepresented in RTC populations.[74]

Not only were children at RTCs increasingly from diverse racial backgrounds, they were also from less affluent backgrounds, a shift fueled by the complex interactions of the child welfare and criminal justice systems over the preceding decades. Many children moved directly from the broader child welfare system, which was increasingly focused on helping underserved children of color, to residential treatment centers.[75] The pathologization of poverty as psychological deprivation had contributed to the medicalization of a large swath of minority children.[76] By the 1980s and 1990s, child mental illness, race, and poverty had become inextricably intertwined.

Meanwhile, RTC professionals were convinced that the children they treated were getting sicker. At the Children's Village, the director told child welfare researchers in 1985 that he believed "the children now being admitted to the program tend to be more needy and have more problems. . . . The schizophrenic child was a rare exception, but is becoming increasingly more common."[77] In response to this need, the Children's Village founded the Tompkins Cottage for children too troubled to live safely among the main group of children at the center. The cottage differentiated itself by having a higher staff-to-child ratio, a highly structured program, and a two-way mirror for individual therapy and play therapy. As the researchers noted, "It is the feeling, among staff, that many other children at the Village could benefit from the more intensive program offered at Tompkins."[78] At least in the minds of RTC professionals, the very children they served were more ill than ever before.

Adding Medication to the Mix

Perhaps partially in response to this, RTC professionals began to turn toward medications as new therapeutic tools. Although medications had been used sparingly in RTCs since Charles Bradley's studies of Benzedrine in the 1930s, they slowly came into more general use in the 1970s and

1980s.[79] This differed from the world of adult psychiatry, where medications had been used since the early twentieth century to control symptoms and had been developed and adopted for more specific conditions such as psychosis and depression in the 1950s. Even when RTC professionals used medications, they often did so reluctantly. A 1985 NIMH study of residential treatment centers noted that many RTC professionals viewed medication as a last resort: "Staff acknowledge that for many of these youth, medication may be necessary, but there is a reluctance to use it unless all other avenues have been explored and failed."[80] At the Children's Village, for example, 60 percent of the children had been on medication at some time but only thirty-three of the approximately three hundred children in residence at the time of the report were actively taking psychotropic medication.[81] A spectrum of use existed; the Whitaker School in North Carolina cared for twenty-four children, only four of whom were taking medication, whereas at the Astor Home for Children in Rhinebeck, New York, 40 percent of children were on medication.[82]

William Bolman, a child psychiatrist who had served as a consultant to many RTCs, reflected in 1995 that, for much of his career, "pharmacotherapy was a relatively minor aspect of residential treatment" used to control "explosive, often violent behavior."[83] In the 1980s, Bolman began to notice that child psychiatrists were increasingly employing medications as an adjunct to the therapeutic milieu. In the case of one six-year-old girl who presented with social withdrawal, a child psychiatrist started her on nortriptyline. Two weeks later, Bolman found that "she became outgoing, enjoyed school, played with other children. . . . She then began to make rapid gains from the milieu."[84] When the selective serotonin reuptake inhibitors appeared on the market in the late 1980s and early 1990s, developed to treat symptoms of anxiety but later marketed as antidepressants with relatively minor side-effect profiles, Bolman found that they helped children who might have otherwise been institutionalized.[85] He recalled the case of a fifteen-year-old boy with a hot temper who was prone to "aggressive outbursts" and "was on the verge of being committed to the long-term juvenile detention facility." Within weeks of starting Prozac, his aggressive behavior stopped and he became a star student, telling Bolman that "things didn't get him ticked off anymore . . . he found he liked to be able to solve problems rather than get upset."[86] In Bolman's experience, medication could complement, rather than replace, the other therapies used in an RTC.

Although both nortriptyline and selective serotonin reuptake inhibitors like Prozac were marketed to treat depression, a disorder that had itself emerged as a diagnostic entity in the late twentieth century, in the cases of these two children they were employed to treat behaviors that were never specifically designated as symptoms of depression.[87] In this way, the behavioral model of understanding and categorizing childhood emotional disturbance continued to guide therapeutic decision making. While the young girl had been withdrawn and the teenage boy aggressive, medications categorized as antidepressants had successfully modified each of their behaviors. Perhaps the fact that nortriptyline and Prozac were antidepressants was less important than the ability of both to modify the child's abnormal behavior.

Of course, not all children treated with psychotropic medications experienced miraculous improvement. Yet by the mid-1990s, the majority of children treated in institutional settings were taking medication. A 1997 study of eighty-three children admitted to a Massachusetts RTC found that only nine of the children had never taken any psychotropic medication and that fifty had taken a combination of two or more medications at some point in their lives.[88] A follow-up study found that 76 percent of the children, who ranged in age from five to nineteen, were taking medication at the time of admission.[89] Even at the psychodynamically oriented Children's Division of the Menninger Clinic (formerly the Southard School), medications had become a standard part of residential treatment. As psychologist and former residential unit director Martin Leichtman recalled, staff members started using anxiolytics, stimulants, and major tranquilizers intermittently in the 1970s while stressing the integrated biopsychosocial model of mental health.[90] This practice increased steadily in the 1980s and 1990s, and by 1993, Children's Division staff members lamented their inability to keep up with the growing demand for medication evaluation and therapy in their outpatient department. Of 511 children seen in consultation as outpatients from1992 to 1993, 196 were evaluated for medications, reflecting what staff members felt was "an ever-expanding market" that they were ill-equipped to serve even with appointments every fifteen to thirty minutes in a newly established outpatient medication clinic.[91]

Even as pharmacologic treatment became routine, medications remained peripheral to the ideals of inpatient and residential treatment. As a review of the residential unit at Menninger explained in 1993, "Psychotropic medications are used as adjuncts to the treatment process."[92] In her now classic 1993 book on inpatient and residential treatment, *Lessons from the Lion's Den*, psychologist Nancy Cotton noted that most of the children at the Child Psychiatry Inpatient Unit at New England Memorial Hospital were taking medication. Yet the use of medication occupied only two pages of the 288-page work, which was based on Cotton's ten years as director of the unit. Cotton made it very clear that medication was only one part of a "comprehensive therapeutic plan" developed for each child.[93] In fact, the majority of the book focused on the same themes emphasized by her predecessors in the 1950s and 1960s: providing milieu therapy in a home-like environment in order to correct pathological development.[94] While her training as a psychologist, rather than as a psychiatrist, may have influenced her decision to limit discussion of medication use, its near absence in a book considered a classic in the field is remarkable.

Indeed, *Lessons from the Lion's Den* brought to mind the exact rhetoric and many of the same day-to-day practices used in RTCs more than forty years prior. Cotton focused not on payment, policy, or diagnostic categories but instead on how relationships between staff and children could be optimally therapeutic. For example, she described multiple cases in which children who had acted out verbally or physically were asked to take a five-minute time-out, after which the clinician, nurse, or milieu worker sat with the child and empathized with his or her feelings, while simultaneously stressing the importance of limits and boundaries. She described the ideal milieu as a supportive environment that was physically durable enough to withstand often destructive children while warm enough to feel comforting and inviting. Like her predecessors at early RTCs, Cotton described her unit's efforts to avoid parent-blaming by focusing on dysfunctional relationships and on minimizing judgmental approaches.[95]

Simply put, *Lessons from the Lion's Den* illustrated how little RTCs had changed since they first came to be, despite a multitude of outside pressures. Perhaps this resistance to change—to adopting a more medical model of childhood mental illness by embracing medications as a central component of treatment—in part accounts for the ultimate rejection of residential treatment as the answer to childhood mental illness. In the 1950s, residential treatment with its progressive milieu and optimistic approach to severe emotional disturbance had seemed the answer to how Americans could deal with their most abnormal children. But by the 1990s, the RTC's resource-heavy, psychoanalytically oriented model was simply out of touch.

From Parent to Advocate

As RTCs fought to stay afloat and adapt to the needs of a changing mental health landscape, mental health advocates and parents focused new attention on the experience of parenting emotionally troubled children. Phyllis Vine's *Families in Pain* told the stories of mentally ill men, women, and children from the point of view of their family members, who fought to secure adequate treatment for their loved ones. Vine painted a detailed portrait of a broken mental health system without enough resources to serve the existing demand and of the family members left to pick up the pieces.[96] In one extended vignette, she told the story of fifteen-year-old Roger Anthony, whose parents brought him to the emergency room when he exhibited psychotic symptoms at home. After he had been on the inpatient psychiatric service for two months, Roger's psychiatrist and social worker refused to tell his parents exactly what was wrong with him, even while they tried to discharge him to a long-term private psychiatric institution. Staying at the hospital was not an option, as he had stayed longer than most. Finding an appropriate institution was difficult as well; his age excluded nearby day hospitals, and most of the institutions that were recommended to his parents were over a thousand miles away.[97]

Moreover, the experience of parenting an emotionally troubled child could be one of doubt, shame, guilt, or even denial. At the long-term hospital Roger was ultimately sent to, his mother enjoyed the supportive atmosphere of group meetings for the parents of patients. Still, she "was flattered when someone . . . asked me if I were one of the doctors" and had "difficulty accepting myself in the role of the parent of a psychotic son."[98] Another mother described her self-doubt in a 1988 booklet for parents of troubled children. "What did we do wrong?" she asked. "No one in our family has ever been mentally ill. Our other kids are normal. We treated them all the same. Why is this kid screwed up? What's the matter with us?"[99] A father of a different child described his ambivalent feelings toward his ill son: "I found myself hating my own kid, wishing he had never been born. . . . I knew he was destroying us and I hated him for it. Yet, deep inside I loved him so strongly."[100] As parents recalled their uncertainty and shame, their published stories brought these difficult experiences into the light where they could be discussed more openly.

As family members shared their experiences, they also sought to change a system that frustrated them. Although parents of emotionally disturbed or mentally ill children had advocated for their children's educational and health needs for decades, groups of parents all over the country formed formal organizations for this purpose on a larger scale in the 1980s and 1990s. In Wisconsin, for example, a number of grassroots parent support and advocacy groups formed in 1985 with the help of CASSP and the Association for Mental Illness (now known as the National Alliance on Mental Illness). In 1987, the groups coalesced into the statewide organization Wisconsin

Family Ties, which still exists today.[101] A 1986 directory of organizations "that offer support, information, and other services to parents of seriously emotionally handicapped children and adolescents" listed contact information for 214 different agencies including organizations in Alaska and Hawaii.[102] The organizations listed in the directory varied greatly, including general parenting support groups, agencies advocating for disabled children, and groups advocating for the mentally ill.

The language of disturbance as an "emotional handicap" was not accidental. When the federal government defined emotional disturbance as a disability in 1960s and 1970s education legislation, parents employed the rhetoric of the broader disability movement to agitate for services for their children.[103] This tactic continued to prove fruitful in the 1980s and 1990s as parents became more organized in their advocacy. In 1988, researchers at Portland State University published *Taking Charge: A Handbook for Parents Whose Children Have Emotional Handicaps*. The 115-page booklet, funded in part by the NIMH and the National Institute on Disability and Rehabilitation Research, featured sections with titles like "Coping with a Handicapped Child" and advocating for special education services, such as an individualized education plan. The booklet instructed parents to make themselves familiar with the Education for All Handicapped Children Act in order to "protect your rights as a parent and to secure an appropriate education for your child."[104] If children were labeled with the wrong diagnosis, the booklet cautioned, they could end up being denied the services they needed.[105]

Not only were parents urged to advocate for their own children, they were also urged to become advocates for all troubled children. A section titled "Becoming an Advocate" boasted that, "historically, mental health services have developed as a result of parents, relatives and friends of the disabled working and pushing for what they needed."[106] Progress had been made, the authors argued, "not so much because of public sympathy or concern for the mentally ill, but because parents and others have applied enough pressure."[107] This rights-based discourse reflected the tactics of the larger disability rights movement and sought to take advantage of its infrastructure by defining emotional disturbance as a disability. On a national stage, groups like the National Parent Network on Disabilities united parents of children with disabilities and agitated on Capitol Hill for causes like inclusion in education.[108] A 1994 *U.S. News & World Report* article glorified mothers who, in fighting for their children's needs, had achieved success on a state or even national level. One of the mothers profiled, Barbara Roberts, took one day off work per week for five months to lobby the

Oregon Legislature to allow her autistic son to attend his local elementary school. As a result, the legislature passed a law guaranteeing the right of all disabled children in Oregon to public education. Roberts, "another militant mother turned canny politician," served as the governor of Oregon from 1991 to 1994.[109]

As one critic pointed out, the expectation that all parents of disabled children could advocate for their needs both locally and nationally was simply unrealistic for many families who were already struggling to meet their children's daily needs.[110] This was especially true for women who could not take a day off work every week to lobby the state legislature, who might be struggling to make ends meet at home, or who were running a single-parent household. This advocacy in some ways dovetailed with those of the disability rights movement to obtain so-called positive rights (in the form of services) for disabled individuals. But at times, parents' activism on behalf of their children with disabilities was paternalistic as they fought to institutionalize their children or separate them from other children, sometimes with the goal of normalizing their own lives or those of their other, "typical" daughters and sons.[111] Most commonly, parents of emotionally disturbed children in the 1980s and 1990s were agitating for additional services and against institutional solutions, in harmony with the goals of the disability rights movement. As one father reflected, "It made me so damned mad that my daughter needed help and there just wasn't any available. . . . Getting mad made me see that something had to be done. . . . No politician was going to care about my child unless I made him do it."[112] If the government wasn't going to step up, mothers and fathers vowed to take the reins and achieve tangible results for their children.

Out of Desperation

At the turn of the twenty-first century, experts continued to decry what they felt was a crisis in child mental health, echoing concerns that had been expressed almost continuously for the last thirty years.[113] Harvard child psychiatrist Michael Jellinek lamented in 1999 that, "despite our impressive scientific gains, [child psychiatry] has been hit by a tsunami of market forces. . . . Many children are floating out to sea unrecognized as being in need, too poor, or in prison, or they are being allocated 'partial' lifesavers."[114] In this reflection, Jellinek drew attention to children neglected by a broken mental health system as well as the unfortunate reality that child psychiatry could not exist apart from the struggling health-care economy. Journalists covered the plight of severely mentally ill "stuck kids" who remained at home or in emergency rooms because no beds were available for them, or who remained in inpatient units because there was no space at a nearby RTC.[115] One *Washington Post* article profiled a Maryland mother whose son suffered from bipolar disorder and attention-deficit/hyperactivity disorder (ADHD) and had tried to commit suicide multiple times. Because of a lack of nearby beds, he had been briefly hospitalized in Virginia and was now back at home, where he was physically attacking members of his family. As his mother explained, "Finding a bed in a residential treatment center is next to impossible."[116] Notably, diagnostic terminology like "ADHD," "depression," and "bipolar disorder"—many of which had been developed in the adult setting and were increasingly codified with every subsequent edition of the *Diagnostic and Statistical Manual of Mental Disorders*—were now being used to characterize troubled children, marking a move away from behavioral descriptors. This was part of a larger shift toward a medicalized model of mental illness in the late twentieth century, with the development of strict diagnostic criteria for a growing list of disorders as proxy for the field's more "scientific" nature.[117]

For many parents, the only way to secure treatment for their children was to relinquish custody to the state. One 1999 article in the *Nation* told the story of Nelson Smith, a seventeen-year-old young man with multiple mental health diagnoses including anxiety, depression, and ADHD. When Smith's insurance refused to continue paying for his mental health costs, state officials promised his mother that if she gave up her custody he could get the help he needed. When she did so, he was briefly sent to a residential program with teens who had recently been released from jail and was then transferred to two different correctional centers where he was physically abused. In another equally tragic case, teenager Randy Oaks's psychiatrist recommended hospitalization for Randy to treat his bipolar disorder. When the managed-care company in charge of his Medicaid plan denied coverage for his care, they recommended that Randy's mother transfer custody to the state so he could be treated. When she did so, he was sent to a filthy, locked facility for teenage criminals.[118] Faced with a seemingly hopeless situation, some parents even called the police themselves and had their children arrested to help them enter "the system." Sadly, many parents found that their children landed in locked correctional facilities where little if any attention was paid to providing mental health care.[119]

Stories like these were not just dramatic tales in the pages of liberal magazines. A 1999 national study of 756 mentally ill children and their parents, conducted by researchers at Virginia Commonwealth University and the National Alliance on Mental Illness, found that 21 percent of parents surveyed were told they would have to give up custody to get mental health care for their child and that 17 percent of them had done so. Moreover, 36 percent of the respondents marked "agree" or "strongly agree" to the statement: "In my opinion, my child has been wrongly placed in the juvenile justice system because the needed services were not available."[120] As one National Mental Health Association representative explained in 2001, "There is a general feeling out there that this is a way to get your kid into treatment. . . . There are case workers out there saying, 'There's nothing I can do unless your child gets arrested." Some mental health providers found themselves recommending these options even though they knew they were less than ideal. One Denver psychologist admitted that he had "occasionally" recommended to "desperate" parents that they relinquish custody or use the criminal justice system. As he explained, "If you had to have something happen fast, the juvenile justice system was quicker."[121]

"Tough Love" and the Return to Punitive Rehabilitation

For parents with more resources, the "tough love" industry promised to "fix" their troubled teens to the tune of more than $15,000 per year. The industry had arisen in the 1980s when a group of untrained individuals who falsely identified themselves as mental health professionals created a variety of programs to help troubled teens. The largest organization, known as Straight, Incorporated, operated a network of programs across the country that forced teens to live in other homes and be monitored by teens who were farther along in the program. Humiliation, food deprivation, and isolation were common "therapeutic" methods used. In the 1990s, the same programmatic approach was applied by the founders of euphemistically named "specialized boarding schools" whose staff often kidnapped children (with their parents' consent) and brought them to prisonlike locations in the United States and abroad.

In these institutions, children were forced to live in squalor and staff members promoted physical and emotional abuse to "straighten them out." Many were operated by the World Wide Association of Specialty Programs, or WWASP, an organization that would become the focus of legal and federal inquiry for the next twenty years. Other programs, often run by the same companies, billed themselves as wilderness boot camps, promising desperate parents that they could straighten out unruly teenagers by taking them on grueling hiking trips.[122] In 1999, the National Association of Therapeutic Schools and Programs was founded as an organizing body for forty-three of these programs; by 2005, there were 135 members. Most of these programs, which frequently billed themselves as "wilderness programs," "boot camps," and "therapeutic schools," were unaccredited, unlicensed, or both.[123] Some existed in tropical locations like the Caribbean, beyond the reach of American jurisdiction.

Although they had existed since the 1980s, tough love programs experienced significant growth and achieved increased public visibility in the late 1990s and early 2000s. Although these programs were not run by mental health professionals and were operated on a for-profit basis, they filled a need that was not being met by RTCs, which were too few in number and struggling to fund themselves; crowded hospital units, which could offer only limited stays; or other resources in a child's community. Many times, parents—who were primarily well-off and white—sent their children to these expensive programs when they had simply had enough. Administrators preyed on overwhelmed parents with advertising and outreach programs that promised to straighten out their troublesome children with strict discipline and hard work.[124] In contrast to nonprofit RTCs, tough love programs represented a return to a punitive model of treatment, in which psychological distress was not acknowledged as a contributing factor to a child's behavior.

In the 2000s, child mental health professionals and parents raised concerns that these programs were staffed by unqualified people and perpetuated a range of abuses against the children they were "treating." An organization of professionals and parents called A START (Alliance for the Safe, Therapeutic, and Appropriate Use of Residential Treatment) argued that these programs were infringing on children's rights by preventing them from seeing their parents for long periods of time and forcing them to police one another. The group also alleged that the programs were physically and emotionally abusive.[125] The former charge was based on evidence that they used physical restraints and that wilderness programs provided "improper protection against the elements" and made "excessive physical demands."[126] Both occurred in the case of one thirteen-year-old boy with asthma who died in a wilderness program where he was restrained and denied his inhaler. Emotional abuse took many forms, including "verbal abuse, humiliation, forced personal self-disclosure followed by mockery, forced re-enactments of traumatic events, and extreme fear inducement."[127] Members of another group founded primarily by alumni of these programs, the Community Alliance for the Ethical Treatment of Youth, declared that "the very youth, who are in most dire need of empathy, care, and holistic treatments, are being bombarded by trauma-inducing interventions within the walls of facilities, masquerading as optimal models of healing and hope."[128] These members, as well as others who had experienced tough love programs, rebranded themselves as survivors and demanded government investigation into the abuses rampant in programs allegedly created to help them.

In response to these allegations, Democratic Congressman George Miller, chair of the House Committee on Education and Labor, asked the Government Accountability Office to investigate unsolved deaths in these programs. He also held an October 2007 hearing to discuss the "nightmare" of for-profit RTCs. By his own account, Miller had failed to persuade former attorneys general John Ashcroft and Alberto Gonzales to look into these abuses, which he alleged had "remained an open secret for years."[129] The hearings revealed that for-profit programs numbered in the hundreds, treated ten to fourteen thousand children per year, and were a billion dollar business.[130] According to Greg Kutz of the Government Accountability Office, the ten deaths his office had investigated had in common "untrained staff, misleading marketing practices, abuse before death and negligent operating practices."[131] Physical and emotional abuse, he found, was widespread and egregious.

At the hearings, distraught parents described how they had sent their troubled children to for-profit programs that had assured them of their expertise and promised their children's safety, only to be notified of their children's death days later. Paul Lewis told of sending his severely depressed son Ryan to Alldredge Academy, a wilderness program recommended by an educational consultant. Only seven days later, he received a call from Alldredge saying Ryan had hung himself. On further investigation, Lewis learned that Ryan had cut himself the day before and had threatened to hurt himself further. Instead of confiscating his knife, the staff gave it back to him and assured him that people who could help would arrive the next day. When program administrators, who were not trained mental health professionals, arrived, they felt that his statements were simply empty threats to help him get discharged from the program. Ryan's father also learned that he had been required to carry a sixty-pound backpack although he was only ninety pounds and that staff had forced water down his throat. To make matters worse, a four-hour window had passed between Ryan's death and the call notifying his father that his son was dead.[132]

Another father, Bob Bacon, told the committee that he and his wife had sent their son Aaron to a wilderness program in Utah, concerned that he was getting involved with a gang and possibly selling drugs. In the program, he was forced to hike eight to ten miles a day with almost nothing to eat and to sleep with only a thin blanket in freezing temperatures. When Aaron asked to see a doctor, staff members thought he was faking his complaints and denied his request; he died the next day. When his parents rushed to the site, they barely recognized his battered body. Bacon told the committee:

> What you cannot see in these photos are the bruises, cuts, lesions, rashes, blisters and open sores that covered Aaron's body from head to toe. These scars of abuse and the dried skin stretched taut over his bones is what his mother and I were left to discover without any warning when the sheet was pulled back in the mortuary. "This," we screamed, "could not be our son," as we grabbed each other and collapsed to our knees, but the scar above his now sunken right eye, told us that it was. It was in that one shocking moment of proof that our lives changed forever.[133]

Other similarly horrific accounts followed. The Government Accountability Office's Greg Kutz concluded: "If you had walked in partway through my presentation, you might have assumed that I was talking about human rights violations in a Third World country."[134] While some of the programs in question had closed, others had merely moved to other states with less regulation.

Over the last ten years, legislators have attempted to regulate these abusive programs with little success. In 2008, the Stop Child Abuse in Residential Programs for Teens Act was introduced in the House to implement federal regulations to protect children's welfare in residential programs.[135] However, the bill died in committee. Since then, the act has been introduced in the U.S. House of Representatives or Senate almost every year and was most recently reintroduced in the House by Representative Adam Schiff (D-CA) in July 2017.[136] Meanwhile, A START still exists and actively works to identify and eliminate abuses in for-profit RTCs and related treatment programs.[137] The website of a group called WWASP Survivors (www.wwaspsurvivors.com) features dozens of testimonies from men and women who formerly participated in programs run by the organization. Lawsuits by parents of children who have died or been abused in these programs have forced several of these programs, like those in Mexico and Guam, to shut down. Despite these legal challenges and advocacy efforts, WWASP has reemerged as Teen Revitalization, another Utah-based organization offering thirteen different residential programs for troubled teens.[138]

What these stories make clear is that, in the absence of sufficient mainstream child mental health resources in the community and at local RTCs and psychiatric hospitals, parents hoping to do the best for their children turned to alternatives. Those without many resources looked to the juvenile justice system, which itself disproportionately targeted poor minority children. Unfortunately, the correctional system had little to offer youth in terms of mental health services and served only as a holding zone at best. For parents with money to spend, therapeutic boarding schools and wilderness programs offered the promise of exotic locations and a tough approach to straightening out kids who have strayed from the beaten path. But as we have seen, many of these programs were (and still are) operated by untrained individuals and promote an abusive environment that only serves to worsen the existing emotional troubles of the children enrolled in them.

These abuses, which were widely covered in the popular press, only compounded residential treatment's ongoing image problems.[139] Now, critics could argue that RTCs (under which they could include traditional nonprofit centers as well as for-profit tough love programs) were not only financially inefficient institutions that separated children from their families but dangerous sites of abuse as well. One child psychiatrist sounded the death knell for residential treatment, arguing that "what started off as being a noble experiment initiated and supported by the American Orthopsychiatric Association 50 years ago, has fallen into the hands of politicians and cost-cutting bureaucrats. . . . Perhaps, it is time that we ended the experiment that started 50 years ago."[140] Had RTCs become mere shadows of their former selves? In some cases, the answer was clearly yes.

Despite these dire warnings, many of the oldest RTCs have been surprisingly resilient. Almost all of the RTCs discussed in this book are in existence today, albeit often in altered form. The Menninger Children's Division has moved to Baylor University in Texas, where its inpatient treatment focuses on adolescents. Bradley Hospital is thriving in Providence, Rhode Island, now associated with the Alpert Medical School of Brown University. Bellefaire in Cleveland offers a variety of inpatient and outpatient programs, including a specialized program for autistic children. Yet these programs are nowhere near what is needed to support the existing population of American children who need help for emotional troubles, both inpatient and outpatient. Nor do we have enough professionals to serve them. The American Academy of Child and Adolescent Psychiatry estimates that there are, on average, 12.9 child psychiatrists per hundred thousand children, 20 percent of whom have some kind of mental illness. Although there has always been a shortage of child psychiatrists, this estimate represents a doubling of the 1969 Joint Commission's estimate that 8–10 percent of children needed psychiatric care.[141] The strain is even worse in poorer and rural areas.[142] The solution is not easy and involves more inpatient and outpatient facilities, more clinicians, and most of all, more money to support child mental health. But until we make a major commitment to addressing this issue, our most vulnerable children will keep falling through the cracks.

EPILOGUE

At the height of their popularity in the 1950s and 1960s, RTCs offered a place to send troubled children who didn't fit in at home or in the community and a new, optimistic approach to helping them. Using an intensive program involving a high staff-to-child ratio, individual psychotherapy, casework with parents, and their most novel contribution—the therapeutic milieu—RTCs gave hope that even the most abnormal child might be made a productive citizen who could abide by basic social norms, learn self-acceptance, and be happy. In the process of treating these children, RTC professionals identified a new kind of person: the emotionally disturbed child. More than simply a term, the emotionally disturbed child functioned as a powerful concept around which resources, political will, and public concern coalesced.

But as we have seen, RTCs were small in size and number and could not accommodate all of America's disturbed children, especially after the Joint Commission on Mental Health of Children had identified almost 1.5 million children in need of psychiatric care in its 1969 report, *Crisis in Child Mental Health.* A focus on community and family-based care, anti-institutional sentiment, and rising costs with diminishing financial resources contributed to the disintegration of emotional disturbance as a galvanizing concept. Residential treatment centers, while they still existed and in fact grew in number until the mid-1980s, were not a viable national solution. Enthusiasm about the promise of community mental health was balanced by poor reimbursement for these programs and their inability to accommodate some of the most severely troubled children. A decentralized system arose that shuffled these children among agencies, hospitals, institutions, and, unfortunately, the criminal justice system. Despite periodic swells of enthusiasm for closing training schools, epitomized by

Jerome Miller's dramatic shutdown of Massachusetts's training schools in the 1970s, institutions like these never disappeared.[1] They remained a viable option, especially for poor and nonwhite children who lacked the resources necessary for a private RTC or a for-profit boot camp. Even now, large numbers of children who might have been labeled emotionally disturbed fifty years ago are confined within the juvenile justice system and its institutions.

Until very recently, the Connecticut Juvenile Training School, which sits just down the road from Wesleyan University in central Connecticut, was one of these institutions. The training school was founded in 2001 as a progressive solution to rehabilitation of juvenile offenders.[2] One year later, state officials were calling it an unsafe environment and pointing to the lack of suicide prevention and clinical services and to excessive and inappropriate use of restraints and seclusion.[3] The boys housed at the training school were not particularly dangerous; only a quarter had committed violent crimes, and the majority had committed misdemeanors or minor felonies, had violated probation, or had done poorly in other state residential placements. A 2002 state report concluded that they were "delinquent boys with serious mental health and behavioral problems who cannot be managed in other Department of Children and Families facilities."[4] Despite their near universal "histories of profound abuse and neglect," boys at the training school were not getting the mental health care they needed.[5] In fact, they were often punished when they attempted self-harm. One boy had severe depression and made multiple suicide attempts. Every time he tried to kill himself, the staff would place him in restraints for twenty-four hours. At one point, he made so many suicidal gestures that he remained in restraints for thirteen days in a row without receiving any psychiatric care.[6]

In 2004, a group of Connecticut teenagers publicized the conditions at the training school in their short film, *CJT$: At What Cost?* The film showed the cells where the boys lived, outfitted with a plastic shelf without a mattress for a bed, tiny slit windows, and an intercom that they could use to speak to staff and request permission to use the bathroom.[7] Four days after the film premiered at New Haven's Arts and Ideas Festival, the Connecticut Office of the Child Advocate, a nonpartisan office tasked with "protect[ing] children's rights and promot[ing] their best interest," released video footage of children being treated harshly at the training school.[8] One boy who refused to swallow his medications was dragged to solitary confinement, while another who threw a milk carton was tackled to the ground by three guards.[9]

In response to widespread criticism, officials at the training school decreased the population, closed its most restrictive unit, added more recreational programs, and brought in a national expert to revamp the institution.[10] Governor M. Jodi Rell condemned these efforts as too little, too late, calling the institution "prisonlike."[11] In 2013, the state established the Pueblo Girls' Unit within the nearby Albert J. Solnit Psychiatric Center. Aimed at girls who had "failed" other state placements, Connecticut's Department of Children and Families promised to provide extensive counseling, substance abuse treatment, and recreation for up to five young women living there at any one time.[12] Only a year after Pueblo opened, the *Hartford Courant* raised concerns about the use of restraints on residents, staff injuries, and insufficient suicide safeguards.[13]

On July 22, 2015, the Office of the Connecticut Child Advocate released a damning report on the training school and the Pueblo Girls' Unit. The result of an eighteen-month investigation, the report found that "the vast majority of children and youth at CJTS [Connecticut Juvenile Training School] and Pueblo have histories of trauma, abuse, neglect, complex psychiatric disorders, and special education needs."[14] No one, it seemed, was attending to their needs. Mental health services were minimal to nonexistent. Between June 2014 and February 2015, at least twenty-four suicide attempts were documented with only sixty-eight to 150 boys living there at any one time.[15] Restraints and seclusion were regularly used as instruments of punishment and control, especially for children who attempted self-harm.[16] This was a far cry from the rehabilitative model promoted by RTCs more than sixty years prior as a corrective to similar abuses at training schools for delinquent children. After multiple attempts to close the training school, the last new admission was accepted on January 1, 2018, and the school closed for good on April 12, 2018.[17] In the meantime, new concerns have emerged about the availability of meaningful community care for troubled children who were or who might have been housed there.[18]

The children who lived at the training school posed little danger to the public and most have been abandoned by both their families and the child welfare system. The 2015 training school annual report found that 19 percent of the children there had a mood disorder, 10 percent had posttraumatic stress disorder or an anxiety disorder, and 43 percent had attention-deficit/hyperactivity disorder.[19] Moreover, the majority of the training school population was nonwhite; 49 percent of the children there were African American and 30 percent were Hispanic.[20] This was out of proportion to the general population of children in Connecticut, which was 11.6 percent African American and 15.4 percent Hispanic or Latino.[21] This imbalance was the result of decades of overrepresentation by racial minorities in the criminal justice system, as well as the limited reach of intensive mental health care for disadvantaged youth.

Today, the juvenile justice system is the largest provider of child mental health care in the United States. Youth engaged with the system disproportionately represent racial minority groups and suffer from psychiatric disorders including ADHD, mood disorders, posttraumatic stress disorder, substance use disorders, and suicidality at higher rates than the general population.[22] Sadly, concluded a group of child mental health professionals, "the juvenile justice system has become the only alternative for many poor and minority youth with psychiatric disorders."[23] But as we have seen in Connecticut, it is a system built on a correctional model, without the capacity to treat serious mental illness.

Should mentally ill children be part of the criminal justice system at all? In 2003, the President's New Freedom Commission on Mental Health declared that "it is important to keep adults and youth with serious mental illnesses who are not criminals out of the criminal justice system." Instead, the report concluded, "Many non-violent offenders with mental illnesses could be diverted to more appropriate and typically less expensive supervised community care."[24] Both the American Academy of Pediatrics and the American Academy of Child and Adolescent Psychiatry have published official policy statements acknowledging the high rates of mental illness among incarcerated juveniles and calling for mental health screening on incarceration, careful management of violent or suicidal behavior that limits the use of restraints, and integrated mental health care that does not rely only on pharmacological interventions.[25]

These organizations have also called for improved diversion programs, which attempt to redirect mentally ill adults and children who have committed minor offenses to community mental health care as an alternative to incarceration. This is an appropriate and effective intervention for a population that is largely nonviolent. Young adults with serious mental illnesses are most commonly incarcerated for nonviolent and status offenses.[26] A multitude of diversion programs have arisen in the United States since the 1990s, and many of these efforts have been very successful. For example, a group of researchers analyzing the Special Needs Diversionary Program in Texas found, in 2006, that when intensive mental health services were provided to low-level juvenile offenders, rearrests and felony rearrests declined dramatically.[27] Moreover, these efforts will likely save money given the high cost of incarceration.[28]

How might we use the lessons learned from RTCs to improve the care of this vulnerable population? Residential treatment centers—small, underfunded, and based on removing a child from his or her home—are certainly not the optimal solution for most children. In an ideal world, many of these children would be diverted from the juvenile justice system and instead receive intensive mental health care in their communities. The current state of affairs is not a new one; since the identification of juvenile delinquency and emotional disturbance as major public health problems in the early and mid-twentieth century, available resources have never matched the urgent need for care. Residential treatment centers, caring for a tiny fraction of troubled children, made only a small dent in a much larger problem. The funneling of many troubled children to the juvenile justice system, mirroring the popularity of reform and training schools a hundred years ago, reflects our fundamental discomfort with deviant behavior and hesitancy to invest in the futures of young people who seem unlike us in many ways.

These treatment centers have an important legacy for child mental health, demonstrating what can be accomplished when enough people decide to commit the resources needed to create change. Residential treatment arose in the 1940s and 1950s during a time of national concern about child welfare. Child mental hygiene experts worried that troubled children would become severely mental ill adults and were willing to invest significant resources into trying to forestall this process. Residential treatment centers represented the pinnacle of these efforts. They were expensive, necessitating significant community and private philanthropy and government support, and they required large staffs to take care of small groups of severely troubled children around the clock for months or even years. These resources enabled staff members to address all of a child's needs: social, emotional, intellectual, and physical. When these needs were met, even children previously deemed incorrigible were able to make progress. In short, RTCs demonstrated the lengths to which communities and governments were willing to go to assist this population. In serving children who had been rejected in all other modes of care, RTCs also symbolized an optimism that even the most challenging children might yet be reached.

Our current child mental health system, underfunded and no longer the focus of the kind of public attention that surrounded RTCs in the 1950s and 1960s, reflects Americans' relative lack of investment in children's mental health. Our warehousing of so many of these children in juvenile justice institutions, I would argue, suggests a therapeutic nihilism about these children's potential for improvement. In part, this is sadly due to the fact that the population of affected children has become more disadvantaged and less white. Yet by heeding the lessons of a time of optimism and investment in children's mental health, the fate of these children need not remain dismal. Armed with the kind of academic, financial, and political influence that allowed RTCs to flourish in the mid-twentieth century, children today can have the same chance as those like Marty, Tommy, and Betty more than sixty years ago.

ACKNOWLEDGMENTS

It is a privilege to have the opportunity to thank all the people who helped make this book—and my unusual career—a reality. I have spent many years reading my mentors' and colleagues' acknowledgments and am honored to have the opportunity to write my own. This book emerged from early work done at the Lauretta Bender papers at Brooklyn College, where Colleen Bradley-Sanders and her staff made me feel welcome. At the Kansas Historical Society, Lin Fredericksen and her colleagues made Topeka feel like home for a week and opened the then-unprocessed Menninger Children's Division papers to me with enthusiasm and unfailing energy. I'm glad the tornado never came, but appreciative that the staff was willing to house me if it did. Nancy Sherbert helped locate and scan a number of photographs that are now housed in a different set of processed folders. At the National Library of Medicine, Crystal Smith and Stephen Greenberg made archival research a breeze. Thanks also to Tara Craig at the Columbia University Rare Book and Manuscript Library; Vicki Catozza, Ann Sindelar, and Heather Robinson-Mooney at the Western Reserve Historical Society; Diana Bachman at the University of Michigan's Bentley Historical Library; Evelyn Taylor at California State University, Channel Islands; Kathie Johnson at the University of Louisville's Kornhauser Health Sciences Library, Rena Schergen at the University of Chicago Special Collections Research Center; and the staffs of the Rhode Island Historical Society and University of California, Los Angeles, Film and Television Archive.

Christine Brown at Bradley Hospital and Deborah Cowan at Bellefaire JCB helped direct me toward resources that illuminated their own institutions' histories. Liz Johnson, Vermetha Polite, and the rest of the Yale University Interlibrary Loan staff brought priceless unpublished work to my doorstep that proved critical to this book. Oral histories with Evelyn

Brownstone, Martin Leichtman, Stanley Leiken, Earle Silber, and Peter Tanguay were illuminating and I thank these individuals for inviting me into their lives and, in a few cases, their homes to share their recollections.

At Yale, the Program in the History of Science and Medicine and the Section of the History of Medicine have been productive, intellectually stimulating environments in which to work. I thank my peer colleagues at Yale and beyond for their support and guidance. In particular, Laura Bothwell, Ziv Eisenberg, Rana Hogarth, Julia Irwin, Heather Varughese John, Chin Jou, Kelly Kennington, and Kelly O'Donnell have been keen listeners and peer mentors. Justin Barr provided incisive editing and good humor, especially as we have both worked on our books during our medical training. Andrés Martin and Linda Mayes at the Yale Child Study Center have welcomed me with open arms and given me a fantastic audience with which to share and shape my work. My colleagues from across the country, and indeed the globe, who convene every spring at the annual meeting of the American Association for the History of Medicine have provided encouragement, support, and fruitful intellectual exchange. In particular, I want to acknowledge the support of Mical Raz. From our first meeting ten years ago at the annual AAHM meeting to our shared residency in internal medicine at Yale, I have treasured our friendship and ongoing "history hotline," which has provided an important opportunity to gripe about the sometimes challenging task of balancing history and clinical medicine.

My successes have all been due to the wisdom and steadfast support of a group of mentors who continue to support me, both intellectually and personally. Scott Podolsky has been a keen listener, who helped me find my place in internal medicine and is a model clinician-historian. Jeremy Greene has mentored me since college, always pushing me to think and do more. Jeff Baker has always lent a helping hand and helped me craft a paper for *Pediatrics* during which I learned the critical tool of writing for a clinical audience. Cindy Connolly lured me into the exciting world of children's health. John Warner's quiet wisdom and encouragement to be intellectually playful have been a constant presence. Glenda Gilmore shaped me as a social, cultural, and political historian of the United States and, in mentoring me, never asked less of me than her nonmedically focused Americanist students. Anne Harrington, whose undergraduate history of psychiatry course changed my career, has challenged me to think deeply about the stories I tell. I feel intellectually refreshed and excited to forge ahead after our conversations.

Naomi Rogers deserves her own paragraph. We have worked together through many bumps in life, at times as mentor and student, at times as colleagues, and even as friend and physician friend. All of these roles have been rewarding. Naomi, you have challenged me to keep making my writing better, to keep asking questions even when I feel my work is done, and to dream bigger. I know of no one else who reads draft after draft, scribbling on pages to the point of illegibility, and has something thoughtful to say about every topic presented at our departmental colloquia. I hope I can be as helpful to you as you have been to me.

In my medical life, members of the Department of Internal Medicine and Section of Medical Oncology have recognized the importance of history to me personally and professionally and have given me the space to continue my historical work even as I learn the challenging new role of clinical trialist. My residency and fellowship colleagues have come to my history lectures, asked questions about my book, and have never made me feel that my "other life," albeit completely unrelated to adult oncology, doesn't fit. My patients and their families keep me grounded every day, and I am so grateful for their openness, honesty, strength, and vulnerability.

At the University of Chicago Press, Karen Darling and my anonymous reviewers have provided detailed, keen analysis and advice. I have done my best to address it and am grateful for your time and attention to this manuscript.

My extended family has been a font of good times and support. In particular, my late Grandma Mimi, who trained as a pediatrician in the 1940s and became a child psychiatrist later in her career, supported me without judgment and always with the tightest hugs. My cousins Ben and Andrea and their children Miles and Bea and my cousins Jasmine and Steve and their daughter Sage make my life and heart full. My Kaufman and Gaines cousins may mostly live a little further away, but I love spending time together whenever we get the chance and watching your children grow up.

My parents, James and Robin Doroshow, are exemplary physician scholars. My dad is a creative clinical investigator, physician, and health administrator whose love of historical biographies is one hint of his past as a history of science undergraduate concentrator at Harvard. My mom, whose pediatric patients are much cuter than my patients, is an astute clinician and fantastic educator who is not afraid to remake her own career to seize new opportunities. Their excitement and professional fulfillment have served as a model for me, even though my puzzle pieces may not fit together quite as logically. Thank you for your support, love, and humor.

Todd Olszewski is quite simply the best. Not only did he make sure the house didn't fall apart during my medical residency, he is caring, patient, and thoughtful. He is my favorite editor and our walks always clear the tangle of brush in my head when my writing is stuck. I am so proud of your historical and teaching work, and am even more proud to be your partner in life.

As another of my mentors, Allan Brandt, said in his own first book: whatever shortcomings and errors remain are, of course, my own damn fault.

KEY TO ARCHIVES AND MANUSCRIPTS

AACAP Archives of the American Academy of Child and Adolescent Psychiatry, Washington, DC

BA Bellefaire Archives, Western Reserve Historical Society, Cleveland, Ohio

CHA Illinois Children's Home and Aid Archives, University of Illinois at Chicago

EG Edward Greenwood papers, Menninger Foundation Corporate Archives, Kansas Historical Society, Topeka, Kansas

LB Lauretta Bender papers, Brooklyn College Library, Brooklyn, New York

KSHS Unprocessed Children's Division papers, Menninger Foundation Corporate Archives, Kansas Historical Society, Topeka, Kansas

Box number abbreviations:

097-02-01-13	IR-CD-1	1
097-02-01-14	IR-CD-1.1	1.1
097-02-01-15	IR-CD-1.2	1.2
097-02-01-16	IR-CD-2	2
097-02-01-20	IR-CD-3	3
097-02-01-26	IR-CD-4.2	4.2
097-02-02-4	IR-CD-5.2	5.2
097-02-02-06	IR-CD-5.4	5.4
097-02-02-07	IR-CD-6	6
097-02-02-11	IR-CD-7.3	7.3
097-02-02-12,	IR-CD-8	8
097-02-02-13	IR-CD-9	9
097-02-02-14	IR-CD-9.1	9.1
118-5-2-16		16

NLM American Child Guidance and Child Psychiatry Movement Interview Collection 1975–1978, National Library of Medicine, Bethesda, Maryland

RES	Robert E. Switzer papers, Menninger Foundation Corporate Archives, Kansas Historical Society, Topeka, Kansas
RIHS	Bradley Hospital miscellaneous publications, Rhode Island Historical Society Library, Providence, Rhode Island
RW	Raymond W. Waggoner papers, Bentley Historical Library, University of Michigan, Ann Arbor, Michigan
UC	University of Chicago School of Social Service Administration Records, 1920–1956, University of Chicago Special Collections Research Center
UL	S. Spafford Ackerly papers, Kornhauser Health Sciences Library, University of Louisville, Louisville, Kentucky
UCLA	University of California, Los Angeles, Film and Television Archive, Los Angeles, California
WR	Wiltwyck School for Boys Records, Rare Book and Manuscript Library, Columbia University, New York, New York

NOTES

INTRODUCTION

1. Lauretta Bender, *Child Psychiatric Techniques; Diagnostic and Therapeutic Approach to Normal and Abnormal Development through Patterned, Expressive, and Group Behaviour* (Springfield, IL: Thomas, 1952), 89.
2. Ibid., 216.
3. Ibid., 89, 216.
4. Ibid., 6.
5. Lauretta Bender, "Group Activities on a Children's Ward as Methods of Psychotherapy," *American Journal of Psychiatry* 93, no. 5 (March 1, 1937): 1156.
6. Ibid., 1160–65; Bender, *Child Psychiatric Techniques*, 216.
7. Bender, *Child Psychiatric Techniques*, 91.
8. Ibid., 216.
9. Historian Kathleen W. Jones suggests that seriously mentally ill children were grouped with the "feebleminded" in the late nineteenth and early twentieth centuries and often institutionalized with a heterogeneous group of children who might be considered intellectually disabled, epileptic, and delinquent by today's standards (*Taming the Troublesome Child: American Families, Child Guidance, and the Limits of Psychiatric Authority* [Cambridge, MA: Harvard University Press, 1999], 26). On the history of intellectual disability in America, see James W. Trent, *Inventing the Feeble Mind: A History of Mental Retardation in the United States*, Medicine and Society 6 (Berkeley: University of California Press, 1994); Peter L. Tyor and Leland V. Bell, *Caring for the Retarded in America: A History* (Westport, CT: Greenwood Press, 1984). On children in state hospitals, see Richard L. Lael, Barbara Brazos, and Margot Ford McMillen, *Evolution of a Missouri Asylum: Fulton State Hospital, 1851–2006* (Columbia, MO: University of Missouri Press, 2007), esp. 159–60 and chap. 13. Lael et al. discuss children beginning with a rise in youth admissions in the late 1950s, but they were likely present in smaller numbers beforehand.
10. American Psychiatric Association, *Psychiatric Inpatient Treatment of Children: Report of the Conference on Inpatient Psychiatric Treatment for Children Held at Washington, D. C., October 17–21, 1956* (Washington, DC: American Psychiatric Association, 1957), xi; Lauretta Bender and Archie A. Silver, "Problems in Community Planning for Disturbed Children as Suggested by Hospital Experience," *Journal of Educational Sociology* 24, no. 9 (May 1951): 1.

11. Joseph H. Reid and Helen R. Hagan, *Residential Treatment of Emotionally Disturbed Children: A Descriptive Study* (New York: Child Welfare League of America, 1952), 39.
12. Steven L. Schlossman, *Love and the American Delinquent: The Theory and Practice of "Progressive" Juvenile Justice, 1825–1920* (Chicago: University of Chicago Press, 1977).
13. Jones, *Taming the Troublesome Child*; Margo Horn, *Before It's Too Late: The Child Guidance Movement in the United States, 1922–1945* (Philadelphia: Temple University Press, 1989).
14. Trent, *Inventing the Feeble Mind*.
15. Steven Schlossman uses case studies to explore juvenile courts and reform institutions for delinquent children (*Love and the American Delinquent*) and David B. Wolcott's *Cops and Kids* explores how delinquency was treated more proximally on the streets (*Cops and Kids: Policing Juvenile Delinquency in Urban America, 1890–1940* [Columbus: Ohio State University Press, 2005]).
16. Horn, *Before It's Too Late*; Jones, *Taming the Troublesome Child*.
17. Ian Hacking, "Making Up People," in *Reconstructing Individualism: Autonomy, Individuality, and the Self in Western Thought*, ed. Thomas C. Heller, Morton Sosna, and David E. Wellbery (Stanford, CA: Stanford University Press, 1986), 222–36.
18. See Anna G. Creadick, *Perfectly Average: The Pursuit of Normality in Postwar America* (Amherst: University of Massachusetts Press, 2010).
19. On nostalgia and the construction of the "good old days" narrative, see Stephanie Coontz, *The Way We Never Were: American Families and the Nostalgia Trap* (New York: Basic Books, 1992). On heterogeneous cultural messages about women's "appropriate" gender roles and the variety of ways women resisted those roles, see Joanne J. Meyerowitz, ed., *Not June Cleaver: Women and Gender in Postwar America, 1945–1960* (Philadelphia: Temple University Press, 1994). On the personal cost of striving for normality, see Wini Breines, *Young, White, and Miserable: Growing up Female in the Fifties* (Boston: Beacon Books, 1992); Elaine Tyler May, *Homeward Bound: American Families in the Cold War Era* (New York: Basic Books, 1988).
20. Deborah Blythe Doroshow, "An Alarming Solution: Bedwetting, Medicine, and Behavioral Conditioning in Mid-Twentieth-Century America," *Isis* 101, no. 2 (June 2010): 312–37. On the slow pace of clinical change more generally, see Joel D. Howell, *Technology in the Hospital: Transforming Patient Care in the Early Twentieth Century* (Baltimore, MD: Johns Hopkins University Press, 1995); Martin S. Pernick, *A Calculus of Suffering: Pain, Professionalism, and Anesthesia in Nineteenth-Century America* (New York: Columbia University Press, 1985); John Harley Warner, *The Therapeutic Perspective: Medical Practice, Knowledge, and Identity in America, 1820–1885* (Cambridge, MA: Harvard University Press, 1986).

CHAPTER 1

1. Albert Deutsch, *Our Rejected Children* (Boston: Little, Brown, 1950), 20.
2. Ibid., 15.
3. Ibid., 50–51.
4. Ibid., 133–34.
5. Ibid., 138–39.
6. As Marshall B. Jones explains, "'dependent' meant 'in need of public or charitable support,' and 'neglected' included abandoned and abused children" ("Decline of the American Orphanage, 1941–1980," *Social Service Review* 67, no. 3 [September 1993]: 462).

7. For example, societies opposing cruelty to children were founded in the 1870s in New York and Boston (Susan E. Lederer, *Subjected to Science: Human Experimentation in America before the Second World War* (Baltimore, MD: Johns Hopkins University Press, 1995). Also see Linda Gordon, *Heroes of Their Own Lives: The Politics and History of Family Violence: Boston, 1880–1960* (New York: Viking, 1988), chap. 2. On orphan trains, see Linda Gordon, *The Great Arizona Orphan Abduction* (Cambridge, MA: Harvard University Press, 1999); Marilyn Irvin Holt, *The Orphan Trains: Placing Out in America* (Lincoln: University of Nebraska Press, 1992); and Stephen O'Connor, *Orphan Trains: The Story of Charles Loring Brace and the Children He Saved and Failed* (Boston: Houghton Mifflin Company, 2001). For an overview of nineteenth-century child welfare reform, see Walter I. Trattner, *From Poor Law to Welfare State: A History of Social Welfare in America,* 6th ed. (New York: Free Press, 1999), chap. 6.
8. Timothy A. Hacsi, *Second Home: Orphan Asylums and Poor Families in America* (Cambridge, MA: Harvard University Press, 1997).
9. LeRoy Ashby, *Saving the Waifs: Reformers and Dependent Children, 1890–1917* (Philadelphia: Temple University Press, 1984), 4; Michael B. Katz, "Review: Child-Saving," *History of Education Quarterly* 26, no. 3 (October 1, 1986): 413–14.
10. Kriste Lindenmeyer, *A Right to Childhood: The U.S. Children's Bureau and Child Welfare, 1912–46* (Urbana: University of Illinois Press, 1997); Nancy Pottishman Weiss, "Save the Children: A History of the Children's Bureau, 1903–1918" (PhD diss., University of California, 1974), and "Mother, the Invention of Necessity: Dr. Benjamin Spock's Baby and Child Care," *American Quarterly* 29, no. 5 (1977): 519–46; Molly Ladd-Taylor, *Mother-Work: Women, Child Welfare, and the State, 1890–1930* (Urbana: University of Illinois Press, 1994), chap. 6.
11. See Linda Gordon, *Pitied but Not Entitled: Single Mothers and the History of Welfare, 1890–1935* (New York: Free Press, 1994), chap. 9.
12. Bernadine Barr, "Spare Children, 1900–1945: Inmates of Orphanages as Subjects of Research in Medicine and in the Social Sciences in America" (PhD diss., Stanford University, 1992), 32, fig. 2.2, cited in Ethan G. Sribnick, "Rehabilitating Child Welfare: Children and Public Policy, 1945–1980" (PhD diss., University of Virginia, 2007), 126.
13. *Proceedings of the Conference on the Care of Dependent Children Held at Washington, D.C., January 25, 26, 1909* (Washington, DC: Government Printing Office, 1909), 57.
14. Ibid., 87–88.
15. Ibid., 5.
16. Ashby, *Saving the Waifs*, 13, 25–30.
17. Steven L. Schlossman, *Love and the American Delinquent: The Theory and Practice of "Progressive" Juvenile Justice, 1825–1920* (Chicago: University of Chicago Press, 1977); Katz, "Review: Child-Saving," 423.
18. Barbara Melosh, *Strangers and Kin: The American Way of Adoption* (Cambridge, MA: Harvard University Press, 2002), 3.
19. Sribnick, "Rehabilitating Child Welfare," 125–27.
20. Bernadine Barr, "Spare Children, 1900–1945," 32, fig. 2.2; Marshall B. Jones, "Crisis of the American Orphanage, 1931–1940," *Social Service Review* 63, no. 4 (1989): 613–29.
21. Henry Dwight Chapin, "Family vs. Institution," *Survey* 55 (January 15, 1926): 485–588, excerpted at Ellen Herman, *The Adoption History Project*, last updated February 24, 2012, http://darkwing.uoregon.edu/~adoption/archive/ChapinFvI.htm.

22. Lauretta Bender and Helen Yarnell, "An Observation Nursery: A Study of 250 Children on the Psychiatric Division of Bellevue Hospital," *American Journal of Psychiatry* 97, no. 5 (March 1, 1941): 1158–74.
23. Ibid., 1169.
24. Ibid., 1172.
25. Timothy Hacsi, "From Indenture to Family Foster Care: A Brief History of Child Placing," *Child Welfare* 74, no. 1 (January 1995): 174; Jones, "Crisis of the American Orphanage."
26. Norman V. Lourie and Rena Schulman, "The Role of the Residential Staff in Residential Treatment," *American Journal of Orthopsychiatry* 24, no. 4 (1952): 800; See also foreword, American Psychiatric Association, *Psychiatric Inpatient Treatment of Children: Report of the Conference on Inpatient Psychiatric Treatment for Children Held at Washington, D. C., October 17–21, 1956* (Washington, DC: American Psychiatric Association, 1957), xii–xiii.
27. Illinois Children's Home and Aid Society, *Plans for an Institution for the Treatment of Emotionally Disturbed Children* (Chicago: Illinois Children's Home and Aid Society, 1946), 1.
28. Jones, "Decline of the American Orphanage." Jones argues that, after World War II, child welfare experts started to realize that the children living in orphanages and foster homes "were more and more frequently disturbed" (ibid., 464).
29. New leaders, like Johns Hopkins University psychiatrist Adolf Meyer, suggested that mental illness might be influenced by both heredity and environment. If a person's early environment could be modified, perhaps mental illness might be prevented entirely. On Meyer's psychobiological approach to mental illness and its practical application to patient treatment, see S. D. Lamb, *Pathologist of the Mind: Adolf Meyer and the Origins of American Psychiatry* (Baltimore, MD: Johns Hopkins University Press, 2014). On mental hygiene and its application to children, see Gerald N. Grob, *Mental Illness and American Society, 1875–1940* (Princeton, NJ: Princeton University Press, 1983), chap. 6; Theresa R. Richardson, *The Century of the Child: The Mental Hygiene Movement and Social Policy in the United States and Canada* (Albany: State University of New York Press, 1989), chap. 4.
30. Schlossman, *Love and the American Delinquent*; Robert M. Mennel, Thorns & Thistles; Juvenile Delinquents in the United States, 1825–1940 (Hanover, NH: University Press of New England, 1973); Eric Schneider, *In the Web of Class: Delinquents and Reformers in Boston, 1810s–1930s* (New York: New York University Press, 1992).
31. Margo Horn, *Before It's Too Late: The Child Guidance Movement in the United States, 1922–1945* (Philadelphia: Temple University Press, 1989), 12.
32. Kathleen W. Jones, *Taming the Troublesome Child*, 32–35; Judith Sealander, *The Failed Century of the Child: Governing America's Young in the Twentieth Century* (Cambridge: Cambridge University Press, 2003), 21–25.
33. Schlossman, *Love and the American Delinquent.*
34. *White House Conference on Child Health and Protection, Preliminary Committee Reports* (New York: Century Co., 1930), 541, http://archive.org/details/whitehouse confe00unse.
35. Horn, *Before It's Too Late*, 25.
36. Ibid., 31, 14–15.
37. Ibid., 57–58.
38. Ibid., 31–33.
39. Horn, *Before It's Too Late*; Jones, *Taming the Troublesome Child.*

40. Leo P. O'Donnell, "Prevision of the Development of the New Children's Unit of Rockland State Hospital," *Psychiatric Quarterly* 9, no. 3 (July 1935): 428.
41. Ibid., 426.
42. Horn, *Before It's Too Late*; Jones, *Taming the Troublesome Child*.
43. White House Conference on Child Health and Protection, *The Delinquent Child; Report of the Committee on Socially Handicapped—Delinquency* (New York: Century, 1932), 297.
44. Herschel Alt, *Residential Treatment for the Disturbed Child: Basic Principles in Planning and Design of Programs and Facilities* (New York: International Universities Press, 1960), 42.
45. Joseph H. Reid and Helen R. Hagan, *Residential Treatment of Emotionally Disturbed Children: A Descriptive Study* (New York: Child Welfare League of America, 1952), 5.
46. O'Donnell, "Prevision of the Development of the New Children's Unit," 427.
47. Albert Q. Maisel, "Bedlam 1946," *Life* 20, no. 18 (May 6, 1946): 102–18.
48. Reid and Hagan, *Residential Treatment of Emotionally Disturbed Children*, 1.
49. *The First Annual Report of the Arthur Brisbane Child Treatment Center at Allaire for the Year Ending June 30, 1948* (Allaire, NJ: The Center, 1948), 1.
50. Bernadine Barr, "Spare Children, 1900–1945," 32, fig. 2.2.
51. Jones, "Decline of the American Orphanage."
52. Reid and Hagan, *Residential Treatment of Emotionally Disturbed Children*, 21.
53. Ibid.; Child Welfare League of America and Council of Jewish Federations and Welfare Funds, *Bellefaire Survey: 1952–1953*, Container 19, Folder 4, BA, 4.
54. Unfortunately, Bellefaire's motives for requesting this study are unclear; it is likely that administrators had already begun to notice changes in the kinds of children being referred there and wanted to formally document these changes.
55. "Bellefaire Trustees' Meeting," April 26, 1942, Container 6, Folder 4, BA, 3.
56. Michael Sharlitt, *Annual Report*, July 20, 1941, in "Meeting of Case Committee at Bellefaire," April 14, 1942, Container 10, Folder 6, BA, 8.
57. "Bellefaire Enlarges Its Service," *Bellefaire Briefs* 3, no. 1 (July 1940): 1, Container 18, Folder 4, BA.
58. Admissions at Bellefaire in 1945 were triple those only five years earlier, and the staff of Bellefaire continued to grow in order to care for children under its developing psychiatric model (Leon H. Richman, *Annual Report of Executive Director*, in "Bellefaire Board of Trustees Minutes of Meeting Held July 8, 1945," Container 6, Folder 7, BA, 3, 23–24).
59. Ibid., 23a.
60. "'Unit Social Worker' Plan Adopted," *Bellefaire Bulletin* 3, no. 1 (Fall 1954): 2, Container 18, Folder 4, BA.
61. *Bellefaire: 25 Years* (Shaker Heights, OH: Bellefaire Jewish Children's Home, 1967), 2, Container 19, Folder 4, BA.
62. Schneider, *In the Web of Class*.
63. David Jay Rothman, *Conscience and Convenience: The Asylum and Its Alternatives in Progressive America* (Boston: Little, Brown, 1980), chap. 8.
64. Alida C. Bowler and Ruth S. Bloodgood, *Institutional Treatment of Delinquent Boys* (Washington, DC: U.S. Children's Bureau, 1935), 2.
65. Ibid., 148, 149, 152–53.
66. American Psychiatric Association, ed., *Training Schools for Delinquent Children: A Guide to Planning with Particular Reference to Clinical Facilities* (Washington, DC: American Psychiatric Association, 1952), 337–59.

67. Ibid., 356.
68. Ibid., 243–58.
69. Bowler and Bloodgood, *Institutional Treatment of Delinquent Boys,* 190.
70. Ibid., 179, 191, 205.
71. Ibid., 195–96, 205.
72. *First Annual Report: Hawthorne School of the Jewish Protectory and Aid Society* (Albany, NY: J. B. Lyon Co., 1908), quoted in Alt, *Residential Treatment for the Disturbed Child,* 11.
73. Ibid., 12, 35.
74. Ibid., 12–13.
75. Alt, *Residential Treatment for the Disturbed Child,* 12.
76. Ibid., 14.
77. Milton J. E. Senn, "Interview with Dr. Herschel Alt, December 12, 1978 in New York City" n.d., 62, Box 1, Folder 4, NLM, 62.
78. Hawthorne School annual report (1927), quoted in Alt, *Residential Treatment for the Disturbed Child,* 15.
79. Ibid., 14–16, 74.
80. Ibid., 19, 72–73.
81. Ibid., 27.
82. Ibid., 19.
83. Ibid., 24–25.
84. Ibid., 27.
85. Ibid., 5.
86. American Psychiatric Association, *Training Schools for Delinquent Children;* U.S. Children's Bureau, *Institutions Serving Delinquent Children: Guides and Goals* (Washington, DC: Government Printing Office, 1957).
87. George H. Weber, *A Report on Some Aspects of Rhode Island's Training Schools* (Washington, DC: U.S. Department of Health, Education, and Welfare, Social Security Administration, Children's Bureau, 1959).
88. Juvenile Delinquency Evaluation Project of the City of New York, *Three New York State Training Schools: A Study of New York State Training School for Boys, Warwick, New York State Training School for Girls, Hudson, Otisville State Training School for Boys* (New York: n.p., 1957).
89. Ibid., 1.
90. August Aichhorn, *Wayward Youth* (New York: Viking Press, 1925), 149.
91. Ibid., 156.
92. Ibid., 157.
93. Ibid., 146.
94. Richard Pollak, *The Creation of Dr. B: A Biography of Bruno Bettelheim* (New York: Simon & Schuster, 1997); Robert Gottlieb, "The Strange Case of Dr. B.," *New York Review of Books,* February 27, 2003, http://www.nybooks.com/articles/archives/2003/feb/27/the-strange-case-of-dr-b/.
95. Sonia Shankman Orthogenic School, *Family Handbook,* accessed October 26, 2016, http://orthogenicschool.uchicago.edu/Admission_Packet_Residential.pdf.
96. Bruno Bettelheim and Emmy Sylvester, "Milieu Therapy: Indications and Illustrations," *Psychoanalytic Review* 36 (1949): 54. On Bettelheim and his troubled legacy, see Pollak, *The Creation of Dr. B;* Nina Sutton, *Bettelheim: A Life and a Legacy* (New York: Basic Books, 1996); Theron Raines, *Rising to the Light: A Portrait of Bruno Bettelheim* (New York: Alfred A. Knopf, 2002).

97. Bruno Bettelheim, *Love Is Not Enough: The Treatment of Emotionally Disturbed Children* (Glencoe, IL: Free Press, 1950), 22.
98. William C. Morse, "Introduction and Perspective," in *Crisis Intervention in Residential Treatment: The Clinical Innovations of Fritz Redl*, ed. William C. Morse (New York: Haworth Press, 1991); Allen L. Otten and Charles B. Seib, "The Case of the Furious Children," *Harper's Magazine*, January 1958.
99. Fritz Redl and David Wineman, *Children Who Hate: The Disorganization and Breakdown of Behavior Controls* (Glencoe IL.: Free Press, 1951), 7.
100. In an address at the Walter Reed Army Medical Center in August 1957, child psychiatrist Earle Silber explained that "most workers in the field of milieu therapy with children, or as it is commonly referred to in most of the recent literature, residential treatment for children, acknowledge August Aichhorn as a pioneer in this method of treatment" (Earle Silber, "Some Aspects of Milieu Treatment with Children," talk given at Walter Reed Army Medical Center, August 1957, transcript provided by Silber, 1). Reid and Hagan also acknowledged Aichhorn in the foreword to their 1952 CWLA study of residential treatment: "August Aichhorn's notable book, 'Wayward Youth,' was perhaps the earliest description of the dynamics of 'milieu' therapy" (*Residential Treatment of Emotionally Disturbed Children*, iii).
101. Milton J. E. Senn, "Interview with Dr. Herschel Alt, December 12, 1978 in New York City," Box 1, Folders 3–4, NLM, 8.
102. John G. Milner, "The Residential Treatment Center," *Annals of the American Academy of Political and Social Science* 355, no. 1 (1964): 99.
103. Earle Silber, interview with the author, March 27, 2011, Chevy Chase, MD.
104. See George Makari, *Revolution in Mind: The Creation of Psychoanalysis* (New York: HarperCollins, 2008), chap. 11. Anna Freud took a more empirical approach, emphasizing winning the child's trust and focusing on traumatic events in the child's life, whereas Melanie Klein argued that even the very young child had unconscious impulses that might be uncovered through play therapy and transference.
105. See Michal Shapira, *The War Inside: Psychoanalysis, Total War, and the Making of the Democratic Self in Postwar Britain* (New York: Cambridge University Press, 2013), chap. 2.
106. Horn, *Before It's Too Late*, 149–54.
107. "Children's Division Time Line," 1978, Menninger Foundation Archives—Children's Division, Box 1, Historical background, KSHS, 1; "The Southard School," 1934, Box 1, Southard School (1934), KSHS.
108. James W. Trent, *Inventing the Feeble Mind: A History of Mental Retardation in the United States*, Medicine and Society 6 (Berkeley: University of California Press, 1994).
109. For an example of such admission criteria, see Joseph H. Reid and Helen R. Hagan, *Residential Treatment of Emotionally Disturbed Children: A Descriptive Study* (New York: Child Welfare League of America, 1952).
110. Earl Saxe, *Report to the Board of Directors of the Southard School*, August 22, 1939, Box 1.1, Southard School, Annual Reports, 1939–46, KSHS.
111. *Annual Report of the Southard School*, 1940, Box 1.1, Southard School, Annual Reports, 1939–46, KSHS, 1–2.
112. "Children's Division Time Line," 2.
113. *Annual Report of the Southard School*, 1940, 14.
114. Ibid.
115. For a synthetic history of the Menninger Foundation and Clinic, see Lawrence Jacob Friedman, *Menninger: The Family and the Clinic* (New York: Knopf, 1990).

116. *Menninger Foundation: Report of Committee on Southard School,* January 16, 1955, Box 1, Annual Reports—1952–56, KSHS, 8.
117. Despite the official name change, many people still referred to the Children's Division as Southard School. I will continue to do so for clarity's sake.
118. "Future Plans for Southard School," n.d. [likely mid-1950s], Box 9, Reorganization Plans, KSHS, 1–2.
119. Ibid., 2. The use of both "disturbed" and "delinquent" in this sentence reflects the fluid connection between the two; even though "delinquent" children were often considered "disturbed" and treated in RTCs, "delinquent" remained a common term and cultural touchstone.
120. Helen D. Sargent, *Progress Report on Study of Southard School,* November 26, 1951, Box 1, Summaries, 1949–52, KSHS, 2.
121. J. Cotter Hirschberg, "A Long Range Plan for Child Psychiatry at the Menninger Foundation," October 1955, Box 1, Annual Reports—1952–56, KSHS, 1.
122. "Help for the Child with Problems," 1954, Box 3, Help for the Child with Problems (1954), KSHS, 1.
123. On Southard and the Boston Psychopathic Hospital, see Elizabeth Lunbeck, *The Psychiatric Persuasion: Knowledge, Gender, and Power in Modern America* (Princeton, NJ: Princeton University Press, 1994).
124. Robert E. Switzer, "The Evolution of a New Program and a New House" (paper presented at the annual meeting of the American Association for Children's Residential Centers, November 5, 1961, Box 118-8-4-56 S-Z Switzer, The Evolution of a New Program and a New House," RES), 1.
125. "Help for the Child with Problems," 1; Southard School Journalism Class, *Don't Forget the Children: A History of Southard School, 1926–1986* (Topeka, KS: Menninger Foundation, 1986).
126. Emma Pendleton Bradley Hospital, *Out of Their Misfortune: 25th Anniversary Report of the Emma Pendleton Bradley Home* (Riverside, RI: The Hospital, 1956).
127. Wrenshall A. Oliver, "A State Hospital Children's Unit," *American Journal of Psychiatry* 106, no. 4 (October 1, 1949): 266.
128. Fritz Redl, "New Ways of Ego Support in Residential Treatment of Disturbed Children," *Bulletin of the Menninger Clinic* 13, no. 2 (March 1949): 64.
129. Louis Lurie and J. Victor Greenebaum, "The Perspectives of the Mental Hygiene Movement in the Jewish Community of Cincinnati," *Cincinnati Journal of Medicine* 39, no. 10 (1958): 505; Alt, *Residential Treatment for the Disturbed Child,* 50; *The Fifth Annual Report of the Arthur Brisbane Child Treatment Center at Allaire for the Year Ending June 30, 1952* (Allaire, NJ: The Center, 1952): 1.
130. Lurie and Greenebaum, "Perspectives of the Mental Hygiene Movement," 505.
131. Georges Lussier, quoted in Reid and Hagan, *Residential Treatment of Emotionally Disturbed Children,* 20.
132. Shirley Camper, "A Follow-up Study of Children Discharged from a Psychiatric Ward," pt. 2, "Factors in Treatment" (MSS thesis, Smith College School for Social Work, 1946), 2–3.
133. *Fifth Annual Report of the Arthur Brisbane Child Treatment Center,* 1.
134. Ibid.
135. Camper, "A Follow-up Study of Children Discharged from a Psychiatric Ward," 8.
136. Dennis A. Doyle, "Black Celebrities, Selfhood, and Psychiatry in the Civil Rights Era: The Wiltwyck School for Boys and the Floyd Patterson House," *Social History of Medicine* 28, no. 2 (May 2015): 332–35.

137. "Certificate of Amendment Extending and Changing the Purposes and Powers of *Wiltwyck School for Boys, Inc.*, January 1955," Box 4, Folder 60, Wiltwyck School for Boys Records, Rare Book and Manuscript Library, Columbia University, New York, NY.
138. Doyle, "Black Celebrities, Selfhood, and Psychiatry."
139. "The Wiltwyck Story," 1966, Box 48, Folder 1120, WR.
140. Ibid.
141. "Ed Sullivan Presents at Philharmonic Hall, Lincoln Center, June 13, 1966: Benefit for the Wiltwyck School for Boys," Box 48, Folder 1115, WR.
142. Fact Sheet about Wiltwyck School for Boys, Inc., ca. 1970, Box 43, Folder 1052, WR, 3.
143. U.S. Children's Bureau, *Residential Treatment Centers for Emotionally Disturbed Children: A Listing* (Washington, DC: Federal Security Agency, Social Security Administration, Children's Bureau, 1952).
144. U.S. Children's Bureau, *Child Welfare Statistics, 1961* (Washington, DC: U.S. Dept. of Health, Education, and Welfare, Social Security Administration, Children's Bureau, 1962), 28, 31, 34.
145. Joseph H. Reid, "Administrative Auspices of Residential Treatment," *Child Welfare,* March 1958, 5.
146. Lourie and Schulman, "The Role of the Residential Staff," 801.
147. Ibid., 101; American Psychiatric Association, *Psychiatric Inpatient Treatment of Children,* xvi.
148. Lourie and Schulman, "The Role of the Residential Staff," 801.
149. Morris Krugman et al., "Symposium, 1953: The Education of Emotionally Disturbed Children," *American Journal of Orthopsychiatry* 23, no. 4 (1953): 667–90.
150. Morris F. Mayer et al., "The Role of Residential Treatment for Children Symposium, 1954," *American Journal of Orthopsychiatry* 25 (1955): 667–719.
151. Martin Leichtman, "Residential Treatment of Children and Adolescents: Past, Present, and Future," *American Journal of Orthopsychiatry* 76, no. 3 (2006): 285–86.
152. American Psychiatric Association, *Psychiatric Inpatient Treatment of Children.* For complete text of the meeting, see *Proceedings of the Conference on In-Patient Psychiatric Treatment for Children,* held under the auspices of the American Psychiatric Association, October 17–21, 1956, Woodner Hotel, Washington DC, in Box 118-8-2-8, RS.
153. Ibid.
154. Helen Hagan and Child Welfare League of America, *Bibliography, Residential Treatment of Emotionally Disturbed Children* (New York: Child Welfare League of America, 1951); Child Welfare League of America, *Residential Treatment of Emotionally Disturbed Children: Selected References,* rev. (New York: Child Welfare League of America, 1957); U.S. Children's Bureau, *Residential Treatment Centers;* Reid and Hagan, *Residential Treatment of Emotionally Disturbed Children.*
155. *The Second Annual Report of the Arthur Brisbane Child Treatment Center at Allaire for the Year Ending June 30, 1949* (Allaire, NJ: The Center, 1949): 9; *Fifth Annual Report of the Arthur Brisbane Child Treatment Center,* 5.
156. "House Planned for Emotionally Disturbed Boys," *Los Angeles Times,* October 4, 1954, A6.
157. "The Wiltwyck School for Boys, Inc., Minutes of the Meeting of the Board of Directors, February 5, 1959," Box 4, Folder 63, WR.
158. Stanislaus A. Szurek, "Child Therapy Procedures," *Psychiatry* 7, no. 1 (1944): 9.
159. U.S. Children's Bureau, *Child Welfare Statistics, 1961,* 7.

160. Charles P. Gershenson, "Residential Treatment of Children," pt. 2, "Research Problems and Possibilities," *Social Service Review* 30, no. 3 (September 1956): 268.
161. Reid, "Administrative Auspices of Residential Treatment," 6.

INTERLUDE: THE ROAD TO RESIDENTIAL

1. Otis Chandler, "Bewildered Children Await Camarillo Mental Therapy," *Los Angeles Times*, August 26, 1955, 2; Wrenshall A. Oliver, "A State Hospital Children's Unit," *American Journal of Psychiatry* 106, no. 4 (October 1, 1949): 265.
2. Samuel Lerner, "Selective Criteria for Admission to Hawthorne-Cedar Knolls School: A Dissertation Based upon an Investigation at the Jewish Board of Guardians, New York City" (MSS thesis, Smith College School for Social Work, 1947), 12; Joseph H. Reid and Helen R. Hagan, *Residential Treatment of Emotionally Disturbed Children: A Descriptive Study* (New York: Child Welfare League of America, 1952), 150; Isaac Zeke Youcha, "A Study of Schizophrenic Children in Cottage Life at the Hawthorne Cedar Knolls School" (master's thesis, New York School of Social Work, Columbia University, 1953), 4. Lee Stringer recounts his own experience at Hawthorne Cedar Knolls in the early 1960s, where he was referred from a juvenile court, in his memoir (*Sleepaway School: Stories from a Boy's Life* [New York: Seven Stories Press, 2004]).
3. Herschel Alt, *Residential Treatment for the Disturbed Child: Basic Principles in Planning and Design of Programs and Facilities* (New York: International Universities Press, 1960), 40.
4. Milton J. E. Senn, "Interview with Dr. Norman Lourie, April 14, 1977 in Harrisburg, Pennsylvania," Box 3, Folder 6, NLM, 8–9
5. Lillian J. Johnson and Joseph H. Reid, *Evaluation of Ten Years Work with Emotionally Disturbed Children* (Seattle: Ryther Child Center, 1947), 3; Lotte Eichenwald Scharfman, "An Examination of Referrals of Emotionally Disturbed Children to a Resident Treatment Center" (MSW thesis, University of Washington, 1951), 1.
6. Reid and Hagan, *Residential Treatment of Emotionally Disturbed Children*, 278.
7. Ibid., 101, 202, 206, 223.
8. These figures were compiled using data from Reid and Hagan, *Residential Treatment of Emotionally Disturbed Children*, 3, 23, 50, 68, 77–78, 96, 122–23, 138, 143–44, 202, 226, 282, 258, 312.
9. For a complete directory of RTCs with admissions qualifications, see U.S. Children's Bureau, *Residential Treatment Centers for Emotionally Disturbed Children: A Listing* (Washington DC: Federal Security Agency, Social Security Administration, Children's Bureau, 1952). It is unclear how RTCs decided which children had "organic" troubles, but many centers specified certain physical or neurological conditions that disqualified children from entry, such as intellectual disability, epilepsy, cerebral palsy, and visual impairment.
10. U.S. Children's Bureau, *Residential Treatment Centers;* Marvin Bloom and Adrian Cabral, "A Description of a Newly Introduced Group Work Program in a Residential Treatment Setting—the Hawthorne Cedar Knolls School" (master's thesis, New York School of Social Work, Columbia University, 1954), 8. At Bellefaire, non-Jewish children were a minority but were regularly accepted. Just as the Jewish children went to synagogue on campus, non-Jewish children at Bellefaire were able to engage in religious practices, through church, religious education, or a visiting minister ("Bellefaire 90th Anniversary 1868–1958," Container 19, Folder 7, BA; "Daily Living," Container 19, Folder 7, BA).

11. U.S. Children's Bureau, *Residential Treatment Centers.*
12. Arthur Madelbaum, "Description of the Southard School: Conference on Inpatient Psychiatric Treatment for Children," Box 16, Children's Div. 1956, KSHS, 14.
13. Reid and Hagan, *Residential Treatment of Emotionally Disturbed Children*, 77.
14. Lydia Hylton, *The Residential Treatment Center: Children, Programs, and Costs* (New York: Child Welfare League of America, 1964), 118.
15. "Notes of Meeting of the Evanston Receiving Home Committee," June 22, 1955, Box 32, Folder 304, CHA, 5.
16. Ibid.
17. Herbert R. Stratford to Robert H. MacRae, February 7, 1956, Box 1, Folder 7, CHA.
18. Ibid.
19. "Notes of Meeting of the Evanston Receiving Home Committee," 2.
20. Jessie E. Peeke, "A Survey of 199 Boys Admitted to the Children's Ward of Bellevue Psychiatric Hospital during the First Six Months of 1943" (master's thesis, New York School of Social Work, Columbia University, 1944), 5; U.S. Children's Bureau, *Residential Treatment Centers*, 75.
21. At Pioneer House in Detroit, "children with problem behavior of an intensity which would warrant 'closed' institutional care were . . . unacceptable" (Vera Kare, "A Study of the Adjustment of a 'Problem' Child in a Group Therapy Home for Pre-Delinquent Boys, Pioneer House, September, 1946–June, 1948." [MSW thesis, Wayne University, 1948], 2).
22. Raymond W. Waggoner and Ralph D. Rabinovitch, "The University of Michigan Plan for the Residential Treatment of Disturbed Children," *Medical Bulletin* 22, no. 3 (1956): 121, and "Practical Approach Successful at Disturbed Children's Unit," *Mental Hospitals* 4 (1953): 4; Reid and Hagan, *Residential Treatment of Emotionally Disturbed Children*, 226.
23. "The Wiltwyck School for Boys, Inc., Minutes of the Meeting of the Board of Directors," October 29, 1956, WR, 3.
24. Ibid., 4.
25. Reid and Hagan, *Residential Treatment of Emotionally Disturbed Children*, 1952, 52; Constance Lilian Blackett, "Parents' Reactions to Their Child's Visits from Residential Treatment: A Dissertation Based upon an Investigation at the Child Guidance Home, Cincinnati, Ohio" (MSW thesis, Smith College School for Social Work, 1962), i.
26. "Topic III: Morning Session, Discussion Group B," in *Proceedings of the Conference on In-Patient Psychiatric Treatment for Children*, held under the auspices of the American Psychiatric Association, October 17–21, 1956, Woodner Hotel, Washington, DC, Box 118-8-2-8, EG, 474, 478.
27. Ibid., 479. Policies like these were not uniform. As Frank Curran, a child psychiatrist at the Children's Service Center in Charlottesville, VA, explained, "In some other institutions . . . parents are more or less told, 'You have been a failure. You have caused this sort of thing. You go home and let us handle it.' . . . The parents are discouraged from staying in town and even discouraged from coming back during regular visiting hours" (ibid., 464).
28. U.S. Children's Bureau, *Residential Treatment Centers.*
29. U.S. Children's Bureau, *Child Welfare Statistics, 1961* (Washington, DC: U.S. Dept. of Health, Education, and Welfare, Social Security Administration, Children's Bureau, 1962), 7.
30. U.S. Children's Bureau, *Child Welfare Statistics, 1965* (Washington, DC: U.S. Dept. of

Health, Education, and Welfare, Social Security Administration, Children's Bureau, 1966), 11.

31. At Bellefaire, for example, the staff tried to keep its population to fifty children ("Conference on In-Patient Psychiatric Treatment for Children, Background Material for Preparatory Committees on Personnel and Treatment," April 24, 1956, Box 1, File 5, LB, 4).
32. "Procedures for the Admission of a New Child to the Southard School, October, 1956," Box 9, Admissions Procedures, 1956, KSHS.
33. Ibid., 1.
34. Reid and Hagan, *Residential Treatment of Emotionally Disturbed Children*, 1952, 57.
35. Alt, *Residential Treatment for the Disturbed Child*, 57.
36. [Josephine], "My First Week Here," *Gold and Blue* (Fall 1954) in *Bellefaire Bulletin*, vol. 2, no. 1 (Fall 1954), Container 18, Folder 4, BA.
37. Roberto R. Sucgang, "Orienting New Students in a Residential Treatment Institution," *Federal Probation*, December 1955, 26–27.
38. Anabel Maxwell, "The Inter-Related Movement of Parent and Child in Resident Treatment," *Quarterly Journal of Child Behavior* 2 (1951): 188.
39. Bruno Bettelheim, *Love Is Not Enough: The Treatment of Emotionally Disturbed Children* (Glencoe, IL: Free Press, 1950), 53–54.
40. Ibid., 56–57.
41. [Jean,] "Welcome, [Flora]," *Bellefaire Bulletin*, vol. 2, no. 2 (Winter 1954), Container 18, Folder 4, BA.
42. Children of Bellefaire, "So you'll know all about . . . Bellefaire," Container 19, Folder 7, BA.
43. [Josephine], "My First Week Here."

CHAPTER 2

1. Othilda Krug, Helen Hayward, and Bernice Crumpacker, "Intensive Residential Treatment of a Nine-Year-Old Girl with an Aggressive Behavior Disorder, Petit Mal Epilepsy and Enuresis," *American Journal of Orthopsychiatry* 22, no. 2 (1952): 405.
2. Ibid., 406–8.
3. Ian Hacking, "Making Up People," in *Reconstructing Individualism: Autonomy, Individuality, and the Self in Western Thought*, ed. Thomas C. Heller, Morton Sosna, and David E. Wellbery (Stanford, CA: Stanford University Press, 1986).
4. Stephanie Coontz, *The Way We Never Were: American Families and the Nostalgia Trap* (New York: Basic Books, 1992); Elaine Tyler May, *Homeward Bound: American Families in the Cold War Era* (New York: Basic Books, 1988); Arlene S. Skolnick, *Embattled Paradise: The American Family in an Age of Uncertainty* (New York: Basic Books, 1991).
5. Bernice Crumpacker, "The Caseworker as Residential Worker: A Dissertation Based upon a Study at the Child Guidance Home, Cincinnati, Ohio" (MSS thesis, Smith College School for Social Work, 1950), 24.
6. Ibid., 25.
7. Ibid., 28.
8. Donald A. Bloch, "Residential Treatment for Disturbed Children," *Nursing Outlook* 5, no. 11 (1957): 637.
9. Menninger Foundation, Children's Division, "The Southard School: A Re-Educational Center for Children" (Topeka, KS, 1950s).

10. J. Franklin Robinson, "The Role of the Resident Professional Worker," *American Journal of Orthopsychiatry* 19, no. 4 (1949): 677.
11. Crumpacker, "The Caseworker as Residential Worker," 19.
12. Barbara L. Smith, "Programming in a Treatment Home for Disturbed Children: An Analysis of Programming at Pioneer House from December 1, 1946 to June 1, 1947, Evaluating the Relationship of Program Activities to Individual and Group Developments" (MSW thesis, Wayne University, 1948), 16; Herschel Alt and Hyman Grossbard, "Professional Issues in the Institutional Treatment of Delinquent Children," *American Journal of Orthopsychiatry* 19, no. 2 (1949): 280.
13. Marvin Bloom and Adrian Cabral, "A Description of a Newly Introduced Group Work Program in a Residential Treatment Setting—the Hawthorne Cedar Knolls School" (master's thesis, New York School of Social Work, Columbia University, 1954), 7; Reid and Hagan, *Residential Treatment of Emotionally Disturbed Children*, v.
14. Illinois Children's Home and Aid Society, *Plans for an Institution for the Treatment of Emotionally Disturbed Children* (Chicago: Illinois Children's Home and Aid Society, 1946), 2.
15. Emma Pendleton Bradley Hospital, *Out of Their Misfortune: 25th Anniversary Report of the Emma Pendleton Bradley Home* (Riverside, RI: The Hospital, 1956), 3.
16. Anna G. Creadick, *Perfectly Average: The Pursuit of Normality in Postwar America* (Amherst: University of Massachusetts Press, 2010).
17. Helen Renner Brookens, "A Study of Five Children Treated under Ryther Child Center's Program for the Care of Children with Personality Problems" (MA thesis, University of Washington, 1944), 25–29.
18. Ibid., 30.
19. Anne Benjamin and Howard E. Weatherly, "Hospital Ward Treatment of Emotionally Disturbed Children," *American Journal of Orthopsychiatry* 17, no. 4 (October 1947): 668.
20. Herschel Alt, *Residential Treatment for the Disturbed Child: Basic Principles in Planning and Design of Programs and Facilities* (New York: International Universities Press, 1960), 30.
21. Evelyn Brownstone, Robert A. Cohn, Margaret Hooks, Herbert Moskowitz, and Phyllis Pfeiffer "Children's Services at the Camarillo State Hospital" (MSW thesis, School of Social Welfare, UCLA, 1952), 54; Brookens, "A Study of Five Children Treated under Ryther Child Center's Program," 66.
22. Brownstone et al., "Children's Services at the Camarillo State Hospital," 25.
23. Benjamin and Weatherly, "Hospital Ward Treatment of Emotionally Disturbed Children," 668.
24. Alt, *Residential Treatment for the Disturbed Child*, 30; "Richman Reports Six Months Service," *Bellefaire Bulletin* 1, no. 2 (February 1953): 2, Container 18, Folder 4, BA.
25. Phyllis E. Pfeiffer, "Group IV. Six Children," in Brownstone et al., "Children's Services at the Camarillo State Hospital," 70.
26. Mr. [Arthur] Mandelbaum, "Presentation for Annual Meeting, October, 1952," Box 16, Annual Meeting—1952, KSHS, 2.
27. Ibid.
28. Ibid., 3.
29. Ibid.
30. On the behavioral interests of general pediatricians in the 1950s, see Sydney A. Halpern, *American Pediatrics: The Social Dynamics of Professionalism, 1880–1980*

(Berkeley: University of California Press, 1988), chap. 7. On the history of adolescent medicine, see Heather Munro Prescott, *A Doctor of Their Own: The History of Adolescent Medicine* (Cambridge, MA: Harvard University Press, 1998).

31. Child psychiatrist J. Franklin Robinson, director of the Children's Service Center of Wyoming Valley in Pennsylvania, explained that treatment "centers on his emotional turmoil rather than his overt behavior," which differentiated RTCs from training and reform schools ("The Use of Residence in Psychiatric Treatment with Children," *American Journal of Psychiatry* 103, no. 6 [1947]: 814).
32. Ibid., 815.
33. Child Psychiatry Service of the Menninger Clinic, the Menninger Foundation, *Child Care Handbook*, May 1957, Box 6, *Child Care Handbook*, May 1957, KSHS, 3.
34. Jonathan Engel, *American Therapy: The Rise of Psychotherapy in the United States* (New York: Gotham Books, 2008); Nathan G. Hale, *Freud and the Americans: The Beginnings of Psychoanalysis in the United States, 1876–1917* (New York: Oxford University Press, 1971).
35. On psychoanalysis's rise to prominence in the United States following World War II, see Nathan G. Hale, *The Rise and Crisis of Psychoanalysis in the United States: Freud and the Americans, 1917–1985* (New York: Oxford University Press, 1995); and Engel, *American Therapy*. On psychology's wartime growth, see Ellen Herman, *The Romance of American Psychology: Political Culture in the Age of Experts* (Berkeley: University of California Press, 1995). For a discussion of psychoanalysis and psychotherapy's influence in popular culture, see Eva S. Moskowitz, *In Therapy We Trust: America's Obsession with Self-Fulfillment* (Baltimore, MD: Johns Hopkins University Press, 2001).
36. Eli Zaretsky, *Secrets of the Soul: A Social and Cultural History of Psychoanalysis* (New York: A. A. Knopf, 2004).
37. See George Makari, *Revolution in Mind: The Creation of Psychoanalysis* (New York: HarperCollins, 2008), chap. 11.
38. Margo Horn, *Before It's Too Late: The Child Guidance Movement in the United States, 1922–1945* (Philadelphia: Temple University Press, 1989), 149–54.
39. Engel, *American Therapy*, chap. 3.
40. Gerald N. Grob, "Origins of DSM-I: A Study in Appearance and Reality," *American Journal of Psychiatry* 148, no. 4 (April 1, 1991): 421–31; Herman, *Romance of American Psychology*.
41. Committee on Nomenclature and Statistics of the American Psychiatric Association, *Diagnostic and Statistical Manual: Mental Disorders* (Washington, DC: American Psychiatric Association, 1952).
42. Alt, *Residential Treatment for the Disturbed Child*, 47.
43. Lotte Eichenwald Scharfman, "An Examination of Referrals of Emotionally Disturbed Children to a Resident Treatment Center" (MSW thesis, University of Washington, 1951), 33.
44. "The New Southard School and Hospital," Box 3, the New Southard School and Hospital (mid-1950s), KSHS.
45. Samuel Lerner, "Selective Criteria for Admission to Hawthorne-Cedar Knolls School: A Dissertation Based upon an Investigation at the Jewish Board of Guardians, New York City" (MSS thesis, Smith College School for Social Work, 1947), 39; Samuel Finestone and Toby Bennett Bieber, "Status at Discharge and Follow-up of Twenty Children with Diagnosis of Primary Behavior Disorder Hospitalized at New

York State Psychiatric Institute and Hospital" (master's thesis, New York School of Social Work, Columbia University, 1946), 13.

46. Jewish Board of Guardians, *Conditioned Environment in Case Work Treatment: A Monograph of Articles on Hawthorne-Cedar Knolls School, Lavenburg Corner House* (New York: Jewish Board of Guardians, 1944), 41.

47. Ibid. The term "psychopathic" was fraught and difficult to distinguish from "delinquency" (itself a vague term) in many cases. Child psychiatrist Ralph D. Rabinovitch, who directed the child psychiatry unit at the University of Michigan, believed that "'psychopathic' [was] still used as a synonym for delinquent behavior regardless of etiology and [had] no more specific or dynamic meaning than listings of behavior such as stealing, truancy or destructiveness" ("Observations on the Differential Study of Severely Disturbed Children," *American Journal of Orthopsychiatry* 22, no. 2 [April 1952]: 230).

48. "The New Southard School and Hospital."

49. For early descriptions of childhood schizophrenia, see Howard W. Potter, "Schizophrenia in Children," *American Journal of Psychiatry* 89, no. 6 (May 1, 1933): 1253–70; J. Louise Despert, "Schizophrenia in Children," *Psychiatric Quarterly* 12, no. 2 (June 1, 1938): 366–71; Lauretta Bender, "Childhood Schizophrenia," *Nervous Child* 1, no. 1 (1941): 138–41; Charles Bradley, *Schizophrenia in Childhood* (New York: Macmillan, 1941); Lauretta Bender, "Childhood Schizophrenia: Clinical Study on One Hundred Schizophrenic Children," *American Journal of Orthopsychiatry* 17, no. 1 (1947): 40–56.

50. Bradley, *Schizophrenia in Childhood*, 33; Despert, "Schizophrenia in Children," 369.

51. E. Janet Allen, "Casework with the Parents at the Child Guidance Home: A Dissertation Based upon an Investigation at the Child Guidance Home, Cincinnati, Ohio" (MSS thesis, Smith College School for Social Work, 1951), 24.

52. Ibid., 25.

53. Ibid.

54. Leo Kanner, "Autistic Disturbances of Affective Contact," *Nervous Child* 2, no. 1943 (1943), 217–50.

55. Jeffrey P. Baker, "Autism in 1959: Joey the Mechanical Boy," *Pediatrics* 125, no. 6 (June 1, 2010): 1101–3.

56. Chloe Silverman, *Understanding Autism: Parents, Doctors, and the History of a Disorder* (Princeton, NJ: Princeton University Press, 2012), 39–40.

57. Crumpacker, "The Caseworker as Residential Worker," 24.

58. Ibid., 25.

59. Alt and Grossbard, "Professional Issues in the Institutional Treatment of Delinquent Children," 281.

60. Lerner, "Selective Criteria for Admission to Hawthorne-Cedar Knolls School," 47.

61. Ibid.

62. Ibid., 52.

63. Reid and Hagan, *Residential Treatment of Emotionally Disturbed Children*, vii.

64. Ibid., 24–25, 145.

65. Lerner, "Selective Criteria for Admission to Hawthorne-Cedar Knolls School," 38.

66. Alt, *Residential Treatment for the Disturbed Child*, 131.

67. Reid and Hagan, *Residential Treatment of Emotionally Disturbed Children*, 254.

68. A. M. Edelman, "Some Observations on Occupational Therapy with Disturbed Chil-

dren in a Residential Program," *American Journal of Occupational Therapy* 7, no. 3 (June 1953): 115.

69. Ibid., 114.
70. Respectively: Scharfman, "An Examination of Referrals of Emotionally Disturbed Children to a Resident Treatment Center," 6; and Thaddeus P. Krush, "State-Subsidized Care and Treatment of Mentally Ill Children in Massachusetts," *American Journal of Psychiatry* 109, no. 11 (May 1, 1953): 819.
71. For example, Kathleen Jones showed how many girls were referred to child guidance clinics for shoplifting or sexual promiscuity while boys were sent for truancy and stealing (*Taming the Troublesome Child*). In the 1910s and 1920s, Elizabeth Lunbeck has argued, women treated in psychopathic hospitals were similarly criminalized and medicalized for their seemingly "hypersexual" behaviors (*The Psychiatric Persuasion: Knowledge, Gender, and Power in Modern America* [Princeton, NJ: Princeton University Press, 1994]).
72. "Bad Boy's Story," *Life*, May 12, 1947, 108–9.
73. Allen L. Otten and Charles B. Seib, "The Case of the Furious Children," *Harper's Magazine*, January 1958, 56.
74. Roger Greene, "'Case of the Furious Children': We Don't Know Why They Hate," *Chicago Daily Tribune*, July 19, 1959. It is notable that the *Harper's* article was described in the *Chicago Tribune*, far away from the NIH campus in Bethesda, Maryland, suggesting that the article was widely read and commented on.
75. Gertrude Samuels, "A New Road for the Juvenile Delinquent," *New York Times*, April 23, 1950, SM6.
76. Lillian J. Johnson, "Making Over Martha," *Parents' Magazine*, March 1948, 26–28; Lillian J. Johnson, "A Girl Named Ann," *Parents' Magazine*, November 1947, 35–37.
77. Joan Beck, "Can 'Bad Kids' Be Saved?," *Chicago Daily Tribune*, February 27, 1955.
78. See Wini Breines, *Young, White, and Miserable: Growing up Female in the Fifties* (Boston: Beacon Books, 1992); Coontz, *The Way We Never Were*; May, *Homeward Bound*; Joanne J. Meyerowitz, ed., *Not June Cleaver: Women and Gender in Postwar America, 1945–1960* (Philadelphia: Temple University Press, 1994); Skolnick, *Embattled Paradise*. On traditional gender roles, their racial connotations, and citizenship, see Ruth Feldstein, *Motherhood in Black and White: Race and Sex in American Liberalism, 1930–1965* (Ithaca, NY: Cornell University Press, 2000).
79. Laslo Benedek, *The Wild One* (Columbia Pictures Corporation, 1954); Richard Brooks, *Blackboard Jungle* (Metro Goldwyn Mayer, 1955). On concerns about juvenile delinquency in the 1950s, see James Burkhart Gilbert, *A Cycle of Outrage: America's Reaction to the Juvenile Delinquent in the 1950s* (New York: Oxford University Press, 1986).
80. See Prescott, *A Doctor of Their Own*, chap. 1.
81. William March, *The Bad Seed* (New York: Rinehart, 1954); Maxwell Anderson, *Bad Seed: A Play in Two Acts* (New York: Dodd, Mead, 1955); Mervyn LeRoy, *The Bad Seed* (Warner Bros. Pictures, 1956).
82. Obviously, this is not a systematic set of case studies. However, I still believe it warrants serious consideration as the sources were all clinical and represented both children who were being presented for academic evaluation (journals, social work theses) but also reviews of unsorted new groups of children who were being admitted to RTCs.
83. Ralph D. Rabinovitch, Janet Bee, and Barbara Outwater, "The Integration of Occu-

pational and Recreational Therapy in the Residential Psychiatric Treatment of Children: A Symposium," *American Journal of Occupational Therapy* 5, no. 1 (1951): 2.

84. Ibid.
85. "Medicine: Psychiatry at Work," *Time Magazine*, June 27, 1955, 55.
86. "Portrait" was the eighth part of *Mr. Muldoon's Hall of Fame*, a series that highlighted the work of local community organizations. *Mr. Muldoon's Hall of Fame*, episode 8, "Portrait of Elaine," written by William D. Ellis, produced by Stuart Buchanan, McCann-Erickson, Inc., Station WNBK, Saturday, January 14, 195?, Container 19, Folder 7, BA.
87. Ibid., 10.
88. Ibid., 15.
89. On journalistic attention to gender (non)conformity, see Joanne J. Meyerowitz, *How Sex Changed: A History of Transsexuality in the United States* (Cambridge, MA: Harvard University Press, 2002).
90. Thomas P. Monahan, "The Trend in Broken Homes among Delinquent Children," *Marriage and Family Living* 19, no. 4 (November 1957): 362–65; Ivan L. Russell, "Behavior Problems of Children from Broken and Intact Homes," *Journal of Educational Sociology* 31, no. 2 (November 1957): 124–29.
91. Bradford W. Wright, *Comic Book Nation: The Transformation of Youth Culture in America* (Baltimore, MD: Johns Hopkins University Press, 2001).
92. Johnson and Reid, *Evaluation of Ten Years Work*, 3; "Bellefaire (the Cleveland Jewish Orphan Home) Report on Examination, December 31, 1947," Container 7, Folder 1, BA, 10.
93. Eva E. Burmeister, *Roofs for the Family* (New York: Columbia University Press, 1954), 18.
94. Smith, "Programming in a Treatment Home for Disturbed Children," 31.
95. Ibid., 32–33.
96. Edna J. Baer, "Study of Seven Schizophrenic Children: Inquiry into Family Background and Current Adjustment of Seven Children Who Were Patients in the Bellevue Children's Ward" (master's thesis, New York School of Social Work, Columbia University, 1943), 11–13.
97. Ibid., 39–40.
98. Ibid., 33–35.
99. Johnson and Reid, *Evaluation of Ten Years Work*, 17.
100. Lucy Freeman, "Delinquency Roll Shifts in Pattern," *New York Times*, July 31, 1949, 38. It is very difficult to trace how the socioeconomic backgrounds of RTC children changed over time. In this article, Hawthorne's chairman attributed the change to the admission of nondelinquent (likely withdrawn or neurotic) children. However, Hawthorne's director in the early 1940s, Herschel Alt, later attributed this change to the school's changing orientation away from children referred by juvenile courts for breaking the law toward those whose problems were noticed by their parents and understood more psychologically (*Residential Treatment for the Disturbed Child*, 32).
101. Reid and Hagan, *Residential Treatment of Emotionally Disturbed Children*.
102. Donald Bloch and Marjorie L. Behrens, *A Study of Children Referred for Residential Treatment in New York State* (Albany: New York State Interdepartmental Health Resources Board, 1959).
103. Robert B. Westbrook, "Fighting for the American Family: Private Interests and Political Obligations in World War II," in *The Power of Culture: Critical Essays in American*

History, ed. Richard Wightman Fox and T. J. Jackson Lears (Chicago: University of Chicago Press, 1993).

104. Elaine Tyler May, *Homeward Bound: American Families in the Cold War Era* (New York: Basic Books, 1988).
105. Coontz, *The Way We Never Were*; Skolnick, *Embattled Paradise*.
106. David Swift, *The Parent Trap* (Walt Disney Productions, 1961); Richard Rodgers and Oscar Hammerstein, *The Sound of Music* (Williamson Music; distributed by Hal Leonard Publishing Corp, 1960); Robert Wise, *The Sound of Music* (Argyle Enterprises, Inc.; Twentieth Century Fox, 1965); Richard Rodgers and Oscar Hammerstein, *South Pacific: A Musical Play* (New York: Random House, 1949); Joshua Logan, *South Pacific* (Twentieth Century Fox, 1958).
107. Johnson and Reid, *Evaluation of Ten Years Work*, 14.
108. Ibid., 16.
109. Deborah Weinstein, *The Pathological Family: Postwar America and the Rise of Family Therapy* (Ithaca, NY: Cornell University Press, 2013).
110. Joseph Lander, "The Role of Residential Treatment for Children Symposium, 1954," pt. 3, "When Does an Agency Refer a Child to a Residential Treatment Center?," *American Journal of Orthopsychiatry* 25, no. 4 (1955): 675.
111. Barbara J. Betz, "A Psychiatric Children's Ward," *American Journal of Nursing* 45, no. 10 (October 1945): 820–21.
112. "The Story of Dorothy M.," *Bellefaire Bulletin* 2 no. 1 (Fall 1954): 2, Container 18, Folder 4, BA.
113. Ibid.
114. Ibid.
115. "Medicine: Psychiatry at Work," 1.
116. Ellis, "Portrait of Elaine," 9.
117. Reid and Hagan, *Residential Treatment of Emotionally Disturbed Children*, 217.
118. Allen, "Casework with the Parents at the Child Guidance Home," 19.
119. "Applications considered by local board, January 25, 1942 to April 26, 1942," in "Bellefaire Trustees' Meeting," April 26, 1942, Container 6, Folder 4, BA, 6.
120. Vera Kare, "A Study of the Adjustment of a 'Problem' Child in a Group Therapy Home for Pre-Delinquent Boys, Pioneer House, September, 1946–June, 1948." (MSW thesis, Wayne University, 1948), 28, 36.
121. Ibid., 28. Most social work graduates who wrote about RTCs in their theses specifically stated that they were not attempting to draw any conclusions, but merely wished to present raw case material. This makes them excellent primary sources for my purposes but also requires the reader to read between the lines. Typically, the student would provide a complete family history and then describe the child's symptoms, drawing an implicit link between the two.
122. Ibid., 84.
123. Marga Vicedo, *The Nature and Nurture of Love: From Imprinting to Attachment in Cold War America* (Chicago: University of Chicago Press, 2013), 24; Michal Shapira, *The War Inside: Psychoanalysis, Total War, and the Making of the Democratic Self in Postwar Britain* (New York: Cambridge University Press, 2013), chap. 2.
124. John Bowlby, *Maternal Care and Mental Health* (Geneva: World Health Organization, 1951); Vicedo, *The Nature and Nurture of Love*, 37.
125. Vicedo, *The Nature and Nurture of Love*, 26.
126. Eduardo Duniec and Mical Raz, "Vitamins for the Soul: John Bowlby's Thesis of

Maternal Deprivation, Biomedical Metaphors and the Deficiency Model of Disease," *History of Psychiatry* 22, no. 1 (2011): 93.

127. Lauretta Bender, "Group Activities on a Children's Ward as Methods of Psychotherapy," *American Journal of Psychiatry* 93, no. 5 (March 1, 1937): 1151.
128. Betz, "A Psychiatric Children's Ward," 821; Helen R. Hagan, "Residential Treatment," *Child Welfare* 31 (1952): 3.
129. Earl Saxe and Jeanetta Lyle, "Function of the Psychiatric Residential School," *Bulletin of the Menninger Clinic* 4, no. 6 (November 1940): 163.
130. Angela Baird, "Behavior and Anxiety in Disturbed Children: A Dissertation Based upon an Investigation at the Child Guidance Home of Cincinnati" (MSS thesis, Smith College School for Social Work, 1951), 36.
131. Ibid., 36–37.
132. Ibid., 38.
133. Burmeister, *Roofs for the Family*, 20.
134. "Can a Child Be Mentally Ill?," folder titled "Can a Child Be Mentally Ill?" (58–59), Box 3, KSHS.
135. Johnson, "Making Over Martha."
136. Ibid., 120.
137. Ibid.
138. Ibid., 122–23.
139. Ibid., 124.
140. Ibid., 125.
141. Ibid., 120, 122.
142. For example, a 1950 story told cautionary tales of mothers who pushed their children to succeed in school and at play so much that the children were not able to learn on their own and test their curiosity (Gladys G. Jenkins, "Watch Your Child's Mental Growth," *Parents' Magazine*, March 1950, 44–45, 128–30).
143. See, e.g., Molly Ladd-Taylor and Lauri Umansky, eds., *"Bad" Mothers: The Politics of Blame in Twentieth-Century America* (New York: New York University Press, 1998); and Rebecca Jo Plant, *Mom: The Transformation of Motherhood in Modern America* (Chicago: University of Chicago Press, 2010).
144. S. A. Szurek, "The Family and the Staff in Hospital Psychiatric Therapy of Children," *American Journal of Orthopsychiatry* 21, no. 3 (1951): 599. Szurek, director of the Langley Porter children's unit, argued that it was "a particularly pervasive and often insidiously disguised misconception . . . [that] to look for conflicts in the parents and to make an effort to help them resolve their conflicts is equated with 'blaming' them for their child's disorder."
145. "New Home Urged to Aid Upset Child," *New York Times*, November 17, 1954, 35.
146. Harris B. Peck, Ralph D. Rabinovitch, and Joseph B. Cramer, "A Treatment Program for Parents of Schizophrenic Children," *American Journal of Orthopsychiatry* 19, no. 4 (1949): 594.
147. Ibid.
148. Szurek, "The Family and the Staff in Hospital Psychiatric Therapy of Children," 601.
149. Allen, "Casework with the Parents at the Child Guidance Home," 19.
150. Krug, Hayward, and Crumpacker, "Intensive Residential Treatment of a Nine-Year-Old Girl," 425.
151. Ibid., 418.

CHAPTER 3

1. Southard School Journalism Class, *Don't Forget the Children: A History of Southard School, 1926–1986* (Topeka, KS: Menninger Foundation, 1986), 26.
2. Milton J. E. Senn, "Interview with Dr. William Goldfarb in New York City, March 17, 1977," n.d., Box 2, Folder 13, NLM, 2.
3. Morris F. Mayer, "The Role of Residential Treatment for Children Symposium, 1954," pt. 1, "Introduction," *American Journal of Orthopsychiatry* 25 (1955): 668.
4. Herschel Alt, *Residential Treatment for the Disturbed Child: Basic Principles in Planning and Design of Programs and Facilities* (New York: International Universities Press, 1960), ix.
5. Ibid.
6. Margo Horn, *Before It's Too Late: The Child Guidance Movement in the United States, 1922–1945* (Philadelphia: Temple University Press, 1989); Kathleen W. Jones, *Taming the Troublesome Child: American Families, Child Guidance, and the Limits of Psychiatric Authority* (Cambridge, MA: Harvard University Press, 1999).
7. Two Hawthorne administrators explained that "with this kind of program, the entire staff must be oriented in the direction of therapy—the people who live with the children and give physical care—the house parents, the cook, the maintenance staff, teachers, recreational workers" (Norman V. Lourie and Rena Schulman, "The Role of the Residential Staff in Residential Treatment," *American Journal of Orthopsychiatry* 24, no. 4 [1952]: 802). Twenty-five years later, one of the authors (Lourie) reflected that "everybody in contact with the children had to be therapeutic, whether it was the pediatrician, or the house parent, or the farmer with whom you might place a child that couldn't sit in the classroom" (Milton J. E. Senn, "Interview with Dr. Norman Lourie, April 14, 1977 in Harrisburg, Pennsylvania," n.d., Box 3, Folder 6, NLM, 10).
8. Robert E. Switzer, "Roles and Functions of Child Psychiatrists in Residential Treatment—What and How," 1962, Box 7.3, SWITZER: Child Psychiatrists in the Residential Treatment of Children, 1963, 36.
9. Ralph D. Rabinovitch, Janet Bee, and Barbara Outwater, "The Integration of Occupational and Recreational Therapy in the Residential Psychiatric Treatment of Children: A Symposium," *American Journal of Occupational Therapy* 5, no. 1 (1951): 2.
10. Erwin Angres, "Therapeutic Techniques Used with a Special Group of Disturbed Children," *Illinois Medical Journal* 89 (March 1946): 133.
11. American Psychiatric Association, *Psychiatric Inpatient Treatment of Children Report of the Conference on Inpatient Psychiatric Treatment for Children Held at Washington, D. C., October 17–21, 1956* (Washington, DC: American Psychiatric Association, 1957), 67.
12. Eva E. Burmeister, *Roofs for the Family* (New York: Columbia University Press, 1954), 62.
13. Hipolito Bravo, "Job Analysis of the Hawthorne Cedar Knolls School Employers" (master's thesis, New York School of Social Work, Columbia University, 1948), 25, 35.
14. Ibid., 29, 35.
15. Emma Pendleton Bradley Hospital, *Out of Their Misfortune: 25th Anniversary Report of the Emma Pendleton Bradley Home* (Riverside, RI: The Hospital, 1956), 13.
16. "Bellefaire Profiles," *Bellefaire Bulletin* 1, no. 1 (Fall 1952): 2, 4, Container 18, Folder 4, BA.
17. Ibid.

18. Ibid., 4.
19. Mignon, "THE STAFF," in Bellefaire Campus Council, "So you'll know all about . . . Bellefaire," mid-1950s, Container 19, Folder 7, BA, 15.
20. Joseph H. Reid and Helen R. Hagan, *Residential Treatment of Emotionally Disturbed Children: A Descriptive Study* (New York: Child Welfare League of America, 1952), 25–26.
21. At Brisbane, there were forty-two full-time and three part-time employees, which included twenty-six noncustodial positions (ibid., 3). Michigan had the equivalent of thirty-nine full-time noncustodial staff members for twenty-five children, (with 105 total staff members recorded five years later in 1957), and Southard School had sixty-six staff members, forty-seven of whom were noncustodial, for twenty children (Reid and Hagan, *Residential Treatment of Emotionally Disturbed Children*, 227–28, 283, "Children's Psychiatric Hospital," 1957, Box 2, General, 1956–60, RW).
22. Reid and Hagan, *Residential Treatment of Emotionally Disturbed Children*, 147, 26, 124.
23. American Psychiatric Association, *Psychiatric Inpatient Treatment of Children*, 55.
24. Joseph H. Reid, "Administrative Auspices of Residential Treatment," *Child Welfare*, March 1958, 8–9.
25. For a more thorough discussion of the child guidance team approach, see Jones, *Taming the Troublesome Child*, chap. 3.
26. Milton J. E. Senn, "Interview with Dr. Maurice Laufer, May 27, 1978 in Providence, R.I.," Box 3, Folder 2, NLM, 24–25.
27. "Training Program in Child Psychiatry, Child Psychiatry Service of the Menninger Clinic, November 1, 1956," Switzer: 118-8-4-3 Subject File A-C, American Board of Psychiatry and Neurology, Child Psychiatry Division, 1959–74, RS.
28. "Interview of Reynold A. Jensen, by S. S. Ackerly, October 20, 1972," UL; Milton J. E. Senn, "Interview with S. Spafford Ackerly, MD, December 4, 1976," Box 1, Folder 1, NLM, 13–15, 22–26.
29. Senn, "Interview with S. Spafford Ackerly," 2; "Interview of Reynold A. Jensen," 3.
30. "Interview of Reynold A. Jensen," 6.
31. Milton J. E. Senn, "Interview with Dr. Lauretta Bender, July 13, 1978 in Baltimore, Maryland," Box 1, Folder 9, NLM, 5–8, and "Interview with Dr. Frank J. Curran, January 12, 1978 in New York City," Box 2, Folder 3, NLM, 2–3; "Interview of Frank Curran, by S. S. Ackerly, May 29, 1973," UL, 2.
32. Milton J. E. Senn, "Interview with Dr. Salvador Minuchin, October 6, 1977 in Philadelphia, PA," n.d., Box 3, Folder 14, NLM, 2, and "Interview with Dr. Lauretta Bender," 51.
33. I have only found one individual, Georges Lussier of the Arthur Brisbane Child Treatment Center, who had experience running a school for the "feebleminded," which should not be conflated with a training school (Reid and Hagan, *Residential Treatment of Emotionally Disturbed Children*, 4).
34. Edward D. Greenwood, "The Psychiatrist's Role in Residence Treatment," in "Some Problems in Group Care Treatment: Round Table 1951," *American Journal of Orthopsychiatry* 22, no. 1 (January 1952): 111–12.
35. Other examples include Eva Burmeister of the Lakeside Children's Center in Milwaukee, Bernice Crumpacker of the Evanston Receiving Home of the Illinois Children's Home and Aid Society, and Lillian Johnson of the Ryther Child Center in Seattle.
36. The 1956 membership directory of the American Academy of Child Psychiatry contained eighty-six male and thirty-nine female members (American Academy of

Child Psychiatry, *American Academy of Child Psychiatry Membership Directory Constitution and By-Laws*, 1956). This proportion was significantly greater than their prevalence in general psychiatry. In 1958, women comprised less than 9 percent of the membership of the American Psychiatric Association (*Biographical Directory of the Fellows & Members of the American Psychiatric Association* [New York: R. R. Bowker Company, 1958]). The statistic on women physicians in the United States is from 1950 (Ellen Singer More, *Restoring the Balance: Women Physicians and the Profession of Medicine, 1850–1995* [Cambridge, MA: Harvard University Press, 1999], 186).

37. Reid and Hagan, *Residential Treatment of Emotionally Disturbed Children*, 99; "Interview of Reynold A. Jensen," 3. In a 1978 interview, Maurice Laufer explained that, when he arrived at Bradley in 1942, he "was still viewing [himself] as a pediatrician" (Milton J. E. Senn, "Interview with Dr. Maurice Laufer, May 27, 1978 in Providence, R.I.," Box 3, Folder 2, NLM, 3).
38. See Sydney A. Halpern, *American Pediatrics: The Social Dynamics of Professionalism, 1880–1980* (Berkeley: University of California Press, 1988).
39. Benjamin Spock, *The Common Sense Book of Baby and Child Care* (New York: Duell, Sloan and Pearce, 1946).
40. Jones, *Taming the Troublesome Child*, 113–19.
41. "Interview of Reynold A. Jensen by S. S. Ackerly," 10.
42. "The History of the American Academy of Child Psychiatry," *Journal of the American Academy of Child Psychiatry* 1, no. 1 (January 1962): 196–202.
43. American Psychiatric Association, *Psychiatric Inpatient Treatment of Children*, 59; Bravo, "Job Analysis of the Hawthorne Cedar Knolls School Employers," 42.
44. Ibid.
45. Reid and Hagan, *Residential Treatment of Emotionally Disturbed Children*, 4–5, 27, 99, 148, 204, 230, 260, 285. "Training Program in Child Psychiatry, Child Psychiatry Service of the Menninger Clinic," November 1, 1956, 118-8-4-3 Subject File A-C, American Board of Psychiatry and Neurology, Child Psychiatry Division, 1959–74, RES, 4. Their limited roles at RTCs did not reflect their expanded involvement in other areas, such as government affairs (see Ellen Herman, *The Romance of American Psychology: Political Culture in the Age of Experts* [Berkeley: University of California Press, 1995]).
46. Social workers occupying positions of authority at RTCs mirrored similar developments in more generalized social welfare agencies, where social workers were increasingly appointed as directors (Walter I. Trattner, *From Poor Law to Welfare State: A History of Social Welfare in America*, 6th ed. [New York: Free Press, 1999], 262–63). On social workers in psychopathic hospitals, see Elizabeth Lunbeck, *The Psychiatric Persuasion: Knowledge, Gender, and Power in Modern America* (Princeton, NJ: Princeton University Press, 1994).
47. Reid and Hagan, *Residential Treatment of Emotionally Disturbed Children*, 26, 147. Milton J. E. Senn, "Interview with Charles Leonard, Robert Evans at High Meadows, Hamden, Connecticut, January 27, 1977," Box 3, Folder 3, NLM. On social workers as traditionally female, see Regina G. Kunzel, *Fallen Women, Problem Girls: Unmarried Mothers and the Professionalization of Social Work, 1890–1945* (New Haven, CT: Yale University Press, 1993); Lunbeck, *The Psychiatric Persuasion*.
48. Bravo, "Job Analysis of the Hawthorne Cedar Knolls School Employers," 41; "Minutes of Case Committee," December 12, 1949, Container 10, Folder 7, BA, 2.
49. Mrs. Steinberg, "Report on Content of Case Worker's Job at Bellefaire," 1949, Container 10, Folder 7, BA, 2.

50. Andrew Abbott, "Boundaries of Social Work or Social Work of Boundaries? The Social Service Review Lecture," *Social Service Review* 69, no. 4 (1995): 545–62.
51. "The Social Worker in the Inpatient Section, Children's Division, Menninger Foundation," n.d., Box 16, Social Work Dept, 1947–56 Child Div., KSHS, 3; Dorothy Wright, "The Social Worker in the Inpatient Section, Children's Division, Menninger Foundation," December 1950, Box 6, Social Work, KSHS, 1–2.
52. Trattner, *From Poor Law to Welfare State,* chap. 12. There is some disagreement regarding the extent to which social work experienced an analytic turn in the 1920s. It appears that the uptake of analytic theory in psychiatric social work was an uneven process that was focused among professional elites and those practicing in the Northeast; one researcher found that social workers at the Illinois Children's Home and Aid Society only began adopting analytic ideologies in the 1940s (Leslie B. Alexander, "Social Work's Freudian Deluge: Myth or Reality?," *Social Service Review* 46, no. 4 [December 1, 1972]: 517–38; Martha Heineman Field, "Social Casework Practice during the 'Psychiatric Deluge,'" *Social Service Review* 54, no. 4 [December 1, 1980]: 482–507).
53. See Kunzel, *Fallen Women, Problem Girls,* chap. 2; Karen Whitney Tice, *Tales of Wayward Girls and Immoral Women: Case Records and the Professionalization of Social Work* (Urbana: University of Illinois Press, 1998).
54. Roy Lubove, *The Professional Altruist: the Emergence of Social Work as a Career, 1880–1930* (Cambridge, MA: Harvard University Press, 1968), 110–17.
55. For a detailed discussion of this issue, see "Psychotherapy and Casework: Symposium of the Boston Psychoanalytic Society and Institute, Inc., February 19 and 20, 1949," special issue of *Journal of Social Casework* 30, no. 6 (June 1949).
56. Andrew Delano Abbott, *The System of Professions: An Essay on the Division of Expert Labor* (Chicago: University of Chicago Press, 1988).
57. For example, Hawthorne's executive director Herschel Alt had an extensive child guidance background, one of Hawthorne's clinical directors, Hyman Grossbard, worked at the Jewish Board of Guardians on an outpatient basis before coming to Hawthorne, and Southard's chief psychiatric social worker Arthur Mandelbaum was first a caseworker at the Denver Mental Hygiene Clinic (Milton J. E. Senn, "Interview with Dr. Herschel Alt, December 12, 1978 in New York City," Box 1, Folders 3–4, NLM, and "Interview with Dr. Hyman Grossbard, June 22, 1977, in New York City," Box 2, Folder 15, NLM, 7; "Training Program in Child Psychiatry, Child Psychiatry Service of the Menninger Clinic," 3).
58. Senn, "Interview with Dr. Norman Lourie," 2–8.
59. High Meadows superintendent Charles Leonard had previously run the Illinois State Training School for Boys in the 1940s, where he had implemented a full child guidance clinic within the institution (Senn, "Interview with Charles Leonard, Robert Evans," 1–2). Southard's Mary Ella Wheeler, a psychiatric social worker with a PhD, had been a public welfare and research analyst for the Children's Bureau before working at two different child guidance clinics, and her colleagues Jennie Wykert and Hazle Corrigan had been on the staffs of a Veterans Affairs hospital and an army hospital, respectively ("Training Program in Child Psychiatry, Child Psychiatry Service of the Menninger Clinic," 3–4). Morris Mayer, a caseworker at Bellefaire who would ultimately become its director, had previously worked at the New York Hebrew Orphan Asylum (a general institution for dependent children) and at Hawthorne Cedar Knolls ("Meeting of Bellefaire Board of Trustees," January 14, 1945, Container 6, Folder 7, BA, 5).

60. "Plenary Session, Saturday Morning, October 20, 1956," in *Proceedings of the Conference on In-Patient Psychiatric Treatment for Children*, held under the auspices of the American Psychiatric Association, October 17–21, 1956, Woodner Hotel, Washington, DC, Box 118-8-2-8, EG, 592.
61. Of thirty social work theses I consulted for this project, there were thirty-two authors (two theses were coauthored), nine of whom were men. Nine theses, two of which were cowritten by two authors, came from students at the New York School of Social Work (later Columbia University), with five of eleven male authors. Twelve came from the Smith College School for Social Work, with two of twelve male authors. Many of the Smith theses were based on fieldwork at the Cincinnati Child Guidance Home, where Krug and the Home's head caseworker were part-time faculty members (Reid and Hagan, *Residential Treatment of Emotionally Disturbed Children*, 70).
62. For example, Helen Brookens spent the spring and summer of 1941 at the Ryther Children's Center while she was a student at the University of Washington School of Social Work, but she ultimately went on to work in the Seattle Public School system (Helen Renner Brookens, "A Study of Five Children Treated under Ryther Child Center's Program for the Care of Children with Personality Problems" [MA thesis, University of Washington, 1944], 2; "Education Calendar," *Washington Education* 74 [1962]: 44). Jean Collard, also a University of Washington social work student, did her field work at Ryther between 1940 and 1941, going on to work at the Neurological Institute of the Columbia-Presbyterian Medical Center in New York (Jean Collard, "A Statistical Description of the 186 Children Admitted to the Institutional Unit of the Ryther Child Center from October 1935 to October 1939" [MA thesis, University of Washington, 1946], 8; Ben Avis Orcutt et al., eds., *Social Work and Thanatology* [New York: Ayer Publishing, 1980]). Evelyn Brownstone, a social work student at UCLA, spent three days per week over the 1951–52 school year working at the Camarillo State Hospital before beginning a career at the Los Angeles Bureau of Social Work and in an outpatient clinic (Evelyn Brownstone, interview with the author, March 20, 2011). New York School of Social Work student Isaac Youcha worked at Hawthorne Cedar Knolls during his field placement and is now affiliated with the Postgraduate Center for Mental Health in New York City and in private practice (Isaac Zeke Youcha, "A Study of Schizophrenic Children in Cottage Life at the Hawthorne Cedar Knolls School" [master's thesis, New York School of Social Work, Columbia University, 1953], 1; Jeffrey L. Kleinberg et al., "Responses to 'Tools of the Trade' by Sabert Basescu," *Group* 14, no. 3 [September 1990]: 166–75).
63. Reid and Hagan, *Residential Treatment of Emotionally Disturbed Children*, 250; "Psychiatric Unit, Children's Hospital, the University of Michigan," n.d., Box 2: General, 1956–60, RW.
64. "Future Plans for Southard School," Box 9, Reorganization Plans, KSHS, 2.
65. All of the twenty-one RTCs Lydia Hylton examined in her 1959–60 study employed in-service training, "a continuous learning experience that permeates the day-to-day work of the staff . . . given through informal staff contacts, through supervision, in case staffings or staff meetings, and in educational seminars" (Lydia Hylton, *The Residential Treatment Center: Children, Programs, and Costs* [New York: Child Welfare League of America, 1964], 25).
66. Charles Bradley, "Education in a Children's Psychiatric Hospital," *Nervous Child* 3 (1944): 330.

67. Herschel Alt, "Responsibilities and Qualifications of the Child Care Worker," pt. 2 of "Symposium, 1953: The Education of Emotionally Disturbed Children," *American Journal of Orthopsychiatry* 23, no. 4 (1953): 672.
68. American Psychiatric Association, *Psychiatric Inpatient Treatment of Children*, 60; Alt, "Responsibilities and Qualifications of the Child Care Worker," 672; Lourie and Schulman, "The Role of the Residential Staff in Residential Treatment," 804.
69. Alt, *Residential Treatment for the Disturbed Child*, 84; Herschel Alt and Hyman Grossbard, "Professional Issues in the Institutional Treatment of Delinquent Children," *American Journal of Orthopsychiatry* 19, no. 2 (1949): 287; Bernice Crumpacker, "The Caseworker as Residential Worker: A Dissertation Based upon a Study at the Child Guidance Home, Cincinnati, Ohio" (MSS thesis, Smith College School for Social Work, 1950), 33.
70. "Plenary Session, Saturday Morning, October 20, 1956," 586.
71. Ibid.
72. Alt and Grossbard, "Professional Issues in the Institutional Treatment of Delinquent Children," 293–94.
73. J. Franklin Robinson, "The Use of Residence in Psychiatric Treatment with Children," *American Journal of Psychiatry* 103, no. 6 (1947): 815.
74. Othilda Krug, "The Application of Principles of Child Psychotherapy in Residential Treatment," *American Journal of Psychiatry* 108, no. 9 (March 1, 1952): 696–97.
75. Reid and Hagan, *Residential Treatment of Emotionally Disturbed Children*, 254; "Bellefaire Trustees' Meeting," April 26, 1942, Container 6, Folder 4, BA, 24.
76. Hylton, *The Residential Treatment Center*, 160.
77. Reid and Hagan, *Residential Treatment of Emotionally Disturbed Children*, 205; Bravo, "Job Analysis of the Hawthorne Cedar Knolls School Employers," 44; J. Franklin Robinson, "The Role of the Resident Professional Worker," *American Journal of Orthopsychiatry* 19, no. 4 (1949): 680; "Handbook for Parents (Early 1950s?)," Box 3, folder titled "Handbook for Parents, 1950's," KSHS, 13. Sometimes, social workers served as residential workers or took on somewhat more prestigious supervisory roles, but this was less common. For example, two of the three residential workers at the Cincinnati Child Guidance Home were social workers (Reid and Hagan, *Residential Treatment of Emotionally Disturbed Children*, 55). At Bellefaire and Southard School, a new group worker and group work supervisor were hired in 1943 and 1956, respectively, both with social work training and experience with children's welfare agencies (Fred Lazarus Jr., "Annual Message to Bellefaire Board of Trustees," 6; "Training Program in Child Psychiatry, Child Psychiatry Service of the Menninger Clinic," 4).
78. Morris F. Mayer, "Some Problems Relative to the Cottage Parent," in "Some Problems in Group Care Treatment: Round Table 1951," *American Journal of Orthopsychiatry* 22, no. 1 (January 1952): 107.
79. Southard School Journalism Class, *Don't Forget the Children*, 23.
80. Ibid.; obituary, Lillabelle Stahl, *Topeka Capital-Journal*, January 3, 2007, http://www.legacy.com/obituaries/cjonline/obituary.aspx?n=lillabelle-stahl&pid=20516934.
81. *Armstrong Circle Theatre*, season 11, episode 3, "The Hidden World," directed by William Corrigan, written by Alvin Boretz, aired November 23, 1960 on CBS.
82. For example, the Children's Service Center of Wyoming Valley required childcare workers to participate in seminars on psychotherapy, casework, and psychology for residential workers, and workers at Hawthorne Cedar Knolls took part in case conferences and individual consultations in addition to formal seminars (Reid and

Hagan, *Residential Treatment of Emotionally Disturbed Children*, 91; Alt, *Residential Treatment for the Disturbed Child*, 93).

83. *Armstrong Circle Theatre*, season 11, episode 3, "The Hidden World."
84. At Southard School, clinical staff met with individual residential workers to discuss individual children, during which "an attempt [was] made to understand the meaning of symptoms and their dynamics" (Arthur Mandelbaum, "Description of the Southard School: Conference on Inpatient Psychiatric Treatment for Children," Box 16, Children's Div. 1956, KSHS, 24). Herschel Alt of Hawthorne Cedar Knolls argued that in-service training opportunities like these were "important not only because they yield additional understanding and great capacity to cooperate with other staff groups, but because they also add to the self-regard of the cottage parent" (Alt, *Residential Treatment for the Disturbed Child*, 93).
85. Youcha, "A Study of Schizophrenic Children in Cottage Life," 5; Alt, *Residential Treatment for the Disturbed Child*, 89, 94.
86. Youcha, "A Study of Schizophrenic Children in Cottage Life," 5.
87. Alt, *Residential Treatment for the Disturbed Child*, 94–95. These wish lists were common across RTCs. Southard School looked for "emotional maturity, a high degree of intellectual curiosity, the wish for creative growth, and the desire to grow in discipline and self-awareness," as well as "individuals who can be spontaneous, warm, and natural people who are not frightened of angry feelings and aggressive behavior" (Child Psychiatry Service of the Menninger Clinic, the Menninger Foundation, *Child Care Handbook*, May 1957, Box 6, *Child Care Handbook*, May 1957, KSHS, 1, 3). The participants of the 1956 American Psychiatric Association conference made an even more elaborate list, including a "warm 'mothering' personality, a basic liking for children, emotional maturity, capacity to work with colleagues and supervisors, a sense of humor, and potential capacity for learning . . . patience and tolerance in handling the children's illogical behavior; ability to function efficiently and comfortably as adult authorities; a warm acceptance of the child's needs; capacity to share functions with other workers and at the same time accept personal responsibilities; ability to avoid emotional involvement in relationships with parents; skill in recording and reporting observations of individual and group behavior; physical as well as emotional health; vitality and energy for work under pressure, and resiliency in recuperating from emotional and physical fatigue" (American Psychiatric Association, *Psychiatric Inpatient Treatment of Children*, 62).
88. Mayer, "Some Problems Relative to the Cottage Parent," 107.
89. Alt, *Residential Treatment for the Disturbed Child*, 95; "Summary Report on Topic IV—Personnel," in *Proceedings of the Conference on In-Patient Psychiatric Treatment for Children*, held under the auspices of the American Psychiatric Association, 126.
90. Helen D. Sargent, "Progress Report on Study of Southard School," November 26, 1951, Box 1, Summaries 1949–52, KSHS, 3.
91. "Salary Information," in "Employees' Roll Book," Box 7.3, KSHS. For historical data on federal minimum wage legislation, see "History of Federal Minimum Wage Rates under the Fair Labor Standards Act, 1938—2009," accessed July 24, 2018, http://www.dol.gov/whd/minwage/chart.htm. Kansas did not enact a state minimum wage law until 1978 (Aline O. Quester, "State Minimum Wage Laws, 1950–1980," in U.S. Minimum Wage Study Commission, *Report of the Minimum Wage Study Commission* [Washington, DC: The Commission, 1981], 2:51).
92. "Conference on In-Patient Psychiatric Treatment for Children, Background Material for Preparatory Committees on Personnel and Treatment," April 24, 1956, Box 1,

Folder 5, LB, 11–12. For historical data on average wages nationally, see "National Average Wage Index," accessed July 24, 2018, http://www.ssa.gov/oact/COLA/AWI .html.

93. Mayer, "Some Problems Relative to the Cottage Parent," 106.
94. American Psychiatric Association, *Psychiatric Inpatient Treatment of Children*, 70.
95. Ibid., 107.
96. "Employees' Roll Book."
97. "Minutes," February 23, 1950, Container 11, Folder 8, BA, 1.
98. "History of Federal Minimum Wage Rates."
99. Morris Kaplan, "School May Close Because of Strike," *New York Times*, February 23, 1962, 20.
100. "Hawthorne School Open Despite Strike," *New York Times*, February 18, 1962, 80; Morris Kaplan, "School May Close Because of Strike," and "44 Child Patients to Be Transferred by Struck School," *New York Times*, February 25, 1962, 68; "Guardian School Settles Walkout," *New York Times*, February 27, 1962, 35.
101. Richard P. Hunt, "Concern Expressed for Children Caught in Social Aides' Strike," *New York Times*, March 5, 1964, 30; Martin Tolchin, "Both Sides Decry Welfare Strike," *New York Times*, March 3, 1964, 37.
102. John B. Geisel, "Looking Back over the Year at Southard School," *Bulletin of the Menninger Clinic* 10, no. 2 (March 1946): 58. Geisel also commented that "this devotion . . . is all the more remarkable when we stop to think that they have been without sufficient guidance and leadership in their work" ("Looking Back over the Year," 4). Geisel's impression was echoed a decade later by visiting psychiatrist and member of the Child Research Council at the University of Colorado School of Medicine John Benjamin, who remarked in a letter to Karl Menninger that "since few of [the childcare workers] had had any previous training, and since in-service training in this profession is a very difficult job, I felt that the quality of these workers spoke very highly for the care, skill and insight with which they had been selected, as well as for their training on the job" (John D. Benjamin to Karl A. Menninger, November 8, 1957, Box 3, Publicity Materials, KSHS, 1).
103. "Summary Report on Topic IV—Personnel," 127–30; Child Welfare League of America and the Council of Jewish Federations and Welfare Funds, "Bellefaire Survey, 1952–1953," Container 19, Folder 4, BA, 39; Gisela Konopka, "The Role of Residential Treatment for Children Symposium, 1954," pt. 4, "The Role of the Group in Residential Treatment," *American Journal of Orthopsychiatry* 25, no. 4 (1955): 680.
104. The historiography on professionalization, and more specifically on professionalization in medicine and related fields, is vast. On how practice shapes professional identity in medicine and social work, see John Harley Warner, *The Therapeutic Perspective: Medical Practice, Knowledge, and Identity in America, 1820–1885* (Cambridge, MA: Harvard University Press, 1986); Kunzel, *Fallen Women, Problem Girls*; Tice, *Tales of Wayward Girls and Immoral Women*. On the development of specialized knowledge and training, see Paul Starr, *The Social Transformation of American Medicine* (New York: Basic Books, 1982); Rosemary Stevens, *American Medicine and the Public Interest* (New Haven, CT: Yale University Press, 1971); George Weisz, *Divide and Conquer: A Comparative History of Medical Specialization* (Oxford: Oxford University Press, 2006). On the power of language in demarcating professional authority, see JoAnne Brown, *The Definition of a Profession: The Authority of Metaphor in the History of Intelligence Testing, 1890–1930* (Princeton, NJ: Princeton University Press, 1992).
105. Collard, "A Statistical Description of the 186 Children Admitted," 37.

106. Robinson, "The Role of the Resident Professional Worker," 680.
107. "Plenary Session, Saturday Morning, October 20, 1956," 573; Alt and Grossbard, "Professional Issues in the Institutional Treatment of Delinquent Children," 288.
108. "Plenary Session, Saturday Morning, October 20, 1956," 587.
109. Alt and Grossbard, "Professional Issues in the Institutional Treatment of Delinquent Children," 288; Alt, "Responsibilities and Qualifications of the Child Care Worker," pt. 2 of "Symposium 1953: The Education of Emotionally Disturbed Children," *American Journal of Orthopsychiatry* 23, no. 4 (1953): 674.
110. Alt, "Responsibilities and Qualifications of the Child Care Worker," 673–74. Staff members from the University of Pittsburgh's Children's Residential Treatment Service reported that "there has been a decisive trend toward sharing pertinent information with the child care worker and including him as full partner in the treatment team" (Henry Maier et al., "The Role of Residential Treatment for Children Symposium, 1954," pt. 7, "Supervision of Child Care Workers in a Residential Treatment Service," *American Journal of Orthopsychiatry* 25, no. 4 [October 1955]: 701).
111. Ibid., 702–3.
112. Ibid.
113. Ibid.
114. Morris Fritz Mayer, "Annual Report of Head Resident," in "Bellefaire Board of Trustees Minutes of Meeting Held July 8, 1945," Container 6, Folder 7, BA, 6.
115. Ibid., 7. Similarly, caseworkers at Hawthorne Cedar Knolls had initially seen cottage parents as "mere custodians and caretakers of children," but by the mid 1940s they were actively trying to "increase the prestige and the authority of the cottage parents" and include them in the decision-making process (Bruno Herbert, "Factors Influencing the Later Adjustment of Girls Discharged from the Hawthorne-Cedar Knolls School: A Dissertation Based upon an Investigation at the Jewish Board of Guardians, New York City" [MSS thesis, Smith College School for Social Work, 1946], 14).
116. "Summary Report on Topic IV—Personnel," 134; Howard Bath, "Henry W. Maier (1919–2005): Influences on His Life and Thinking; an Interview by Howard Bath," *Cyc-Online*, no. 138 (August 2010), http://www.cyc-net.org/cyc-online/cyconline-aug2010-maier.html.
117. "Training Course for Houseparents of Children's Institutions, 1953–1955, April 4–May 6, 1955," Box 15, Folder 1, UC.
118. Lourie and Schulman, "The Role of the Residential Staff in Residential Treatment," 804.
119. Susan Reverby, *Ordered to Care: The Dilemma of American Nursing, 1850–1945* (New York: Cambridge University Press, 1987); Charles E. Rosenberg, *The Care of Strangers: The Rise of America's Hospital System* (New York: Basic Books, 1987), chap. 9.
120. Ursula Weiss Moore, a social work student, commented that at Langley Porter "the nurses act as 'good mothers' and maintain a continuity of relationship with the children. . . . The nurses are encouraged to treat the children as 'normal' using spontaneous techniques of customary child raising" ("A Study of Children with Primary Behavior Disorders Treated at Langley Porter Clinic: Results of In-Patient and Out-Patient Care" [MSW thesis, University of California, Berkeley, 1949], 35–36). At the Illinois Neuropsychiatric Institute, two nurses described their role as "a parent-substitute, an adult to whom the child clings in his dependency and emotional deprivation . . . some of the children have picked one or the other of the nurses for

their parent and openly call her 'Mother'" (Ruth J. L. Gilbertson and Helen Sutton, "A Children's Psychiatric Service," *American Journal of Nursing* 43, no. 6 [1943]: 571).

121. Joan Beck, "Can 'Bad Kids' Be Saved?," *Chicago Daily Tribune*, February 27, 1955, K19.
122. Anne Benjamin and Howard E. Weatherly, "Hospital Ward Treatment of Emotionally Disturbed Children," *American Journal of Orthopsychiatry* 17, no. 4 (October 1947): 667.
123. Ibid., 670.
124. Helen A. Sutton, "Some Nursing Aspects of a Children's Psychiatric Ward," *American Journal of Orthopsychiatry* 17, no. 4 (1947): 675.
125. Ibid., 681.
126. Ibid., 681–82.
127. Also see Gilbertson and Sutton, "A Children's Psychiatric Service."
128. Reverby, *Ordered to Care*.
129. Nathan W. Ackerman, "A Plan for Maladjusted Children," *Bulletin of the Menninger Clinic* 1, no. 3 (January 1937): 68; Mary Faust, "The Parents' Role in a Child's Residential Treatment: A Dissertation Based upon an Investigation at the Institute for Juvenile Research, Chicago, Illinois" (MSS thesis, Smith College School for Social Work, 1949), 12; Samuel Finestone and Toby Bennett Bieber, "Status at Discharge and Follow-up of Twenty Children with Diagnosis of Primary Behavior Disorder Hospitalized at New York State Psychiatric Institute and Hospital" (master's thesis, New York School of Social Work, Columbia University, 1946), 1; Fritz Redl and David Wineman, *Children Who Hate: The Disorganization and Breakdown of Behavior Controls* (Glencoe, IL.: Free Press, 1951), 42; Joseph Harold Reid, "The Evolution of a Treatment Center for Problem Children: A History of the Ryther Child Center" (MSW thesis, University of Washington, 1950), 21.
130. Senn, "Interview with Dr. Norman Lourie," 9; Morris F. Mayer, "Casework within an Institution," *Children* 1, no. 2 (1954): 65.
131. "Interview of Edward David Greenwood, by Spafford Ackerly, October 20, 1972," n.d., William E. Gardner Collection, History Collections, Kornhauser Health Sciences Library, University of Louisville.
132. On interdisciplinarity in modern child mental health, see Margaret Bourdeaux Arbuckle and Charlotte Anne Herrick, *Child & Adolescent Mental Health: Interdisciplinary Systems of Care* (Sudbury, MA: Jones and Bartlett, 2005).
133. Morris Fritz Mayer, "Report of the Head Resident," in "Minutes, Board of Trustees," July 18, 1948, Container 7, Folder 1, BA, 2; "Minutes," September 30, 1956, Container 7, Folder 2, BA, 5.
134. *Child Care Handbook*, May 1957, 5.
135. "Bellefaire Annual Report," 1952–53, Container 7, Folder 2, BA, 2.
136. "Unit Social Worker Project Bringing Results," *Bellefaire Bulletin* 3, no. 2 (Spring 1955): 2, Container 18, Folder 4, BA.
137. Senn, "Interview with Charles Leonard, Robert Evans at High Meadows, Hamden, Connecticut, January 27, 1977," 9, 15, 17.
138. Bradley, "Education in a Children's Psychiatric Hospital," 330.
139. Abraham J. Simon, "Residential Treatment of Children: I. Unanswered Questions," *Social Service Review* 30, no. 3 (1956): 261, 264.
140. "Handbook for Parents (Early 1950s?)," 7.
141. Raymond W. Waggoner and Ralph D. Rabinovitch, "The University of Michigan

Plan for the Residential Treatment of Disturbed Children," *Medical Bulletin* 22, no. 3 (1956): 125.

142. Robert E. Switzer, "The Evolution of a New Program and a New House" (paper presented at the annual meeting of the American Association for Children's Residential Centers, November 5, 1961), Box 118-8-4-56 S-Z Switzer, The Evolution of a New Program and a New House," RES, 14–15.
143. Alt and Grossbard, "Professional Issues in the Institutional Treatment of Delinquent Children," 285.
144. Senn, "Interview with Charles Leonard, Robert Evans," 6.
145. Reid and Hagan, *Residential Treatment of Emotionally Disturbed Children*, 110–11.
146. Senn, "Interview with Dr. Norman Lourie," 10.
147. Helen R. Hagan, "Residential Treatment," *Child Welfare* 31 (1952): 6.
148. Change of Shift Log, July 1958–July 1961, Box 7.3, KSHS.
149. Mandelbaum, "Description of the Southard School," 11.
150. Reid and Hagan, *Residential Treatment of Emotionally Disturbed Children*, 298; Mandelbaum, "Description of the Southard School," 49.
151. American Psychiatric Association, *Psychiatric Inpatient Treatment of Children*, 75–76.
152. Lurie, "Some Problems in Group Care Treatment: Round Table 1951," 112.
153. Benjamin to Menninger, November 8, 1957, 2.
154. E. D. Greenwood, "The Role of Residential Treatment for Children Symposium, 1954," pt. 6, "The Role of Psychotherapy in Residential Treatment," *American Journal of Orthopsychiatry* 25, no. 4 (October 1955): 692–98; Mayer, "The Role of Residential Treatment for Children Symposium, 1954," pt. 1, "Introduction,"694–95.
155. Mayer, "The Role of Residential Treatment for Children Symposium, 1954," pt. 1, "Introduction," 695.
156. Florence Clothier, "Institutional Needs in the Field of Child Welfare," *Nervous Child* 7 (1948): 169.
157. Konopka, "The Role of Residential Treatment for Children Symposium, 1954," pt. 4, "The Role of the Group in Residential Treatment," 680.
158. Krug, "The Application of Principles of Child Psychotherapy in Residential Treatment," 698.
159. Ibid.
160. Konopka, "The Role of Residential Treatment for Children Symposium, 1954," pt. 4, "The Role of the Group in Residential Treatment," 684.
161. "Conference on In-Patient Psychiatric Treatment for Children," 14; Mayer, "Report of the Head Resident," 4.

INTERLUDE: THERAPEUTICS IN RESIDENTIAL TREATMENT

1. Herschel Alt, *Residential Treatment for the Disturbed Child: Basic Principles in Planning and Design of Programs and Facilities* (New York: International Universities Press, 1960), 307–12.
2. Ibid., 307.
3. Ibid.
4. American Psychiatric Association, *Psychiatric Inpatient Treatment of Children Report of the Conference on Inpatient Psychiatric Treatment for Children Held at Washington, D. C., October 17–21, 1956* (Washington, DC: American Psychiatric Association, 1957), 2.
5. Allegra Larson, "Mother's Image of Her Relationship with Maternal Grandmother as a Factor in Her Own Mothering" (MSS thesis, Smith College School for Social Work,

1963), 13. As Jerome M. Goldsmith of Hawthorne reflected in 1953, "The total life of the child, including his group living experiences, relationships with adults and children, his school classes, work assignments and recreational activities become part of the . . . tools of the therapist . . . the experiential aspects of the childs [*sic*] life are . . . intermeshed with the process of individual therapy" (Jerome M. Goldsmith et al., "Integrating Clinical Processes with Planned Living Experience," unpublished report, February 17, 1953, in Isaac Zeke Youcha, "A Study of Schizophrenic Children in Cottage Life at the Hawthorne Cedar Knolls School" [master's thesis, New York School of Social Work, Columbia University, 1953], 8).

6. Although most RTCs used this model, treatment at the Children's Service Center of Wyoming Valley was centered solely on the child's individual psychotherapy. Residential treatment there allowed the staff more regular access to the child in the occasion that consistent outpatient therapy was impossible (J. Franklin Robinson, "The Use of Residence in Psychiatric Treatment with Children," *American Journal of Psychiatry* 103, no. 6 [1947]: 814, 817).
7. Othilda Krug, "The Application of Principles of Child Psychotherapy in Residential Treatment," *American Journal of Psychiatry* 108, no. 9 (March 1, 1952): 695.
8. Bernice Crumpacker, "The Caseworker as Residential Worker: A Dissertation Based upon a Study at the Child Guidance Home, Cincinnati, Ohio" (MSS thesis, Smith College School for Social Work, 1950), 14.
9. Joseph H. Reid and Helen R. Hagan, *Residential Treatment of Emotionally Disturbed Children: A Descriptive Study* (New York: Child Welfare League of America, 1952), 58.
10. S. A. Szurek, "The Family and the Staff in Hospital Psychiatric Therapy of Children," *American Journal of Orthopsychiatry* 21, no. 3 (1951): 602–3.
11. Wrenshall A. Oliver, "A State Hospital Children's Unit," *American Journal of Psychiatry* 106, no. 4 (October 1, 1949): 267.
12. Arthur Mandelbaum, "Description of the Southard School: Conference on Inpatient Psychiatric Treatment for Children," Box 16, Children's Div. 1956, KSHS, 36.
13. "The Big 'R' at Bellefaire School," *Bellefaire Voice and Views* (Spring 1958), Container 18, Folder 4, BA, 1.
14. Lillian Johnson, *Monograph on Organization and Operation*, Monograph/Ryther Child Center, no. 2 (Seattle: The Center, 1948), 9; Eva E. Burmeister, *Roofs for the Family* (New York: Columbia University Press, 1954), 142.
15. For example, two disconnected sources used almost identical terminology to describe the process. Othilda Krug of the Cincinnati Child Guidance Home explained in 1952 that "within the security of the therapeutic relationship the child's emotional development is recapitulated in a new, corrective manner for meeting his needs for both dependency and growth" ("The Application of Principles of Child Psychotherapy in Residential Treatment," 696). Almost identically, the 1953 Southard annual report stated that, "within the security of a meaningful living experience, the child's emotional development can, through therapy, be recapitulated in a new and corrective manner which will allow for healthy growth and development" ("Annual Report, Department of Child Psychiatry of the Menninger Foundation, July 1, 1951 to July 1, 1953," Box 1, Annual Reports—1952–56, KSHS, 1–2). Most likely, the author of the Menninger annual report was citing Krug's paper from the year before. It is notable that he or she found the recapitulation metaphor representative enough to repeat it almost word for word, suggesting that many RTCs shared this psychoanalytic concept of leading disturbed people through each stage of development to rectify any past traumas. For an excellent discussion of the use of recollec-

tion as catharsis, see Anne Harrington, "The Body That Speaks," chap. 2 of *The Cure Within: A History of Mind-Body Medicine* (New York: W. W. Norton, 2008).

16. Fred C. Kelly, "Solving the Problem Child," *Reader's Digest*, November 1939, 113.
17. On the history of somatic therapies, see Joel T. Braslow, *Mental Ills and Bodily Cures: Psychiatric Treatment in the First Half of the Twentieth Century* (Berkeley: University of California Press, 1997); Deborah Blythe Doroshow, "Performing a Cure for Schizophrenia: Insulin Coma Therapy on the Wards," *Journal of the History of Medicine and Allied Sciences* 62, no. 2 (April 2007): 213–43; Jack David Pressman, *Last Resort: Psychosurgery and the Limits of Medicine* (Cambridge: Cambridge University Press, 1998); Mical Raz, "Between the Ego and the Icepick: Psychosurgery, Psychoanalysis, and Psychiatric Discourse," *Bulletin of the History of Medicine* 82, no. 2 (2008): 387–420; Jonathan Sadowsky, "Beyond the Metaphor of the Pendulum: Electroconvulsive Therapy, Psychoanalysis, and the Styles of American Psychiatry," *Journal of the History of Medicine and Allied Sciences* 61, no. 1 (January 2006): 1–25.
18. On the history of psychopharmacology, see David Healy, *The Creation of Psychopharmacology* (Cambridge, MA: Harvard University Press, 2002); David L. Herzberg, *Happy Pills in America: From Miltown to Prozac* (Baltimore, MD: Johns Hopkins University Press, 2009); Susan L. Speaker, "From 'Happiness Pills' to 'National Nightmare': Changing Cultural Assessment of Minor Tranquilizers in America, 1955–1980," *Journal of the History of Medicine and Allied Sciences* 52, no. 3 (July 1997): 338–76; Andrea Tone, *The Age of Anxiety: A History of America's Turbulent Affair with Tranquilizers* (New York: Basic Books, 2009).
19. Elizabeth Bromley, "Stimulating a Normal Adjustment: Misbehavior, Amphetamines, and the Electroencephalogram at the Bradley Home for Children," *Journal of the History of the Behavioral Sciences* 42, no. 4 (Fall 2006): 379–98; Madeleine P. Strohl, "Bradley's Benzedrine Studies on Children with Behavioral Disorders," *Yale Journal of Biology and Medicine* 84, no. 1 (March 2011): 27–33.
20. Lauretta Bender, "100 Cases of Childhood Schizophrenia Treated with Electric Shock," *Transactions of the American Neurological Association* 72 (1947): 165–69, and "D-Lysergic Acid in the Treatment of the Biological Features of Childhood Schizophrenia," *Diseases of the Nervous System* 7 suppl., no. 7 (July 1966): 43–46.
21. Howard W. Potter, "The Treatment of Problem Children in a Psychiatric Hospital," *American Journal of Psychiatry* 91, no. 4 (January 1, 1935): 878; Raymond W. Waggoner to Claude Uhler, August 20, 1948, Box 4, Children's Centers, 1946–4?, RW; *First Annual Report of the Arthur Brisbane Child Treatment Center at Allaire for the Year Ending June 30, 1948* (Allaire, NJ: The Center, 1948), 1.
22. "Topic III: Morning Session, Discussion Group B," in *Proceedings of the Conference on In-Patient Psychiatric Treatment for Children*, held under the auspices of the American Psychiatric Association, October 17–21, 1956, Woodner Hotel, Washington, DC, Box 118-8-2-8, EG, 491.
23. Ibid., 492.
24. Archie A. Silver, "Report on Somatic Therapies," June 25, 1956, Conference on Psychiatric Inpatient Treatment for Children, Preparatory Document for the Committees on Personnel and Treatment, Box 1, File 5, LB, 1. Each RTC tended to use a given somatic therapy for one indication. Bradley Hospital, which had pioneered the use of amphetamines in children in the 1930s, employed them only for hyperactive children, while Bellevue used them for hypersexual ones (Silver, "Report on Somatic Therapies," 2). On the early history of amphetamine use at Bradley Hospital, see Strohl, "Bradley's Benzedrine Studies on Children with Behavioral Disor-

ders." Chlorpromazine, the most transformative psychopharmaceutical for hospitalized patients in the 1950s, was used by seven RTCs specifically for schizophrenic children, and then only rarely (Silver, "Report on Somatic Therapies," 1–2).

25. As Southard School director Cotter Hirschberg explained to his Board of Trustees, "our goal is always the eventual return of a stronger, healthier child to his own community, his own home, and his parents" (Cotter Hirschberg, "Presentation for Annual Meeting, October 1952," Box 16, Annual Meeting—1952, KSHS, 2).
26. Krug, "The Application of Principles of Child Psychotherapy in Residential Treatment," 695.
27. Morris F. Mayer, "Casework within an Institution," *Children* 1, no. 2 (1954): 65–66.
28. "Topic III: Morning Session, Discussion Group B," in *Proceedings of the Conference on In-Patient Psychiatric Treatment for Children*, held under the auspices of the American Psychiatric Association, October 17–21, 1956, Woodner Hotel, Washington, DC, Box 118-8-2-8, EG, 482. Mandelbaum continued: "There are children who it is better not to return to the family until they have acquired enough inner strength and outer support to be able to endure whatever contaminating effect the family has upon the child" ("Topic III: Morning Session, Discussion Group B," 483).
29. American Psychiatric Association, *Psychiatric Inpatient Treatment of Children*, 84.
30. Brochures for Southard School in 1954 and 1964, respectively, explained that "normal social adjustment is an aim for *each* child in the School" and that "the ultimate goal for each child in inpatient treatment is normal family and social adjustment" (Don Lawder, "Help for the Child with Problems," Box 3, May 1954, Help for the Child with Problems [1954], KSHS; "Help for the Child with Problems," 1964, folder titled "Help for the Child with Problems [1964]," KSHS).
31. Henry I. Klopp, "The Children's Institute of the Allentown State Hospital," *American Journal of Psychiatry* 88, no. 6 (May 1, 1932): 1110.
32. At the Cincinnati Child Guidance Home, the Evanston Children's Home, and Pioneer House, e.g., most children attended local public schools (Othilda Krug, "A Concept of Education in the Residential Treatment of Emotionally Disturbed Children," pt. 5 of "Symposium, 1953: The Education of Emotionally Disturbed Children," *American Journal of Orthopsychiatry* 23, no. 4 (1953): 694; Reid and Hagan, *Residential Treatment of Emotionally Disturbed Children*, 133; Barbara L. Smith, "Programming in a Treatment Home for Disturbed Children: An Analysis of Programming at Pioneer House from December 1, 1946 to June 1, 1947, Evaluating the Relationship of Program Activities to Individual and Group Developments" (MSW thesis, Wayne University, 1948, 13). For children at the Ryther Child Center and at the Southard School, attending public school was a sign that the child was improving and getting ready to go home ("Bad Boy's Story," *Life*, May 12, 1947, 113; E. M. Leitch and E. R. Geleerd, "Residential Psychiatric School," *Nervous Child* 3 [1944]: 22; Adah Jean Mears, "A Follow up Study of Students Who Were Discharged from the Southard School in the Period between January 1, 1940 and December 31, 1944" [MSW thesis, Washington University, 1945], 7).
33. "Children's Work Program, 1-9-63," Container 1, Folder 10, BA, 2.
34. Child Welfare League of America, Inc., "Report to the Illinois Children's Home and Aid Society Regarding the Evanston Receiving Home," February 1955, Box 32, Folder 304, CHA, 1.
35. "Report of Executive Director," in "Bellefaire Minutes of the Annual Meeting Held July 1, 1951," Container 7, Folder 2, BA, 8.
36. Psychiatrist Nathan Ackerman of Southard School stated that "above all else our aim

is to make of every child a happy child," and Shirley Camper of the Illinois Neuropsychiatric Institute explained that their unit's goal was "to effect such changes in the emotional adjustments of the individual child that in approximately a year he will be relatively happy and able to learn (i.e. assimilate new personality and intellectual growth material)" (Nathan W. Ackerman, "A Plan for Maladjusted Children," *Bulletin of the Menninger Clinic* 1, no. 3 [January 1937]: 68; Shirley Camper, "A Follow-up Study of Children Discharged from a Psychiatric Ward," pt. 2, "Factors in Treatment" [MSS thesis, Smith College School for Social Work, 1946], 1).

37. "At Bellefaire, Unhappy Children Learn to Face the World," *Woman's World*, vol. 5, no. 6 (December 1955), Container 19, Folder 7, BA.
38. A 1958 fundraising pamphlet celebrating Bellefaire's ninetieth anniversary declared that "Bellefaire's goal is to help [children], through treatment and sympathetic understanding, to discover for themselves that life can be worthwhile" ("Bellefaire 90th Anniversary 1868–1958," Container 19, Folder 7, BA, 4).
39. John G. Milner, "The Residential Treatment Center," *Annals of the American Academy of Political and Social Science* 355, no. 1 (1964): 100–101.
40. The Southard staff measured internal change by a child's level of self-acceptance. Through establishing healthy relationships with staff members, they believed that "a child can gradually learn to live with his problems" and gain "a sense of dependable acceptance of himself as an individual regardless of his level of deviation from the norm" (Mandelbaum, "Description of the Southard School," 56–57).
41. "Goodby to Bellefaire!" *Bellefaire Bulletin* 4, no. 1 (Fall 1955): 1, Container 18, Folder 4, BA.

CHAPTER 4

1. Arthur Mandelbaum, "Presentation for Annual Meeting, October, 1952," Box 16, Annual Meeting—1952, KSHS, 3. This description of Tommy's behavior is based on Rudolf Ekstein, "The Space Child's Time Machine: On Reconstruction in the Psychotherapeutic Treatment of a Schizophrenoid Child," *American Journal of Orthopsychiatry* 24, no. 3 (July 24, 1954): 492; Rudolf Ekstein and Dorothy Wright, "The Space Child: A Note on the Psychotherapeutic Treatment of a 'Schizophrenoid' Child," *Bulletin of the Menninger Clinic* 16 (1952): 212, and "Comments on a Psychotherapeutic Session with the Space Child," *International Record of Medicine and General Practice Clinics* 167, no. 11 (November 1954): 593; and Mandelbaum, "Presentation for Annual Meeting, October, 1952," 2–3.
2. Ekstein and Wright, "The Space Child," 211.
3. Ibid.
4. Dr. Fuller, "Presentation for Annual Meeting, October, 1952," Box 16, Annual Meeting—1952, KSHS, 1.
5. Mrs. Wright, "Presentation for Annual Meeting, October, 1952," Box 16, Annual Meeting—1952, KSHS, 1; Ekstein and Wright, "The Space Child," 212.
6. The words "psychotherapy" and "casework" were used interchangeably; for simplicity's sake, I will use the term "psychotherapy," which more clearly describes the individual interview technique and reflects its grounding in the analytic tradition.
7. American Psychiatric Association, *Psychiatric Inpatient Treatment of Children: Report of the Conference on Inpatient Psychiatric Treatment for Children Held at Washington, D. C., October 17–21, 1956* (Washington, DC: American Psychiatric Association, 1957), 92–93; Lydia Hylton, *The Residential Treatment Center: Children, Programs, and Costs* (New York: Child Welfare League of America, 1964), 129. Seven of the

twenty-one schooles Hylton studied had "a few" children not in therapy, which Hylton attributed to those who had just arrived and had not yet started therapy and to those children who "were not considered capable of sustaining any type of formal therapeutic relationship."

8. American Psychiatric Association, *Psychiatric Inpatient Treatment of Children*, 92–93. The report did not note the number of RTCs studied.
9. Hylton, *The Residential Treatment Center*, 52–53.
10. Ibid., 18, 52–53.
11. Joseph H. Reid and Helen R. Hagan, *Residential Treatment of Emotionally Disturbed Children: A Descriptive Study* (New York: Child Welfare League of America, 1952), 31.
12. Ibid., 207.
13. Shirley Camper, "A Follow-up Study of Children Discharged from a Psychiatric Ward," pt. 2, "Factors in Treatment" (MSS thesis, Smith College School for Social Work, 1946), 11, 36.
14. Reid and Hagan, *Residential Treatment of Emotionally Disturbed Children*, 128.
15. Kevin J. O'Connor, *The Play Therapy Primer*, 2nd ed. (New York: John Wiley & Sons, 2000), 11–12.
16. Samuel Finestone and Toby Bennett Bieber, "Status at Discharge and Follow-up of Twenty Children with Diagnosis of Primary Behavior Disorder Hospitalized at New York State Psychiatric Institute and Hospital" (master's thesis, New York School of Social Work, Columbia University, 1946), 9.
17. Ibid., 10.
18. Allen L. Otten and Charles B. Seib, "The Case of the Furious Children," *Harper's Magazine*, January 1958, 58.
19. Earle Silber, interview with the author, Bethesda, MD, March 27, 2011.
20. Otten and Seib, "The Case of the Furious Children," 58–59.
21. *Third Annual Report of the Arthur Brisbane Child Treatment Center at Allaire for the Year Ending June 30, 1950* (Allaire, NJ: The Center, 1950), 2.
22. Ibid., 13.
23. *Fourth Annual Report of the Arthur Brisbane Child Treatment Center at Allaire for the Year Ending June 30, 1951* (Allaire, NJ: The Center, 1951), 4.
24. Reid and Hagan, *Residential Treatment of Emotionally Disturbed Children*, 8.
25. Evelyn Brownstone, Robert A. Cohn, Margaret Hooks, Herbert Moskowitz, and Phyllis Pfeiffer, "Children's Services at the Camarillo State Hospital" (MSW thesis, UCLA School of Social Welfare, 1952), 15.
26. Lillian Johnson, *Monograph on Organization and Operation*, Monograph/Ryther Child Center, no. 2 (Seattle: The Center, 1948), 4–5.
27. Herschel Alt and Hyman Grossbard, "Professional Issues in the Institutional Treatment of Delinquent Children," *American Journal of Orthopsychiatry* 19, no. 2 (1949): 285.
28. Camper, "A Follow-up Study of Children Discharged from a Psychiatric Ward," 37.
29. Bruno Bettelheim, *Love Is Not Enough: The Treatment of Emotionally Disturbed Children* (Glencoe, IL: Free Press, 1950), 244.
30. Reid and Hagan, *Residential Treatment of Emotionally Disturbed Children*, 234.
31. Charles Bradley, "Education in a Children's Psychiatric Hospital," *Nervous Child* 3 (1944): 331.
32. Group for the Advancement of Psychiatry, Committee on Psychiatry and Law, *Confidentiality and Privileged Communication in the Practice of Psychiatry* (New York: Group for the Advancement of Psychiatry, 1960), 105, 111–12.

33. Ibid., 106.
34. Mandelbaum, "Description of the Southard School," 32.
35. *Child Care Handbook*, May 1957, Box 6, *Child Care Handbook*, May 1957, KSHS, 5.
36. John D. Benjamin to Karl A. Menninger, November 8, 1957, Box 9, Evaluation of Southard School (Benjamin), KSHS, 2.
37. J. Franklin Robinson, "Resident Psychiatric Treatment of Children," *American Journal of Orthopsychiatry* 17 (1947): 459.
38. Lotte Eichenwald Scharfman, "An Examination of Referrals of Emotionally Disturbed Children to a Resident Treatment Center" (MSW thesis, University of Washington, 1951), 39.
39. Othilda Krug, Helen Hayward, and Bernice Crumpacker, "Intensive Residential Treatment of a Nine-Year-Old Girl with an Aggressive Behavior Disorder, Petit Mal Epilepsy and Enuresis," *American Journal of Orthopsychiatry* 22, no. 2 (1952): 408.
40. Stephen Eliot, *Not the Thing I Was: Thirteen Years at Bruno Bettelheim's Orthogenic School* (New York: St. Martin's Press, 2003), 94.
41. Ibid., 280.
42. Krug, Hayward, and Crumpacker, "Treatment of a Nine-Year-Old Girl," 413.
43. Bettelheim, *Love Is Not Enough*, 249.
44. Morris F. Mayer, "Some Problems Relative to the Cottage Parent," in "Some Problems in Group Care Treatment: Round Table 1951," *American Journal of Orthopsychiatry* 22, no. 1 (January 1952): 110.
45. Bettelheim, *Love Is Not Enough*, 249.
46. Scharfman, "An Examination of Referrals of Emotionally Disturbed Children to a Resident Treatment Center," 39.
47. For example, see Morris F. Mayer, "Casework within an Institution," *Children* 1, no. 2 (1954): 68; Othilda Krug, "A Concept of Education in the Residential Treatment of Emotionally Disturbed Children," pt. 5 of "Symposium, 1953: Education of Emotionally Disturbed Children," *American Journal of Orthopsychiatry* 23, no. 4 (1953): 691.
48. "Handbook for Parents (Early 1950s)," Box 3, folder titled "Handbook for Parents," KSHS, 8.
49. Herschel Alt, *Residential Treatment for the Disturbed Child: Basic Principles in Planning and Design of Programs and Facilities* (New York: International Universities Press, 1960), 315, 318.
50. Ibid., 315. Alt described children who might use therapy to "talk—as the price of concessions including release from the institution. Often the discussions may sound revealing, the youngster may express appreciation at learning these things about himself. . . . But there is little emotional content and his real feelings remain untouched" (ibid., 316).
51. Ibid., 327.
52. Ibid., 328–38.
53. Ibid., 152.
54. Bettelheim, *Love Is Not Enough*, 246.
55. "Robert E. Switzer, Roles and Functions of Child Psychiatrists in Residential Treatment—What and How," 1962, Box 7.3, SWITZER: Child Psychiatrists in the Residential Treatment of Children, 1963, KSHS, 37–38.
56. Reid and Hagan, *Residential Treatment of Emotionally Disturbed Children*, 126.
57. Ibid., 152, 103.
58. Ibid., 128, 208.

59. The account that follows in the text is based on Gene Gordon and Leonard Siegel, "The Evolution of a Program of Individual Psychotherapy for Children with Aggressive Acting-Out Disorders in a New Residential Treatment Unit," *American Journal of Orthopsychiatry* 27, no. 1 (1957): 59–68.
60. Ibid., 64.
61. Ibid., 66.
62. Children of Bellefaire, "So you'll know all about . . . Bellefaire," Container 19, Folder 7, BA, 16.
63. Eliot, *Not the Thing I Was*, 91.
64. Lee Stringer, *Sleepaway School: Stories from a Boy's Life* (New York: Seven Stories Press, 2004), 107.
65. Ekstein, "The Space Child's Time Machine," 492.
66. Ekstein and Wright, "The Space Child," 214.
67. Dr. Ekstein, "Presentation for Annual Meeting, October, 1952," Box 16, Annual Meeting—1952, KSHS, 1. In this case, "autistic" is an adjective used to describe Tommy's self-involved behavior. This word was commonly used as such and did not refer necessarily to the emerging diagnostic category of autism.
68. Ekstein and Wright, "The Space Child," 213.
69. Mrs. Wright, "Presentation for Annual Meeting," 1; Ekstein, "The Space Child's Time Machine," 492–93.
70. Ekstein and Wright, "The Space Child," 215.
71. Ibid.
72. Ibid., 216.
73. Ibid.
74. Mrs. Wright, "Presentation for Annual Meeting," 1.
75. Ekstein, "The Space Child's Time Machine," 496.
76. Ibid., 499.
77. Ibid.
78. Ekstein and Wright, "The Space Child," 218.
79. Ibid., 221.
80. Ibid., 221–22.
81. Rudolf Ekstein, *The Language of Psychotherapy* (Philadelphia: John Benjamins Publishing, 1989), 208.
82. Ekstein and Wright, "The Space Child," 224.
83. Ibid., 223.
84. Ekstein, *The Language of Psychotherapy*, 208–9.
85. "Annual Report Department of Child Psychiatry of the Menninger Foundation, July 1, 1951 to July 1, 1953," Annual Reports—1952–56, Box 1, KSHS, 12.
86. Ibid., 13.
87. Hylton, *The Residential Treatment Center*, 55–57.
88. Ibid., 146–47. Hylton found that 457 fathers and 672 mothers in her sample participated in therapy. Just as both parents were implicated in the etiology of emotional disturbance, both were sought for participation in individual therapy. Menninger social worker Arthur Mandelbaum reflected that, "in the past, the mother alone was involved in casework not only because of her emotional closeness to the child, but to secure her important cooperation in the treatment to follow." But times were changing: "In the last decade, the treatment of the disturbed child has shifted from a focus on the mother-child relationship exclusively to an attemtp [*sic*] to understand the interaction of the child within his entire family. . . . This narrow focus on

the mother-child relationship has given way to include the consideration of the important influence of the father on family life and especially his impact upon the disturbed child" (Mandelbaum, "Casework with the Parents of Disturbed Children," September 2, 1958, Box 7.3, Mandelbaum, Arthur E.: Casework with the Parents of a Disturbed Child, KSHS).

89. J. Franklin Robinson, Anabel Maxwell, and Kathryn E. Dominguez, "Resident Psychiatric Treatment with Children," *American Journal of Orthopsychiatry* 17, no. 3 (July 1947): 461; Anabel Maxwell, "The Inter-Related Movement of Parent and Child in Resident Treatment," *Quarterly Journal of Child Behavior* 2 (1951): 185.
90. "Topic III: Morning Session, Discussion Group B," in *Proceedings of the Conference on In-Patient Psychiatric Treatment for Children,* held under the auspices of the American Psychiatric Association, October 17–21, 1956, Woodner Hotel, Washington DC, Box 118-8-2-8, RS, 463. J. Franklin Robinson had also commented in an article nine years prior that a child could not be considered an independent entity but "must be considered in relation to a complementary parental force" ("The Use of Residence in Psychiatric Treatment with Children," *American Journal of Psychiatry* 103, no. 6 [1947]: 814).
91. Anabel Maxwell, "The Parents' Role in Resident Treatment," *News-Letter of the American Association of Psychiatric Social Workers* 15, no. 3 (Winter 1945): 40.
92. S. A. Szurek, "The Family and the Staff in Hospital Psychiatric Therapy of Children," *American Journal of Orthopsychiatry* 21, no. 3 (1951): 602.
93. American Psychiatric Association, *Psychiatric Inpatient Treatment of Children,* 84.
94. Mary Faust, "The Parents' Role in a Child's Residential Treatment: A Dissertation Based upon an Investigation at the Institute for Juvenile Research, Chicago, Illinois" (MSS thesis, Smith College School for Social Work, 1949), 18.
95. Camper, "A Follow-up Study of Children Discharged from a Psychiatric Ward," 28.
96. Faust, "The Parents' Role in a Child's Residential Treatment," 18, 26.
97. Charles Bradley, "Indications for Residential Treatment of Children with Severe Neuropsychiatric Problems," *American Journal of Orthopsychiatry* 19 (1949): 431; Child Welfare League of America and the Council of Jewish Federations and Welfare Funds, "Bellefaire Survey, 1952–1953," Container 19, Folder 4, BA, 31–33.
98. Reid and Hagan, *Residential Treatment of Emotionally Disturbed Children,* 160.
99. Maxwell, "The Parents' Role in Resident Treatment," 41–42. Also see Constance Lilian Blackett, "Parents' Reactions to Their Child's Visits from Residential Treatment: A Dissertation Based upon an Investigation at the Child Guidance Home, Cincinnati, Ohio" (MSW thesis, Smith College School for Social Work, 1962), 4; "Social Work Therapy at the Southard School," Box 6, Social Work, KSHS, 1.
100. Ursula Weiss Moore, "A Study of Children with Primary Behavior Disorders Treated at Langley Porter Clinic: Results of In-Patient and Out-Patient Care." (MSW thesis, University of California, Berkeley, 1949), 102–4.
101. Ibid., 102.
102. Ibid., 103.
103. Ibid., 103, 105.
104. Ibid., 103.
105. Ibid., 105.
106. Maxwell, "The Inter-Related Movement of Parent and Child in Resident Treatment," 191.
107. Eva E. Burmeister, *Roofs for the Family* (New York: Columbia University Press, 1954), 40.

108. Ibid.
109. Louis J. Wise et al., "Residential Treatment of a Ten-Year-Old Boy: Problems in the Differential Diagnosis and Treatment of Marked Destructive Behavior," *Case Studies in Childhood Emotional Disabilities* 1, no. 1 (1953): 332. Although the boy was referred to as Tommy in the forty-page case history of him published in *Case Studies in Emotional Disabilities,* I have chosen to call him Charlie here so as not to confuse the reader with nine-year-old Tommy, the "Space Child."
110. Ibid., 335.
111. Ibid., 341.
112. Ibid., 351.
113. Ibid., 361.
114. Ibid., 360.
115. Reid and Hagan, *Residential Treatment of Emotionally Disturbed Children,* 110; "Visiting Arrangements for Parents," 1950s, Container 1, Folder 11, BA; Howard W. Potter, "A Service for Children in a Psychiatric Hospital," *Psychiatric Quarterly* 8, no. 1 (March 1, 1934): 29; Blackett, "Parents' Reactions to Their Child's Visits from Residential Treatment"; "Visiting Arrangements for Parents," 1–4, 12–15.
116. "Handbook for Parents (Early 1950s?)," 22.
117. Faust, "The Parents' Role in a Child's Residential Treatment," 14.
118. Ibid.
119. "Child's Contacts with Parents and Family during Placement," 1950s, Container 1, Folder 11, BA.
120. Potter, "A Service for Children in a Psychiatric Hospital," 33; Blackett, "Parents' Reactions to Their Child's Visits from Residential Treatment," ii, 54.
121. Maxwell, "The Inter-Related Movement of Parent and Child in Resident Treatment," 192.
122. E. Janet Allen, "Casework with the Parents at the Child Guidance Home: A Dissertation Based upon an Investigation at the Child Guidance Home, Cincinnati, Ohio" (MSS thesis, Smith College School for Social Work, 1951), 29–30.
123. Ibid., 31.
124. "Handbook for Parents (Early 1950s?)," 23.
125. "Procedures for the Admission of a New Child to the Southard School, October, 1956," Box 9, Admissions Procedures, 1956, KSHS, 3.
126. "Visiting," 1950s, Container 1, Folder 11, BA, 4.
127. Ibid., 3–4.
128. Ibid., 1, 3.
129. Blackett, "Parents' Reactions to Their Child's Visits from Residential Treatment," 33–42.
130. Ibid., 38–39.
131. Menninger Foundation Activities, "The Southard School," *Bulletin of the Menninger Clinic* 6, no. 4 (July 1942): 130.
132. Morris Mayer, "Report of the Head Resident, 7-18-48," in Minutes, Board of Trustees, July 18, 1948, Container 7, Folder 1, BA, 4.
133. Harris B. Peck, Ralph D. Rabinovitch, and Joseph B. Cramer, "A Treatment Program for Parents of Schizophrenic Children," *American Journal of Orthopsychiatry* 19, no. 4 (1949): 597. The children were all current or past patients on the child psychiatry unit at Bellevue.
134. Ibid., 593.
135. Ibid., 595.

136. Ibid., 594.
137. Ibid.
138. Ibid., 598.
139. Ibid., 597.
140. League for Emotionally Disturbed Children, "The League Idea," Box 2, File 10, LB, 1.
141. Ibid.; "Child-Aid Agency Widens Its Scope," *New York Times*, March 7, 1954, 44; "League Fights to Help Mentally Ill Children," *Washington Post*, August 9, 1955, 29; "Dr. Norman Laurie Is Speaker at Second Annual LEDC Meeting," *Pittsburgh Courier*, February 4, 1956, A31; "Panel Will Discuss the Emotionally Disturbed Child," *Pittsburgh Courier*, March 22, 1958, A17; "Child Group Aids 7 Schools," *New York Times*, February 13, 1959, 29.
142. League for Emotionally Disturbed Children, "The League Idea," 1; "Children's Group to Gain by Fetes," *New York Times*, December 11, 1956.
143. Ibid.; "Benefit Is Slated at Art Display: Modern Painting Exhibition to Aid Disturbed Youths—Other Shows Listed," *New York Times*, 1958.
144. Irving Kaye, "Aid for Disturbed Children," *New York Times*, 1955, 30. On groups for parents of intellectually disabled children, see Katherine Castles, "'Nice, Average Americans': Postwar Parents' Groups and the Defense of the Normal Family," in*Mental Retardation in America: A Historical Reader*, ed. Steven Noll and James W. Trent (New York: New York University Press, 2004).
145. "Children's Group to Gain by Fetes," 47; "Mayor's Wife Will Give Tea on Tuesday to Aid League for Disturbed Children," *New York Times*, April 8, 1956, 114; "Dec. 8 Concert by Elman to Aid Children's Group," *New York Times*, November 18, 1958, 45; "Child Care Unit to Gain May 14 by Theatre Fete," *New York Times*, March 15, 1959, 106.
146. The league still exists as the League Education and Treatment Center, which offers day, residential, and educational treatment for children "with psychiatric and developmental disabilities" (www.leaguecenter.org, accessed April 14, 2012).
147. David Hallowitz, "Presentation for Annual Meeting, October, 1952," Box 16, Annual Meeting—1952, KSHS, 1.
148. Mrs. Wright, "Presentation for Annual Meeting," 2.
149. Ibid.

CHAPTER 5

1. David Hallowitz, Presentation for Annual Meeting, October 1952, Box 16, Annual Meeting—1952, KSHS, 1.
2. Ibid.
3. Stephen Eliot, *Not the Thing I Was: Thirteen Years at Bruno Bettelheim's Orthogenic School* (New York: St. Martin's Press, 2003), 7.
4. Stephen J. Whitfield, *The Culture of the Cold War* (Baltimore, MD: Johns Hopkins University Press, 1991). Several historians have wisely cautioned that postwar culture ought not to be equated with Cold War culture (Peter J. Kuznick and James Gilbert, eds., *Rethinking Cold War Culture* (Washington, DC: Smithsonian Institution Press, 2001).
5. Jackson Lears, "A Matter of Taste: Corporate Cultural Hegemony in a Mass-Consumption Society," in *Recasting America: Culture and Politics in the Age of Cold War*, ed. Lary May (Chicago: University of Chicago Press, 1989). Lears suggests that this perception was a hegemonic view that crowded out the realities of numerous rich subcultures.

6. Traditionally, Elaine Tyler May has been invoked as a straw woman who argued in her 1988 *Homeward Bound* that American families adopted conformity as a form of domestic containment, while Joanne Meyerowitz's 1994 collection *Not June Cleaver* is said to have convincingly demonstrated that messages about womanly behavior were complex and that women in postwar America proudly took on roles that deviated from the middle-class homemaker norm. However, I would argue that May actually demonstrated the intense cultural pressure that men and women felt to conform, simultaneously showing how fractured and troubled their marriages often became in pursuit of this perfection. Larger cultural messages about "good" families, wives, and mothers were of course not perfectly uniform but I think it is an overcorrection to dismiss the pressure individuals felt to conform to an almost nonexistent ideal (Elaine Tyler May, *Homeward Bound: American Families in the Cold War Era* [New York: Basic Books, 1988]; Joanne J. Meyerowitz, ed., *Not June Cleaver: Women and Gender in Postwar America, 1945–1960* [Philadelphia: Temple University Press, 1994]). Wini Breines argued in *Young, White, and Miserable* (Boston: Beacon Books, 1992) that these pressures were so great that they gave rise to second-wave feminism by pushing young women in the 1950s to resist the terms of their oppression. Even transgender individuals, who were particularly deviant in the eyes of the American public, were obliged to feign personalities aligning with the traditional interests (sexual and otherwise) of their gender identity (Joanne J. Meyerowitz, *How Sex Changed: A History of Transsexuality in the United States* [Cambridge, MA: Harvard University Press, 2002]). Sexuality was similarly policed by groups, including State Department officials, who expunged suspected homosexuals from its ranks during the Lavender Scare, psychiatrists, who deemed homosexuality a perverse disease and attempted to treat it using psychoanalysis, and experts on sexuality (as well as a significant portion of the American public), who looked at the Kinsey Reports as threatening evidence of just how deviant regular Americans were (David K. Johnson, *The Lavender Scare: The Cold War Persecution of Gays and Lesbians in the Federal Government* [Chicago: University of Chicago Press, 2004]; Jennifer Terry, *An American Obsession: Science, Medicine, and Homosexuality in Modern Society* [Chicago: University of Chicago Press, 1999]; Carolyn Herbst Lewis, *Prescription for Heterosexuality: Sexual Citizenship in the Cold War Era* [Chapel Hill: University of North Carolina Press, 2010]; Miriam G. Reumann, *American Sexual Character: Sex, Gender, and National Identity in the Kinsey Reports*[Berkeley: University of California Press, 2005]).
7. Anna G. Creadick, *Perfectly Average: The Pursuit of Normality in Postwar America* (Amherst: University of Massachusetts Press, 2010).
8. Ibid., 66–70.
9. Lizabeth Cohen, *A Consumer's Republic: The Politics of Mass Consumption in Postwar America* (New York: Knopf, 2003).
10. Thomas J. Sugrue, *The Origins of the Urban Crisis: Race and Inequality in Postwar Detroit* (Princeton, NJ: Princeton University Press, 1996).
11. Creadick, *Perfectly Average*, 83–84.
12. Ibid., 15, 20.
13. James Burkhart Gilbert, *A Cycle of Outrage: America's Reaction to the Juvenile Delinquent in the 1950s* (New York: Oxford University Press, 1986).
14. Ken Smith, *Mental Hygiene: Classroom Films, 1945–1970* (New York: Blast Books, 1999).
15. Angela Baird, "Behavior and Anxiety in Disturbed Children: A Dissertation Based

upon an Investigation at the Child Guidance Home of Cincinnati" (MSS thesis, Smith College School for Social Work, 1951), 3.

16. Herschel Alt, "Responsibilities and Qualifications of the Child Care Worker," pt. 2 of "Symposium, 1953: The Education of Emotionally Disturbed Children," *American Journal of Orthopsychiatry* 23, no. 4 (1953): 673; Donald A. Bloch, "Residential Treatment for Disturbed Children," *Nursing Outlook* 5, no. 11 (1957): 636.
17. Gisela Konopka, "Social Group Work for In-patients," in Emma Pendleton Bradley Hospital, *Out of Their Misfortune: 25th Anniversary Report of the Emma Pendleton Bradley Home* (Riverside, RI: The Hospital, 1956), 35.
18. Alt, "Responsibilities and Qualifications of the Child Care Worker," 673; Bloch, "Residential Treatment for Disturbed Children," 636; Emma Pendleton Bradley Hospital, *Out of Their Misfortune*, 35. Earle Silber of the NIH Child Psychiatry Unit differentiated between the milieu, which consisted of "the emotional climate of the setting itself and the attitudes of the responsible adults in these settings," and milieu therapy, which consciously sought to use the milieu as a therapeutic tool (Earle Silber, "Some Aspects of Milieu Treatment with Children" [paper presented at Walter Reed Army Medical Center, August 1957]; copy obtained from Silber).
19. "Handbook for Parents," printed March 20, 1959, discarded August 30, 1962, Box 3, folder titled "Handbook for Parents, 1950's," KSHS, 16.
20. "Topic III: Afternoon Session, Discussion Group B," in *Proceedings of the Conference on In-Patient Psychiatric Treatment for Children*, held under the auspices of the American Psychiatric Association, October 17–21, 1956, Woodner Hotel, Washington, DC, Box 118-8-2-8, EG, 309.
21. American Psychiatric Association, *Psychiatric Inpatient Treatment of Children Report of the Conference on Inpatient Psychiatric Treatment for Children Held at Washington, D. C., October 17–21, 1956* (Washington, DC: American Psychiatric Association, 1957), 88.
22. On the York Retreat in England, one of the first institutions of its kind, see Anne Digby, *Madness, Morality, and Medicine: A Study of the York Retreat, 1796–1914* (Cambridge: Cambridge University Press, 1985). On the development of similar institutions in the United States, see Nancy Tomes, *A Generous Confidence: Thomas Story Kirkbride and the Art of Asylum-Keeping, 1840–1883* (Cambridge: Cambridge University Press, 1984); Ellen Dwyer, *Homes for the Mad: Life inside Two Nineteenth-Century Asylums* (New Brunswick, NJ: Rutgers University Press, 1987).
23. John A. Mills and Tom Harrison, "John Rickman, Wilfred Ruprecht Bion, and the Origins of the Therapeutic Community," *History of Psychology* 10, no. 1 (February 2007): 22–43; Tom Harrison and David Clarke, "The Northfield Experiments," *British Journal of Psychiatry: The Journal of Mental Science* 160 (May 1992): 698–708; Stuart Whiteley, "The Evolution of the Therapeutic Community," *Psychiatric Quarterly* 75, no. 3 (2004): 233–48.
24. Gerald N. Grob, *The Mad among Us: A History of the Care of America's Mentally Ill* (New York: Free Press, 1994), 227.
25. Herschel Alt, *Residential Treatment for the Disturbed Child: Basic Principles in Planning and Design of Programs and Facilities* (New York: International Universities Press, 1960), 45; Joseph H. Reid and Helen R. Hagan, *Residential Treatment of Emotionally Disturbed Children: A Descriptive Study* (New York: Child Welfare League of America, 1952), iii.
26. For a contemporary analysis of the role of milieu therapy, see Yvonne Smith and

Matthew C. Spitzmueller, "Worker Perspectives on Contemporary Milieu Therapy: A Cross-Site Ethnographic Study," *Social Work Research* 40, no. 2 (June 2016): 105–16.

27. Earl Saxe and Jeanetta Lyle, "Function of the Psychiatric Residential School," *Bulletin of the Menninger Clinic* 4, no. 6 (November 1940): 167.
28. Barbara J. Betz, "A Psychiatric Children's Ward," *American Journal of Nursing* 45, no. 10 (October 1945): 821; Bernice Crumpacker, "The Caseworker as Residential Worker: A Dissertation Based upon a Study at the Child Guidance Home, Cincinnati, Ohio" (MSS thesis, Smith College School for Social Work, 1950), 3.
29. Crumpacker, "The Caseworker as Residential Worker," 13. Crumpacker reflected that "this statement is in essence the goal of a residential treatment program as the writer conceives it."
30. "Handbook for Parents," 8; "At Bellefaire, Unhappy Children Learn to Face the World," *Woman's World* 5, no. 6 (December 1955), Container 6, Folder 7, BA; Arthur Mandelbaum, "Description of the Southard School: Conference on Inpatient Psychiatric Treatment for Children," Box 16, Children's Div. 1956, KSHS, 21. Developing positive relationships with staff members was seen as a necessary first step to forming good relationships with parents (Joseph H. Reid and Helen R. Hagan, *Residential Treatment of Emotionally Disturbed Children: A Descriptive Study* [New York: Child Welfare League of America, 1952], 59).
31. On new psychotherapies in the 1950s, see Jonathan Engel, *American Therapy: The Rise of Psychotherapy in the United States* (New York: Gotham Books, 2008), chap. 4.
32. Alt, *Residential Treatment for the Disturbed Child*, 377–402.
33. Ibid., 385. Although Alt presented several case histories, included in his 1960 text, he credited social worker Rena Schulman for compiling them and noted that, in most cases, she had worked intensely with the children herself (ibid., 305).
34. Bruno Herbert, "Factors Influencing the Later Adjustment of Girls Discharged from the Hawthorne-Cedar Knolls School: A Dissertation Based upon an Investigation at the Jewish Board of Guardians, New York City" (MSS thesis, Smith College School for Social Work, 1946), 13.
35. As Erwin Angres of the Illinois Neuropsychiatric Institute's child unit explained, "Our first problem is to provide an environment which approximates, as closely as possible, that of a family, and a healthy atmosphere in which the child can grow" ("Therapeutic Techniques Used with a Special Group of Disturbed Children," *Illinois Medical Journal* 89 [March 1946]: 133).
36. Othilda Krug, "Child Guidance Home—1958," *Cincinnati Journal of Medicine* 39 (1958): 571, and "A Concept of Education in the Residential Treatment of Emotionally Disturbed Children" pt. 5 of "Symposium 1953: The Education of Emotionally Disturbed Children," *American Journal of Orthopsychiatry* 23, no. 4 (1953): 692; Helen R. Hagan, "Residential Treatment," *Child Welfare* 31 (1952): 3; Reid and Hagan, *Residential Treatment of Emotionally Disturbed Children*, 138.
37. Emma Pendleton Bradley Hospital, *Out of Their Misfortune*, 6.
38. Krug, "A Concept of Education," 692; Herschel Alt and Hyman Grossbard, "Professional Issues in the Institutional Treatment of Delinquent Children," *American Journal of Orthopsychiatry* 19, no. 2 (1949): 284; Lauretta Bender, "Group Activities on a Children's Ward as Methods of Psychotherapy," *American Journal of Psychiatry* 93, no. 5 (March 1, 1937): 1156; Isaac Zeke Youcha, "A Study of Schizophrenic Children in Cottage Life at the Hawthorne Cedar Knolls School" (master's thesis, New York School of Social Work, Columbia University, 1953), 20.

39. Norman V. Lourie and Rena Schulman, "The Role of the Residential Staff in Residential Treatment," *American Journal of Orthopsychiatry* 24, no. 4 (1952): 804.
40. Anne Benjamin and Howard E. Weatherly, "Hospital Ward Treatment of Emotionally Disturbed Children," *American Journal of Orthopsychiatry* 17, no. 4 (October 1947): 674; Bruno Bettelheim and Emmy Sylvester, "A Therapeutic Milieu," *American Journal of Orthopsychiatry* 18 (1948): 192, and "Milieu Therapy: Indications and Illustrations," *Psychoanalytic Review* 36 (1949): 67.
41. Benjamin and Weatherly, "Hospital Ward Treatment of Emotionally Disturbed Children," 674.
42. Alt, *Residential Treatment for the Disturbed Child*, 55.
43. Charles Bradley, "Education in a Children's Psychiatric Hospital," *Nervous Child* 3 (1944): 328–29; Charles Bradley, "Indications for Residential Treatment of Children with Severe Neuropsychiatric Problems.," *American Journal of Orthopsychiatry* 19 (1949): 428.
44. Marvin Bloom and Adrian Cabral, "A Description of a Newly Introduced Group Work Program in a Residential Treatment Setting—the Hawthorne Cedar Knolls School" (master's thesis, New York School of Social Work, Columbia University, 1954), 35.
45. This was a daunting task for a population with such a troubled past. Reflected Bellefaire's resident director Morris Fritz Mayer, "It was our goal to find a recreational outlet and some fun for every child at Bellefaire, even if sometimes it was hard to bring pleasure into the lives of some of the children who had been so greatly damaged before they came to us" ("Annual Report of the Resident Director," in Minutes, September 11, 1955, Container 7, Folder 2, BA, 4–5). Their view that play was a right of all children was a popular one, having been decreed by the delegates at the 1930 White House Conference on Child Health and Protection. Howard Chudacoff has demonstrated that, although adults (child experts and otherwise) paid increased attention to play and its purposes in the first half of the twentieth century, their interests mostly diverged from those of children in that period as well. Adults felt that play should help a child practice key skills he would need to use as an adult, while children rejected this purposeful interpretation (*Children at Play: An American History* [New York: New York University Press, 2007], chap. 4). On the idea that play could and should be purposeful, see Chudacoff, *Children at Play*, chap. 5.
46. Gertrude Samuels, "A New Road for the Juvenile Delinquent," *New York Times*, April 23, 1950, 37.
47. Charles Bradley, "Children's Hospital for Neurologic and Behavior Disorders," *Journal of the American Medical Association* 107, no. 9 (August 29, 1936): 651.
48. For example, see Allegra Larson, "Mother's Image of Her Relationship with Maternal Grandmother as a Factor in Her Own Mothering" (MSS thesis, Smith College School for Social Work, 1963), 12; James D. Newman, "A Descriptive Study of Emma Pendleton Bradley Hospital" (Specialist in Education thesis, George Peabody College for Teachers, 1964), 25; Reid and Hagan, *Residential Treatment of Emotionally Disturbed Children*, 23. In his memoir of his stay at Hawthorne in the early 1960s, Lee Stringer re-created his own reaction to the center's unusual campus: "And Cottage Five is just up the slope from the entrance. By my estimate, a mere matter of seconds to be out of here on a quick trot. There are no bars. Or fences. No physical barriers of any kind to keep you in. Just the dense rash of pines that surround the place" (*Sleepaway School: Stories from a Boy's Life* [New York: Seven Stories Press, 2004], 53).

49. Benjamin and Weatherly, "Hospital Ward Treatment of Emotionally Disturbed Children," 665; Reid and Hagan, *Residential Treatment of Emotionally Disturbed Children*, 223; Allen L. Otten and Charles B. Seib, "The Case of the Furious Children," *Harper's Magazine* (January 1958), 56.
50. Helen A. Sutton, "Some Nursing Aspects of a Children's Psychiatric Ward," *American Journal of Orthopsychiatry* 17, no. 4 (1947): 679.
51. On this general trend, see Gerald N. Grob, *Mental Illness and American Society, 1875–1940* (Princeton, NJ: Princeton University Press, 1983); Grob, *The Mad among Us*; Shorter, *A History of Psychiatry*.
52. Albert Deutsch, *The Shame of the States* (New York: Harcourt, Brace, 1948). See also Albert Q. Maisel, "Bedlam 1946," *Life* 20, no. 18 (May 6, 1946): 102–18; "Halfway Up from Bedlam," *Time* 43 (April 17, 1944): 90; "This Shame," *Time* 48 (November 11, 1946): 76; "Herded Like Cattle," *Time* 52 (December 20, 1948): 69.
53. *The Snake Pit*, directed by Anatole Litvak (Twentieth Century Fox, 1948).
54. For example, the 1957 American Psychiatric Association/American Academy of Child Psychiatry report stated of the milieu that "the child is helped to express his own natural inclinations in a permissive atmosphere" (American Psychiatric Association, *Psychiatric Inpatient Treatment of Children*, 89). The director of Napa State Hospital's children's unit stated that its "general atmosphere is permissive," a social work student called the Cincinnati Child Guidance Home a "permissive, accepting atmosphere," and a *Chicago Tribune* reporter called the University of Michigan's Child Psychiatric Hospital "surprisingly permissive" (Wrenshall A. Oliver, "A State Hospital Children's Unit," *American Journal of Psychiatry* 106, no. 4 [October 1, 1949]: 265; E. Janet Allen, "Casework with the Parents at the Child Guidance Home: A Dissertation Based upon an Investigation at the Child Guidance Home, Cincinnati, Ohio" [MSS thesis, Smith College School for Social Work, 1951], 27; Joan Beck, "Can 'Bad Kids' Be Saved?," *Chicago Daily Tribune*, February 27, 1955, K19).
55. This approach would be made famous by Benjamin Spock in his 1946 bestselling book *The Common Sense Book of Baby and Child Care* (New York: Duell, Sloan and Pearce, 1946). One of the first seminal texts on permissive child rearing was C. Anderson Aldrich and Mary Aldrich, *Babies are Human Beings: An Interpretation of Growth* (New York: MacMillan, 1938). Following soon after was the more widely read book by Yale University child psychologists Arnold Gesell and Frances L. Ilg, *Infant and Child in the Culture of Today: The Guidance of Development in Home and Nursery School* (New York: Harper and Row, 1943). For a general overview of the history of permissive parenting techniques, see Julia Grant, *Raising Baby by the Book: The Education of American Mothers* (New Haven, CT: Yale University Press, 1998), chap. 7; and Rima D. Apple, *Perfect Motherhood: Science and Childrearing in America* (New Brunswick, NJ: Rutgers University Press, 2006), Ch. 5.
56. For a general overview of the history of permissive parenting techniques see Grant, *Raising Baby by the Book*, chap. 7; and Apple, *Perfect Motherhood*, chap. 5.
57. Mandelbaum, "Description of the Southard School," 25.
58. Bradley, "Indications for Residential Treatment of Children," 429–30.
59. Bruno Bettelheim, *Love Is Not Enough: The Treatment of Emotionally Disturbed Children* (Glencoe, IL: Free Press, 1950), 41.
60. Ibid., 63.
61. Ibid., 57.
62. Howard W. Potter, "The Treatment of Problem Children in a Psychiatric Hospital," *American Journal of Psychiatry* 91, no. 4 (January 1, 1935): 873.

63. Earle Silber, interview with the author, Bethesda, MD, March 27, 2011.
64. Bloch, "Residential Treatment for Disturbed Children," 637.
65. Shirley Camper, "A Follow-up Study of Children Discharged from a Psychiatric Ward," pt. 2, "Factors in Treatment" (MSS thesis, Smith College School for Social Work, 1946), 18.
66. Ibid., 1; Vera Kare, "A Study of the Adjustment of a 'Problem' Child in a Group Therapy Home for Pre-Delinquent Boys, Pioneer House, September, 1946-June, 1948." (MSW thesis, Wayne University, 1948), 6.
67. Explained Shirley Camper of the Illinois Neuropsychiatric Institute, "The adults' therapeutic role in the current ward methodology is to fill the child's day with experiences which are free from inhibiting restrictions and prohibitions, from traumatizing hostile or retaliatory attitudes and from anxiety-provoking situations or uncertainties" (Camper, "A Follow-up Study of Children Discharged from a Psychiatric Ward," 1).
68. Angres, "Therapeutic Techniques Used with a Special Group of Disturbed Children," 134.
69. Ibid., 135.
70. A 1950s Southard handbook for parents explained, "Each child is helped to fit into his group with the assistance of adults who, by their attitudes, show acceptance and permissiveness and at the same time offer firm control and support when the child's feelings and frustrations cause him to behave in a way harmful to himself and to others in his group" ("Handbook for Parents," 7).
71. Othilda Krug, "The Application of Principles of Child Psychotherapy in Residential Treatment," *American Journal of Psychiatry* 108, no. 9 (March 1, 1952): 696; A. M. Edelman, "Some Observations on Occupational Therapy with Disturbed Children in a Residential Program," *American Journal of Occupational Therapy* 7, no. 3 (June 1953): 116; Crumpacker, "The Caseworker as Residential Worker," 15–16.
72. Krug, "The Application of Principles of Child Psychotherapy in Residential Treatment," 699.
73. Louis J. Wise et al., "Residential Treatment of a Ten-Year-Old Boy: Problems in the Differential Diagnosis and Treatment of Marked Destructive Behavior," *Case Studies in Childhood Emotional Disabilities* 1, no. 1 (1953): 338.
74. "Annual Report and Annual Meeting 1956–1957," Box 16, KSHS, 5–6.
75. "Children's Hospital Psychiatric Unit," June 29, 1953, Box 2, Planning Committee, 1953–56, RW.
76. Raymond W. Waggoner, "The New Children's Psychiatric Hospital, University of Michigan," Box 2, Planning Committee, 1953–56, RW, 3–4.
77. Raymond W. Waggoner and Ralph D. Rabinovitch, "The University of Michigan Plan for the Residential Treatment of Disturbed Children," *Medical Bulletin* 22, no. 3 (1956): 124.
78. Ibid., 121–24.
79. "Menninger Builds Houses for Children," reprinted from *Architectural Record* (November 1963), Box 3, Menninger Builds Houses for Children (1963), KSHS.
80. "Medicine: Children's Mental Hospital," *Time*, February 20, 1956, http://www.time.com/time/magazine/article/0,9171,808177,00.html; "Psychiatric Unit, Children's Hospital, University of Michigan," undated pamphlet, Box 2: General, 1956–60, RW.
81. "Committee on Planning Children's Hospital," April 23, 1953, Box 2, Planning Committee, 1953–56, RW.

82. Morris Fritz Meyer, "Annual Report of the Resident Director," in "Minutes," September 11, 1955, Container 7, Folder 2, BA, 1–2; Mandelbaum, "Description of the Southard School," 10–11; Arthur D. Sorosky, Norbert I. Rieger, and Peter E. Tanguay, "Furnishing a Psychiatric Unit for Children," *Hospital and Community Psychiatry* 20, no. 11 (November 1, 1969): 334–36.
83. On the mass-produced ranch home and its encapsulation of American middle-class family ideals, see Clifford E. Clark Jr., "Ranch-House Suburbia: Ideals and Realities," in *Recasting America*, ed. May.
84. Reid and Hagan, *Residential Treatment of Emotionally Disturbed Children*, 1952, 51, 121.
85. *The First Annual Report of the Arthur Brisbane Child Treatment Center at Allaire for the Year Ending June 30, 1948* (Allaire, NJ: The Center, 1948), 1; Mandelbaum, "Description of the Southard School," 8.
86. Crumpacker, "The Caseworker as Residential Worker," 1.
87. Jewish Board of Guardians, *Conditioned Environment in Case Work Treatment: A Monograph of Articles on Hawthorne-Cedar Knolls School, Lavenburg Corner House* (New York: Jewish Board of Guardians, 1944), 35.
88. Stringer, *Sleepaway School*, 53.
89. Lillian Johnson, *Monograph on Organization and Operation*, Monograph/Ryther Child Center, no. 2 (Seattle: The Center, 1948), 9.
90. Morris Mayer, "Bellefaire Annual Report of Head Resident," January 12, 1947, in Minutes: Board of Trustees, January 12, 1947, Container 7, Folder 1, BA, 1; Brian C. Jones, *Bradley Hospital: Legacy of Hope* (Warwick, RI: Emma Pendleton Bradley Hospital, 2006), 58.
91. Mandelbaum, "Description of the Southard School," 10.
92. Otten and Seib, "The Case of the Furious Children," 60.
93. Joseph D. Noshpitz, "Youth Pervades Half-Way House at NIMH," *Psychiatric Services* 10, no. 5 (May 1959): 26.
94. Greene, "'Case of the Furious Children': We Don't Know Why They Hate," *Chicago Daily Tribune*, July 19, 1959; Otten and Seib, "The Case of the Furious Children," 60.
95. Carly Wharton, "Report to the Board on the Purchase of Furniture and Furnishings for the Wiltwyck School," February 22, 1954, in "Wiltwyck School for Boys, Inc., Minutes of the Meeting of the Board of Directors Held on Monday, January 4, 1954 at 8:30 P.M. at the Home of Mrs. Alfred M. Lindau, 262 Central Park West, N.Y.C.," Box 4, Folder 59, WR, 1.
96. Wharton, "Report to the Board on the Purchase of Furniture and Furnishings for the Wiltwyck School," 2.
97. Benjamin and Weatherly, "Hospital Ward Treatment of Emotionally Disturbed Children," 665; Reid and Hagan, *Residential Treatment of Emotionally Disturbed Children*, 201; Waggoner, "The New Children's Psychiatric Hospital, University of Michigan," 2.
98. Waggoner, "The New Children's Psychiatric Hospital, University of Michigan"; "Psychiatric Unit, Children's Hospital, the University of Michigan."
99. Camper, "A Follow-up Study of Children Discharged from a Psychiatric Ward," 17–18.
100. Eva E. Burmeister, *Roofs for the Family* (New York: Columbia University Press, 1954), 138–39.
101. "Bobby Describes THE CAMPUS," in "So you'll know all about . . . Bellefaire," Container 19, Folder 7, BA.

102. Joan Beck, "Can 'Bad Kids' Be Saved?"
103. Burmeister, *Roofs for the Family*, 126.
104. Camper, "A Follow-up Study of Children Discharged from a Psychiatric Ward," 16.
105. Reid and Hagan, *Residential Treatment of Emotionally Disturbed Children*, 129.
106. Burmeister, *Roofs for the Family*, 26.
107. Alt, *Residential Treatment for the Disturbed Child*, 88. Alt simply states, "These couples did not remain for long," implying that they were either fired or chose not to remain because their methods did not align with the institution's new approach.
108. Pioneering child psychiatrist Howard Potter of the children's unit at the New York State Psychiatric Institute stated in 1935 that "the nurse is essentially a mother surrogate" (Potter, "The Treatment of Problem Children in a Psychiatric Hospital," 873).
109. Sutton, "Some Nursing Aspects of a Children's Psychiatric Ward," 678.
110. Jewish Board of Guardians, *Conditioned Environment in Case Work Treatment*, 13.
111. Ibid., 676.
112. Joan Beck, "Can 'Bad Kids' Be Saved?," K19.
113. "Bad Boy's Story," *Life*, May 12, 1947, 111, 113.
114. Alt, *Residential Treatment for the Disturbed Child*, 85.
115. Eliot, *Not the Thing I Was*, 83.
116. Ibid., 138. It is not clear if Diana's departure was required because she had gotten married. I have not identified RTCs that required women staff members to be single, and of course RTCs with cottage parents employed married couples.
117. Ibid., 84.
118. Lourie and Schulman, "The Role of the Residential Staff in Residential Treatment," 805.
119. Alt, *Residential Treatment for the Disturbed Child*, 90.
120. Crumpacker, "The Caseworker as Residential Worker," 61. Punctuation is as appears in the original.
121. "Volunteer Workshops Underway," in *Bellefaire Bulletin* 1, no. 2 (February 1953): 2, Container 18, Folder 4, BA.
122. "Suggestions to Improve Individual Big Brother Assignments," 1944, Container 1, Folder 10, BA, 1; "Big Sister Shopping Service Manual," effective January 15, 1958; "Teen-Agers Put on Fashion Show," *Bellefaire Bulletin* 2, no. 1 (Fall 1953): 1, Container 18, Folder 4, BA.
123. "Bellefaire," late 1940s, Container 19, Folder 7, BA, 3.
124. Crumpacker, "The Caseworker as Residential Worker," 8; Otten and Seib, "The Case of the Furious Children," 60.
125. Reid and Hagan, *Residential Treatment of Emotionally Disturbed Children*, 291.
126. Burmeister, *Roofs for the Family*, 181.
127. Ibid., 193.
128. American Psychiatric Association, *Psychiatric Inpatient Treatment of Children*, 39–40.
129. Bettelheim, *Love Is Not Enough*, 17.
130. Morris F. Mayer, "Some Problems Relative to the Cottage Parent," in "Some Problems in Group Care Treatment: Round Table 1951," *American Journal of Orthopsychiatry* 22, no. 1 (January 1952): 105–6.
131. J. Franklin Robinson, Anabel Maxwell, and Kathryn E. Dominguez, "Resident Psychiatric Treatment with Children," *American Journal of Orthopsychiatry* 17, no. 3 (July 1947): 465.
132. Burmeister, *Roofs for the Family*, 45–48.

133. By the 1950s, the Children's Bureau was urging training schools to avoid locations that were too rural. In a 1954 booklet titled *Tentative Standards for Training Schools* (U.S. Dept. of Health, Education, and Welfare, Social Security Administration, Children's Bureau, 1954), superintendent of the Illinois Training School for Boys (and later of the RTC High Meadows in Connecticut) Charles Leonard argued that training schools in rural areas had difficulty hiring and retaining high-quality staff members, especially clinical ones, and that their location made visits from family members difficult, if not impossible (21). Even a 1962 Children's Bureau publication, also written by Leonard, urged training schools to interact more with the communities around them, even if just by letting the public visit during special events or speaking openly with members of the press (U.S. Children's Bureau, in cooperation with the National Association of Training Schools and Juvenile Agencies, *Institutions Serving Delinquent Children: Guides and Goals*, 2nd ed. [Washington, DC: Government Printing Office, 1962], 33).

134. Alt, *Residential Treatment for the Disturbed Child*, 9, 32, 56.

135. Milton J. E. Senn, "Interview with Dr. Maurice Laufer, May 27, 1978 in Providence, R.I.," Box 3, Folder 2, NLM, 7.

136. "Annual Report of the Southard School (1940)," Box 1.1, Southard School. Annual Reports, 1939–46, KSHS, 14; "Executive Committee Meeting—November 15, 1941," Box 1.1, Southard School Corp. Executive Comm., Notes, 1931–46, KSHS, 1.

137. Alt, *Residential Treatment for the Disturbed Child*, 9, 32, 56.

138. Senn, "Interview with Dr. Maurice Laufer," 7; "Annual Report of the Southard School (1940)," Box 1.1, Southard School, Annual Reports, 1939–46, KSHS, 14–15.

139. American Psychiatric Association, *Psychiatric Inpatient Treatment of Children*, 14.

140. Ibid.

141. *The First Annual Report of the Arthur Brisbane Child Treatment Center at Allaire for the Year Ending June 30, 1948* (Allaire, NJ: The Center, 1948), 5.

142. When one such conference was offered at the University of Michigan in 1953, the faculty organizers expected 150 participants but were surprised to find "560 at the luncheon meeting alone with a total attendance of approximately 700" (Raymond W. Waggoner to Robert Felix, September 29, 1953, Box 2, Emotionally Disturbed Children Conference, 1953, UM). Southard School had offered a similar program in 1939, just as the center was turning its attention away from intellectual disability and toward emotional disturbance ("Southard School Mental Hygiene Institute," *Bulletin of the Menninger Clinic* 3, no. 5 [September 1939]: 157–59).

143. "Annual Report, Department of Child Psychiatry of the Menninger Foundation," July 1, 1951 to July 1, 1953, Box 1, Annual Reports—1952–56, KSHS, 18–19, 33, 35; untitled timeline, n.d., Switzer 118-8-4-3 Subject File A-C, Community Child Psychiatry in Topeka, RES; "Interview of Edward David Greenwood, by Spafford Ackerly, October 20, 1972," UL.

144. Ackerly, "Interview of Edward David Greenwood," 21.

145. *More Than Half a Chance*, brochure, 1952(?), Container 19, Folder 7, BA.

146. Ibid.

147. "Bellefaire Annual Report," 1952–53, Container 7, Folder 2, BA, 4.

148. "We Are Celebrating," in *Bellefaire Voice and Views* (Spring 1958): 2, Container 18, Folder 4, BA.

149. *Focus on Sanity*, no. 1, rebroadcast June 25, 1958 on KNXT Los Angeles (original broadcast date July 17, 1957), UCLA.

150. Ibid.

151. *Focus on Sanity*, episode titled "Mentally Disturbed Children," no. 4, rebroadcast July 16, 1958 on KNXT Los Angeles (original broadcast date August 7, 1957), UCLA.
152. Krug, "Child Guidance Home—1958," 573; Reid and Hagan, *Residential Treatment of Emotionally Disturbed Children*, 56.
153. *The First Annual Report of the Arthur Brisbane Child Treatment Center*, 5.
154. Reid and Hagan, *Residential Treatment of Emotionally Disturbed Children*, 256–57.
155. Norma H. Goodhue, "Group Aids Camarillo Children," *Los Angeles Times*, July 23, 1954, B1.
156. Martin Gula, "Study and Treatment Homes for Troubled Children," *Child* 12, no. 5 (November 1947): 69; Morris F. Mayer, "Report of the Head Resident," June 15, 1947, in "Bellefaire Minutes Board of Trustees," June 15, 1947, Container 7, Folder 1, BA, 2–3; J. Franklin Robinson, "Educational Procedures in a Resident Setting," pt. 6 of "Symposium, 1953: The Education of Emotionally Disturbed Children," *American Journal of Orthopsychiatry* 23, no. 4 (1953): 704; J. Franklin Robinson, Anabel Maxwell, and Kathryn E. Dominguez, "Resident Psychiatric Treatment with Children," *American Journal of Orthopsychiatry* 17, no. 3 (July 1947): 458, 463.
157. Martin Gula, "Study and Treatment Homes for Troubled Children," 69.
158. Milton J. E. Senn, "Interview with Dr. Frank J. Curran, January 12, 1978 in New York City," Box 2, Folder 3, NLM, 19.
159. Reported the CWLA's Reid and Hagan of Hawthorne Cedar Knolls: "Following an incident, such as a serious theft by a child, there may be some resentment demonstrated in the community to which, it was reported, the staff always give serious attention and find the community responsive to their interpretation" (*Residential Treatment of Emotionally Disturbed Children*, 143).
160. "Wiltwyck School for Boys, Report of the Executive Director to the Board of Directors, July 1951 to June (May) 1952," Box 4, Folder 57, WR, 4.
161. Ibid., 6.
162. "Wiltwyck School for Boys, Inc., Report of the Executive Director to the Board of Directors, March 14, 1955," Box 4, Folder 60, WR, 2.
163. James P. Fitzgerald, "Annual Report and Evaluation of Summer Program," April 29, 1967, Box 43, Folder 1049, WR, 1.
164. "Wiltwyck School for Boys, Report—November, 1967," Box 44, Folder 1073, WR, 2.
165. "Case in Point," *Bellefaire Voice and Views* (Spring 1958), 2, Container 18, Folder 4, BA.
166. Reid and Hagan, *Residential Treatment of Emotionally Disturbed Children*, 70–71.
167. Ibid., 137.
168. On the Arthur Brisbane Child Treatment Center in New Jersey and University of Michigan child psychiatry unit, see ibid., 19, 233. For the Children's Service Center of Wyoming Valley and Southard School, see ibid., 92, 301.
169. American Psychiatric Association, *Psychiatric Inpatient Treatment of Children*, 46–47.
170. "Wiltwyck School for Boys, Income Budget," Box 4, Folder 58, WR.

CHAPTER 6

1. Report of Executive Director, in Bellefaire minutes of the Annual meeting held July 1, 1951, Container 7, Folder 2, BA, 8.
2. Herschel Alt, *Residential Treatment for the Disturbed Child: Basic Principles in Planning and Design of Programs and Facilities* (New York: International Universities Press, 1960), 361.

3. Barbara J. Betz, "A Psychiatric Children's Ward," *American Journal of Nursing* 45, no. 10 (October 1945): 818–19; Bruno Bettelheim and Benjamin Wright, "The Role of Residential Treatment for Children Symposium, 1954," pt. 8, "Staff Development in a Treatment Institution," *American Journal of Orthopsychiatry* 25, no. 4 (October 1955): 668; Lauretta Bender, "Group Activities on a Children's Ward as Methods of Psychotherapy," *American Journal of Psychiatry* 93, no. 5 (March 1, 1937): 1159; Charles Bradley, "Education in a Children's Psychiatric Hospital," *Nervous Child* 3 (1944): 329; Gisela Konopka, "The Role of Residential Treatment for Children Symposium, 1954," pt. 4, "The Role of the Group in Residential Treatment," *American Journal of Orthopsychiatry* 25, no. 4 (1955): 684; Fritz Redl and David Wineman, *Children Who Hate: The Disorganization and Breakdown of Behavior Controls* (Glencoe IL.: Free Press, 1951), 68–69.
4. See Steven Mintz, *Huck's Raft: A History of American Childhood* (Cambridge, MA: Belknap Press of Harvard University Press, 2004), chap. 14; Rebecca Jo Plant, *Mom: The Transformation of Motherhood in Modern America* (Chicago: University of Chicago Press, 2010).
5. Ken Smith, *Mental Hygiene: Classroom Films, 1945–1970* (New York: Blast Books, 1999).
6. Anna G. Creadick, *Perfectly Average: The Pursuit of Normality in Postwar America* (Amherst: University of Massachusetts Press, 2010).
7. Jackson Lears, "A Matter of Taste: Corporate Cultural Hegemony in a Mass-Consumption Society," in *Recasting America: Culture and Politics in the Age of Cold War*, ed. Lary May (Chicago: University of Chicago Press, 1989).
8. Jamie Cohen-Cole, "The Creative American: Cold War Salons, Social Science, and the Cure for Modern Society," *Isis* 100, no. 2 (June 1, 2009): 219–62.
9. Ibid., 219.
10. When writing about children, historians have had particular difficulty representing their subjects' points of view, especially because sources produced by children are difficult to find and remembrances from later life are problematic. Those that do exist have often been produced by adolescents, on whom a good deal of research has been done (see, e.g., Heather Munro Prescott, *A Doctor of Their Own: The History of Adolescent Medicine* [Cambridge, MA: Harvard University Press, 1998]). Because of these limitations, it has been difficult to go beyond what adults have thought about or done to children. Histories of children's health in particular tend to focus on the role of medical experts and parents, despite calls for attention to children's own experiences (Russell Viner and Janet Golden, "Children's Experiences of Illness," in *Medicine in the Twentieth Century*, ed. Roger Cooter and John Pickstone [London: Harwood International, 2001], 575–88). A small number of books have already attempted to do this. Most successfully, Chris Feudtner's *Bittersweet*, a history of Type I diabetes, uses extensive sets of correspondence between young patients and their doctor, Elliott Joslin, to demonstrate how insulin, a panacea to many, could also cause significant disruption in a child's life (*Bittersweet: Diabetes, Insulin, and the Transformation of Illness* [Chapel Hill: University of North Carolina Press, 2003]).
11. Vera Kare, "A Study of the Adjustment of a 'Problem' Child in a Group Therapy Home for Pre-Delinquent Boys, Pioneer House, September, 1946–June, 1948." (MSW thesis, Wayne University, 1948), 47. Kare used pseudonyms for all the children she discussed.
12. Kare, "A Study of the Adjustment of a 'Problem' Child," 45.

13. Arthur Mandelbaum, "Description of the Southard School: Conference on Inpatient Psychiatric Treatment for Children," Box 16, Children's Div. 1956, KSHS, 27.
14. William C. Morse, ed., *Crisis Intervention in Residential Treatment: The Clinical Innovations of Fritz Redl* (New York: Haworth Press, 1991), 5; see chap. 3 for a fuller discussion of the life-space interview.
15. Fritz Redl, "New Ways of Ego Support in Residential Treatment of Disturbed Children," *Bulletin of the Menninger Clinic* 13, no. 2 (March 1949): 62.
16. Bruno Bettelheim, *Love Is Not Enough: The Treatment of Emotionally Disturbed Children* (Glencoe, IL: Free Press, 1950), 34.
17. *Child Care Handbook*, May 1957, Child Psychiatry Service of the Menninger Clinic, the Menninger Foundation, Box 6, *Child Care Handbook*, May 1957, KSHS," 7.
18. Bender, "Group Activities on a Children's Ward," 1155; Bettelheim, *Love Is Not Enough*, chap. 7.
19. *Child Care Handbook*, May 1957, 8.
20. Bettelheim, *Love Is Not Enough*, 176–78; Stephen Eliot, *Not the Thing I Was: Thirteen Years at Bruno Bettelheim's Orthogenic School* (New York: St. Martin's Press, 2003), 35.
21. "Conference on In-Patient Psychiatric Treatment for Children, Background Material for Preparatory Committees on Personnel and Treatment," April 24, 1956, Box 1, Folder 5, LB, 5.
22. "Handbook for Parents (Early 1950s?)," Box 3, folder titled "Handbook for Parents, 1950s," KSHS, 17.
23. Joseph H. Reid and Helen R. Hagan, *Residential Treatment of Emotionally Disturbed Children: A Descriptive Study* (New York: Child Welfare League of America, 1952), 236.
24. Bettelheim, *Love Is Not Enough*, 173.
25. Ibid., 174–75.
26. Isaac Zeke Youcha, "A Study of Schizophrenic Children in Cottage Life at the Hawthorne Cedar Knolls School" (master's thesis, New York School of Social Work, Columbia University, 1953), 21.
27. Bettelheim, *Love Is Not Enough*, 190–91.
28. In the examples from the Orthogenic School, Bettelheim analyzed records kept by residential workers, which he cited in *Love is Not Enough*.
29. Howard Whitman, "Spare the Child," *Collier's*, August 2, 1947, 12. The most egregious events were reported in the popular press. In 1948, three boys at Bellevue climbed over the protective fence of their rooftop playground and walked around the ledge of the hospital building. The arrival of multiple fire trucks excited them more, and they were persuaded to come back inside only after a teacher climbed over the fence and offered them as many lollipops as they wanted ("Lollipops Lure Boys to Safety," *New York Times*, 1948; "3 Boy Patients Frolic on Ledge Eight Floors Up," *New York Herald*, October 15, 1948, Box 17, File 11, LB; "Coax 3 Boys off Hospital Ledge," *News*, October 15, 1948, Box 17, File 11, LB).
30. Suzy, 2/24/60, 10:30pm, Change of Shift Log, July 1958–July 1961, Box 7.3, KSHS.
31. Beth, 11pm, 11/27[/60], ibid.
32. Phyl Fry, March 14th [1960], ibid.
33. Phyl Fry, 4/12/60, ibid.
34. Lee Stringer, *Sleepaway School: Stories from a Boy's Life* (New York: Seven Stories Press, 2004), 84–86.
35. Marvin Bloom and Adrian Cabral, "A Description of a Newly Introduced Group Work Program in a Residential Treatment Setting—the Hawthorne Cedar Knolls

School" (master's thesis, New York School of Social Work, Columbia University, 1954), 44.

36. Ibid.
37. Ibid., 46.
38. Suzy + Roy, 3/22[/60], Change of Shift Log.
39. "Using a Group to Help a Child," Box 7.3, Residential Treatment of Children, KSHS, 11–12.
40. Bender, "Group Activities on a Children's Ward," 1151.
41. Solomon E. Asch, "Effects of Group Pressure upon the Modification and Distortion of Judgments," in *Groups, Leadership and Men: Research in Human Relations*, ed. Harold Guetzkow (Pittsburgh: Carnegie Press, 1951); Solomon E. Asch, "Opinions and Social Pressure," *Scientific American* 193, no. 2 (November 1955): 31–35.
42. Morris Fritz Meyer, "Annual Report of the Resident Director," in "Minutes, September 11, 1955," Container 7, Folder 2, BA, 5.
43. Reid and Hagan, *Residential Treatment of Emotionally Disturbed Children*, 158.
44. "A School for Problem Children," *Life*, March 14, 1938, 52.
45. Douglas W. Orr, "Notes on the Psychoanalytic Orientation of the Southard School," *Bulletin of the Menninger Clinic* 3 (1939): 85.
46. Though the group was "spontaneously" formed, the children were no doubt influenced by the military images and propaganda with which all Americans were confronted during World War II.
47. Helen A. Sutton, "Some Nursing Aspects of a Children's Psychiatric Ward," *American Journal of Orthopsychiatry* 17, no. 4 (1947): 678.
48. Bettelheim, *Love Is Not Enough*, 50.
49. There is very little scholarship on the history of group therapy; most of it is written by practitioners and traces its origins to a diverse set of largely psychoanalytic practitioners in the 1920s, 1930s, and 1940s. See e.g., Scott Simon Fehr, *Introduction to Group Therapy: A Practical Guide* (New York: Haworth Press, 1999); Diane Gibson, *Group Process and Structure in Psychosocial Occupational Therapy* (New York: Haworth Press, 1988); Bill Roller, "Group Therapy Marks Fiftieth Birthday," *Small Group Research* 17, no. 4 (November 1986): 472–74.
50. Kathleen K. Stewart and Pearl L. Axelrod, "Group Therapy on a Children's Psychiatric Ward," *American Journal of Orthopsychiatry* 17, no. 2 (1947): 312–25.
51. Bloom and Cabral, "A Description of a Newly Introduced Group Work Program," 35.
52. Ibid., 56.
53. Ibid., 35.
54. *The First Annual Report of the Arthur Brisbane Child Treatment Center at Allaire for the Year Ending June 30, 1948* (Allaire, NJ: The Center, 1948), 2–3.
55. Reid and Hagan, *Residential Treatment of Emotionally Disturbed Children*, 1952, 35; Meyer, "Annual Report of the Resident Director," in Minutes, September 11, 1955; "Arnold talks about ACTIVITIES," in "So you'll know all about . . . Bellefaire," 22–30, "322 Recreation," Container 1, Folder 11, BA.
56. "Arnold talks about ACTIVITIES," 22.
57. Southard School Journalism Class, *Don't Forget the Children: A History of Southard School, 1926–1986* (Topeka, KS: Menninger Foundation, 1986), 23.
58. Reid and Hagan, *Residential Treatment of Emotionally Disturbed Children*, 237.
59. Kare, "A Study of the Adjustment of a 'Problem' Child," 9.
60. See Howard P. Chudacoff, *Children at Play: An American History* (New York: New York University Press, 2007), chaps. 4–6.

61. Illinois Children's Home and Aid Society, *Plans for an Institution for the Treatment of Emotionally Disturbed Children* (Chicago: Illinois Children's Home and Aid Society, 1946), 16; Edward Linn, "Wiltwyck: Home of the Wild Ones," *Reader's Digest*, condensed from *New York World-Telegram* and *Sun Saturday Feature Magazine*, February 1958, 194.
62. Bettelheim, *Love Is Not Enough*, 218; Bradley, "Education in a Children's Psychiatric Hospital," 334; Meyer, "Annual Report of the Resident Director," in Minutes, September 11, 1955, 4; "Report to the Menninger Foundation on the Activities of the Southard School," October 6, 1942, Box 1.1, Southard School Corp. Executive Comm., Notes, 1931–46, KSHS, 2.
63. Annual Report (untitled), 1946, Box 1.1, Southard School Annual Reports, 1939–46, 6.
64. Milton J. E. Senn, "Interview with Dr. Maurice Laufer, May 27, 1978 in Providence, R.I." n.d., Box 3, Folder 2, NLM., 7.
65. Reid and Hagan, *Residential Treatment of Emotionally Disturbed Children*, 1952, 10.
66. Ibid., 154.
67. Ibid., 238.
68. Ibid., 105–6, 238, 291.
69. Ibid., 60.
70. Ralph D. Rabinovitch, Janet Bee, and Barbara Outwater, "The Integration of Occupational and Recreational Therapy in the Residential Psychiatric Treatment of Children: A Symposium," *American Journal of Occupational Therapy* 5, no. 1 (1951): 2–3.
71. New generations of toys for children and a growing teen consumer culture reinforced seemingly essential differences between boys and girls and reflected the kind of adults they were ultimately supposed to become (Mintz, *Huck's Raft*, 283–86).
72. Alt, *Residential Treatment for the Disturbed Child*, 377.
73. Ibid.
74. Ibid., 395.
75. Ibid., 385–86.
76. Ibid., 395–96.
77. Ibid., 397–99.
78. Ibid., 406–8.
79. Ibid., 410–11.
80. "Children's Hospital Psychiatric Unit Conference Notes," November 25, 1953, Box 2, Planning Committee, 1953–56, RW, 1–2.
81. "Children's Hospital Psychiatric Unit Conference Notes," December 2, 1953, Box 2, Planning Committee, 1953–56, RW.
82. "Report of the Building Committee, Department of Child Psychiatry," July 1, 1956, Box 16, Annual Report and Annual Meeting 1956–57, KSHS, 8.
83. "Southard School, Children's Division of Menninger Foundation," Box 1.1, Southard School Corp., Executive Comm., Notes, 1931–46, KSHS, 1; Reid and Hagan, *Residential Treatment of Emotionally Disturbed Children*, 291.
84. Frank J. Curran, "Art and the Problem Child," Box 17, File 9, LB, 2–3; Rabinovitch, Bee, and Outwater, "The Integration of Occupational and Recreational Therapy," 4.
85. Rabinovitch, Bee, and Outwater, "The Integration of Occupational and Recreational Therapy," 4.
86. Curran, "Art and the Problem Child," 2; Lauretta Bender, "Art and Therapy in the Mental Disturbances of Children," *Journal of Nervous and Mental Disease* 86, no. 3 (1937): 251.

87. Untitled Southard School pamphlet, ca. 1938, obtained from Sterling Memorial Library, Yale University.
88. Bender, "Art and Therapy in the Mental Disturbances of Children," 251. Ralph Rabinovitch of the University of Michigan offers a description of the craft shop: "A warm, informal atmosphere is strived for and the closeness of physical contact aids in this. The general tone is relaxed and usually fairly gay with spontaneous singing, joking and imaginative play" (Rabinovitch, Bee, and Outwater, "The Integration of Occupational and Recreational Therapy," 3).
89. C. F. Menninger to Sidney Vere Smith, July 8, 1936, Box 1.1, Correspondence: Shaw, Ruth Faison, 1936–38, 1947, KSHS, 1–2.
90. Veronica Mayer, "Rediscovering Ruth Faison Shaw and Her Finger-Painting Method," *Art Education* 58, no. 5 (2005): 6–11; Mary Ann Stankiewicz, "Self-Expression or Teacher Influence: The Shaw System of Finger-Painting," *Art Education* 37, no. 2 (March 1984): 20–24. On the history of art in education, see Foster Wygant, *School Art in American Culture, 1820–1970* (Cincinnati, OH: Interwood Press, 1993).
91. Eva E. Burmeister, *Roofs for the Family* (New York: Columbia University Press, 1954), 22–24, 31.
92. Rabinovitch, Bee, and Outwater, "The Integration of Occupational and Recreational Therapy," 4.
93. Jeanetta Lyle and Ruth Faison Shaw, "Encouraging Fantasy Expression in Children," *Bulletin of the Menninger Clinic* 1, no. 3 (1937): 78–79.
94. Ibid., 79–80.
95. Lydia Hylton, *The Residential Treatment Center: Children, Programs, and Costs* (New York: Child Welfare League of America, 1964), 24.
96. Reid and Hagan, Residential Treatment of Emotionally Disturbed Children, 1952, 242.
97. Bender, "Group Activities on a Children's Ward," 1160; Lauretta Bender and Adolf G. Woltmann, "The Use of Puppet Shows as a Psychotherapeutic Method for Behavior Problems in Children," *American Journal of Orthopsychiatry* 6, no. 3 (1936): 341–54; "'Beat Her Up!' Problem Child Yells to Puppet, Baring His Emotions," *New York World-Telegram*, February 29, 1936, Box 17, Folder 12, LB; "Now Willie's Pals Debate His 'Crimes,'" *New York Journal*, March 20, 1936, Box 7, File 12, LB; "Puppet Shows Used in Psychiatric Work," *New York Times*, March 10, 1936, Box 17, File 12, LB.
98. "'Beat Her Up!' Problem Child Yells."
99. Ibid.
100. "Puppet Show Used as Psychiatric Aid."
101. Bender and Woltmann, "The Use of Puppet Shows as a Psychotherapeutic Method," 352.
102. Susan Steel, "Music Therapy on Psychiatric Children's Ward," Box 17, File 9, LB, 3. On music therapy at Bellevue, also see Bender, "Group Activities on a Children's Ward," 1161–62; "The World of Science: Problem Children Swing to Normal after 'Treatment' with Rhythm and Song—Music Doctor's Aid," Saturday March 20, 1937, Box 17, File 8, LB; Frances McFarland to Lauretta Bender, February 15, 1937, Box 17, File 9, LB.
103. Steel, "Music Therapy on Psychiatric Children's Ward," 2.
104. 8/9/1946 Summary, Music therapy handwritten daily notes, 1946, Box 7, File 9, LB.
105. 7/16/46, Music therapy handwritten daily notes.
106. 8/9/1946 Summary, Music therapy handwritten daily notes.

107. Ibid.

108. *The Seventh Annual Report of the Arthur Brisbane Child Treatment Center at Allaire for the Year Ending June 30, 1954* (Allaire, NJ: The Center, 1954), 1; Reid and Hagan, *Residential Treatment of Emotionally Disturbed Children*, 240.

109. "Handbook for Parents," 9; Alt, *Residential Treatment for the Disturbed Child*, 102–4.

110. Bradley, "Education in a Children's Psychiatric Hospital," 333.

111. Robert L. Osgood, *The History of Inclusion in the United States* (Washington, DC: Gallaudet University Press, 2005), 36–42; Robert L. Osgood, *The History of Special Education: A Struggle for Equality in American Public Schools* (Westport, CT: Praeger, 2008), 84.

112. M. A. Winzer, *From Integration to Inclusion: A History of Special Education in the 20th Century* (Washington, DC: Gallaudet University Press, 2009), 129–30.

113. Kathleen W. Jones, "Education for Children with Mental Retardation: Parent Activism, Public Policy, and Family Ideology in the 1950s," in *Mental Retardation in America: A Historical Reader*, ed. Steven Noll and James W. Trent (New York: New York University Press, 2004), 322–50; and Katherine Castles, "'Nice, Average Americans': Postwar Parents' Groups and the Defense of the Normal Family," in *Mental Retardation in America*, ed. Noll and Trent, 351–70.

114. Osgood, *The History of Inclusion in the United States*, 76–79.

115. These RTCs included the Cincinnati Guidance Home, Evanston Receiving Home, Lakeside Children's Center, Pioneer House, and Children's Service Center of Wyoming Valley (Burmeister, *Roofs for the Family*, 61; Othilda Krug, "A Concept of Education in the Residential Treatment of Emotionally Disturbed Children," pt. 5 of "Symposium, 1953: The Education of Emotionally Disturbed Children," *American Journal of Orthopsychiatry* 23, no. 4 (1953): 694; Reid and Hagan, *Residential Treatment of Emotionally Disturbed Children*, 133; J. Franklin Robinson, Anabel Maxwell, and Kathryn E. Dominguez, "Resident Psychiatric Treatment with Children," *American Journal of Orthopsychiatry* 17, no. 3 (July 1947): 458; Barbara L. Smith, "Programming in a Treatment Home for Disturbed Children: An Analysis of Programming at Pioneer House from December 1, 1946 to June 1, 1947, Evaluating the Relationship of Program Activities to Individual and Group Developments" (MSW thesis, Wayne University, 1948), 13).

116. These RTCs included the Bradley Hospital, Arthur Brisbane Child Treatment Center, Camarillo State Hospital, Illinois Neuropsychiatric Institute, Langley Porter, University of Michigan, National Institutes of Health, New York State Psychiatric Institute, the Orthogenic School, Southard School, and Wiltwyck. *The Second Annual Report of the Arthur Brisbane Child Treatment Center at Allaire for the Year Ending June 30, 1949* (Allaire, NJ: The Center, 1949), 4; Mandelbaum, "Description of the Southard School," 29; "Wiltwyck's Unquiet Ones," *Newsweek*, January 31, 1949; Bradley, "Education in a Children's Psychiatric Hospital"; Otis Chandler, "Bewildered Children Await Camarillo Mental Therapy," *Los Angeles Times*, August 26, 1955, 2; Anne Benjamin and Howard E. Weatherly, "Hospital Ward Treatment of Emotionally Disturbed Children," *American Journal of Orthopsychiatry* 17, no. 4 (October 1947): 666; Bettelheim, *Love Is Not Enough*; Claude Brown, *Manchild in the Promised Land* (New York: Macmillan, 1965), 74; Samuel Finestone and Toby Bennett Bieber, "Status at Discharge and Follow-up of Twenty Children with Diagnosis of Primary Behavior Disorder Hospitalized at New York State Psychiatric Institute and Hospital" (master's thesis, New York School of Social Work, Columbia University, 1946), 9; Ursula Weiss Moore, "A Study of Children with Primary Behavior

Disorders Treated at Langley Porter Clinic: Results of In-Patient and Out-Patient Care." (MSW thesis, University of California, Berkeley, 1949), 35; Harold L. Raush, Allen T. Dittmann, and Thaddeus J. Taylor, "The Interpersonal Behavior of Children in Residential Treatment," *Journal of Abnormal and Social Psychology* 58, no. 1 (1959): 10; Reid and Hagan, *Residential Treatment of Emotionally Disturbed Children*, 239; Raymond W. Waggoner and Ralph D. Rabinovitch, "The University of Michigan Plan for the Residential Treatment of Disturbed Children," *Medical Bulletin* 22, no. 3 (1956): 1210.

117. "Conference on In-Patient Psychiatric Treatment for Children, Background Material for Preparatory Committees on Personnel and Treatment," 8–9; Bloom and Cabral, "A Description of a Newly Introduced Group Work Program," 5; Jewish Board of Guardians, *Conditioned Environment in Case Work Treatment: A Monograph of Articles on Hawthorne-Cedar Knolls School, Lavenburg Corner House* (New York: Jewish Board of Guardians, 1944), 35.
118. M. F. Mayer and C. M. Wolfenstein, "Diagnostic Criteria for Intramural and Extramural Schooling of Disturbed Children in a Residential Treatment Center," *American Journal of Orthopsychiatry* 24, no. 2 (1954): 351–67; "Bellefaire Minutes of the Annual Meeting held July 1, 1951," Container 7, Folder 2, BA, 5, 7; Bellefaire Annual Report 1952–53, Container 7, Folder 2, BA, 2; Alan S. Geismer, "Annual Report of the President, September 11, 1955," in Minutes, September 11, 1955, Container 7, Folder 2, BA, 3; Morris Fritz Meyer, "Annual Report of the Resident Director," 3–4; "Minutes (September 30, 1956)," Container 7, Folder 2, BA, 3.
119. Reid and Hagan, *Residential Treatment of Emotionally Disturbed Children*, 11–12, 108–9; James D. Newman, "A Descriptive Study of Emma Pendleton Bradley Hospital" (Specialist in Education thesis, George Peabody College for Teachers, 1964), 47–48.
120. Bettelheim, *Love Is Not Enough*, 169; Shirley Camper, "A Follow-up Study of Children Discharged from a Psychiatric Ward," pt. 2, "Factors in Treatment" (MSS thesis, Smith College School for Social Work, 1946), 30; "Conference on In-Patient Psychiatric Treatment for Children, Background Material for Preparatory Committees on Personnel and Treatment," 8.
121. Bradley, "Education in a Children's Psychiatric Hospital," 333.
122. Ibid., 333–34; "Handbook for Parents," 9.
123. Camper, "A Follow-up Study of Children Discharged from a Psychiatric Ward," 31.
124. Ibid., 19, 31–32.
125. Leonard Kornberg, *A Class for Disturbed Children: A Case Study and Its Meaning for Education* (New York: Bureau of Publications, Teachers College, Columbia University, 1955), 50; Alt, *Residential Treatment for the Disturbed Child*, 109–10.
126. Bettelheim, *Love Is Not Enough*, 135.
127. Alt, *Residential Treatment for the Disturbed Child*, 114.
128. Kornberg, *A Class for Disturbed Children*, 109–10. Kornberg was also a student at the Columbia University Teachers' College; he went on to become a professor of education at Queens College (A. Harry Passow, ed., *Education in Depressed Areas* [New York: Teachers College Press, 1963], ix, http://archive.org/details/educationindepre028394mbp).
129. Alt, *Residential Treatment for the Disturbed Child*, 113.
130. Bettelheim, *Love Is Not Enough*, 134.
131. Ibid., 142.
132. Ibid., 144.
133. Ibid., 142–44.

134. Albert Deutsch, *Our Rejected Children* (Boston: Little, Brown, 1950), 15, 21–33, 42–43, 48–50.
135. Brown, *Manchild in the Promised Land*, 85.
136. "Wiltwyck's Unquiet Ones."
137. Linn, "Wiltwyck: Home of the Wild Ones," 195.
138. Alt, *Residential Treatment for the Disturbed Child*, 24–25.
139. Reid and Hagan, *Residential Treatment of Emotionally Disturbed Children*, 36.
140. Ibid., 107.
141. "Freedom and Limits (Behavior Problems)," 1950s, Residential Treatment of Children, Box 7.3 KSHS, 9.
142. Reid and Hagan, *Residential Treatment of Emotionally Disturbed Children*, 239; *Child Care Handbook*, May 1957, 3.
143. Diana Kahn dictation, July 14, 1963, in Eliot, *Not the Thing I Was*, 277.
144. Robert E. Switzer, "Roles and Functions of Child Psychiatrists in Residential Treatment—What and How," 1962, SWITZER: Child Psychiatrists in the Residential Treatment of Children, 1963, RES, 29.
145. Ibid., 30.

INTERLUDE: HOMEWARD BOUND

1. Shirley Camper, "A Follow-up Study of Children Discharged from a Psychiatric Ward," pt. 2, "Factors in Treatment" (MSS thesis, Smith College School for Social Work, 1946), 38–39; Mary Faust, "The Parents' Role in a Child's Residential Treatment: A Dissertation Based upon an Investigation at the Institute for Juvenile Research, Chicago, Illinois" (MSS thesis, Smith College School for Social Work, 1949), 35–36.
2. Jean Collard, "A Statistical Description of the 186 Children Admitted to the Institutional Unit of the Ryther Child Center from October 1935 to October 1939" (MA thesis, University of Washington, 1946), 37; Joseph H. Reid and Helen R. Hagan, *Residential Treatment of Emotionally Disturbed Children: A Descriptive Study* (New York: Child Welfare League of America, 1952), 140.
3. Arthur Mandelbaum, "Description of the Southard School: Conference on Inpatient Psychiatric Treatment for Children," Box 16, Children's Div. 1956, KSHS, 39–40.
4. Reid and Hagan, *Residential Treatment of Emotionally Disturbed Children*, 89.
5. "Discharges," 1952, Container 7, Folder 2, BA, 6.
6. Ibid., 2.
7. "Conference on In-Patient Psychiatric Treatment for Children, Background Material for Preparatory Committees on Personnel and Treatment," April 24, 1956, Box 1, Folder 5, LB, 10; Reid and Hagan, *Residential Treatment of Emotionally Disturbed Children*, 114, 163–64, 214, 247; Mandelbaum, "Description of the Southard School," 36; Adah Jean Mears, "A Follow up Study of Students Who Were Discharged from the Southard School in the Period between January 1, 1940 and December 31, 1944" (MSW thesis, Washington University, 1945), 23.
8. "Discharges," in "Bellefaire Annual Report 1952–1953," Container 7, Folder 2, BA, 3.
9. "Conference on In-Patient Psychiatric Treatment for Children, Background Material for Preparatory Committees on Personnel and Treatment," 10; Helen M. Frostenson, "Familial Study of Nine Children Diagnosed as Schizophrenic in the Children's Ward at Bellevue Hospital" (master's thesis, New York School of Social Work,

Columbia University, 1944); Reid and Hagan, *Residential Treatment of Emotionally Disturbed Children*, 114. For example, in 1956 Lauretta Bender stated that 50 percent of children at Bellevue returned home while 12 percent went to state mental hospitals and 15 percent were discharged to schools for intellectually disabled children ("Conference on In-Patient Psychiatric Treatment for Children, Background Material for Preparatory Committees on Personnel and Treatment," 10).

10. "Discharges," in "Bellefaire Annual Report 1952–1953," Container 7, Folder 2, BA: 2; Reid and Hagan, *Residential Treatment of Emotionally Disturbed Children*, 44, 163–64, 214, 247. Reid and Hagan stated of Hawthorne that most children were discharged home "even though this is not always the agency's plan for them," implying that the child's and family's wishes at times overrode those of the RTC (*Residential Treatment of Emotionally Disturbed Children*, 164).
11. Mandelbaum, "Description of the Southard School," 41; Reid and Hagan, *Residential Treatment of Emotionally Disturbed Children*, 114.
12. Reid and Hagan, *Residential Treatment of Emotionally Disturbed Children*, 41, 91.
13. Ibid., 69, 214, 248; "Children's Psychiatric Hospital," n.d., Box 2: General, 1956–60, RW.
14. Herschel Alt, *Residential Treatment for the Disturbed Child: Basic Principles in Planning and Design of Programs and Facilities* (New York: International Universities Press, 1960), 81–82; Samuel Lerner, "Selective Criteria for Admission to Hawthorne-Cedar Knolls School: A Dissertation Based upon an Investigation at the Jewish Board of Guardians, New York City" (MSS thesis, Smith College School for Social Work, 1947), 19–20; Reid and Hagan, *Residential Treatment of Emotionally Disturbed Children*, 166.
15. Lerner, "Selective Criteria for Admission to Hawthorne-Cedar Knolls School," 21; Reid and Hagan, *Residential Treatment of Emotionally Disturbed Children*, 166.
16. Helen A. Sutton, "Some Nursing Aspects of a Children's Psychiatric Ward," *American Journal of Orthopsychiatry* 17, no. 4 (1947): 678.
17. Robin Bennett, personal communication with the author, August 3, 2010.
18. Lee Stringer, *Sleepaway School: Stories from a Boy's Life* (New York: Seven Stories Press, 2004), 222.
19. Claude Brown, *Manchild in the Promised Land* (New York: Macmillan, 1965), 119.
20. Ibid., 120.
21. See Brown, *Manchild in the Promised Land*, chaps. 4 and 5.
22. On the history of adjustment in American psychiatry, see S. D. Lamb, *Pathologist of the Mind: Adolf Meyer and the Origins of American Psychiatry* (Baltimore, MD: Johns Hopkins University Press, 2014).
23. Anne Benjamin and Howard E. Weatherly, "Hospital Ward Treatment of Emotionally Disturbed Children," *American Journal of Orthopsychiatry* 17, no. 4 (October 1947): 668.
24. Bruno Herbert, "Factors Influencing the Later Adjustment of Girls Discharged from the Hawthorne-Cedar Knolls School: A Dissertation Based upon an Investigation at the Jewish Board of Guardians, New York City" (MSS thesis, Smith College School for Social Work, 1946), 43.
25. Ibid., 44.
26. Lillian J. Johnson and Joseph H. Reid, *Evaluation of Ten Years Work with Emotionally Disturbed Children* (Seattle: Ryther Child Center, 1947), 8.
27. Ibid., 10.

28. Ibid., 12.
29. Benjamin and Weatherly, "Hospital Ward Treatment of Emotionally Disturbed Children," 668.
30. John G. Milner, "The Residential Treatment Center," *Annals of the American Academy of Political and Social Science* 355, no. 1 (1964): 101; Camper, "A Follow-up Study of Children Discharged from a Psychiatric Ward," 2.
31. Camper, "A Follow-up Study of Children Discharged from a Psychiatric Ward," 52.
32. Ibid., 59–60.
33. Johnson and Reid, *Evaluation of Ten Years Work with Emotionally Disturbed Children,* 4.
34. Othilda Krug, "Child Guidance Home—1958," *Cincinnati Journal of Medicine* 39 (1958): 573.
35. Reid and Hagan, *Residential Treatment of Emotionally Disturbed Children,* 165.
36. Eunice Mary Leitch, "The Southard School Annual Report," 1944, Box 1.1, Southard School Annual Reports, 1949–46, 3.
37. John B. Geisel, "The Southard School Annual Report," 1945, Box 1.1, Southard School Annual Reports, 1939–46, 6; Edward D. Greenwood, untitled annual report, 1946, Box 1.1, Southard School Annual Reports, 1949–46, 3.
38. C. F. Ramsay to Raymond W. Waggoner, October 25, 1948, Box 4, Children's Centers, 1946–4?, RW.
39. "Minutes," Board of Trustees meeting, July 18, 1948, Container 7, Folder 1, BA, 5.
40. "Goodbye from [Jacob]," *Bellefaire Bulletin* 1, no. 1 (Fall 1952): 4, Container 18, Folder 4, BA.
41. Edward Linn, "Wiltwyck: Home of the Wild Ones," *Reader's Digest,* condensed from the *New York World-Telegram and Sun Saturday Feature Magazine,* February 1958, 196.
42. Child Welfare League of America and the Council of Jewish Federations and Welfare Funds, "Bellefaire Survey, 1952–1953," Container 19, Folder 4, BA, 54.
43. Johnson and Reid, *Evaluation of Ten Years Work with Emotionally Disturbed Children,* 14.
44. Stephen Eliot, *Not the Thing I Was: Thirteen Years at Bruno Bettelheim's Orthogenic School* (New York: St. Martin's Press, 2003), 103.
45. Ibid.
46. Doctor Easson to Doctor Switzer, Doctor Hirschberg and Doctor Morrow, March 23, 1965, Box 118-8-4-56 S-Z Switzer, "You Wouldn't Believe It," Folder I, RES, 2.

CHAPTER 7

1. Abraham A. Ribicoff, foreword to Joint Commission on Mental Health of Children, *Crisis in Child Mental Health: Challenge for the 1970's: Report* (New York: Harper & Row, 1970), xv–xvi.
2. Reginald S. Lourie, "The Joint Commission on Mental Health of Children," *American Journal of Psychiatry* 122, no. 11 (May 1966): 1280; "Interview of Reginald Lourie, by Spafford Ackerly," n.d., UL: 4; Melodie Bowsher, "Disturbed Children: Care of Mentally Ill among Young Is Called Far Short of the Need," *Wall Street Journal,* September 30, 1968, 1.
3. Joint Commission on Mental Health of Children, *Crisis in Child Mental Health,* 5.
4. Ibid., 5, 7.
5. Murray Illson, "500,000 Children Need Special Care," *New York Times,* November 11, 1953, 25; Murray Illson, "10% of Pupils in Nation's Schools Are Found Emotionally Disturbed: 10% of Pupils Held Mentally Upset," *New York Times,* February 22, 1954, 1.

6. U.S. Warren Commission, *Report of the President's Commission on the Assassination of President John F. Kennedy* (Washington, DC: Government Printing Office, 1964), 671, http://www.archives.gov/research/jfk/warren-commission-report/.
7. Ibid., 673.
8. Ibid., 675.
9. Ibid., 378–79.
10. Ibid., 379.
11. Ibid., 380.
12. Ibid.
13. Ibid., 382.
14. "Oswald 'Disturbed,' Psychiatrist Recalls," *Washington Post*, December 3, 1963, A9; Martin Tolchin, "Judges Asked Aid for Oswald at 13," *New York Times*, December 3, 1963, 34; U.S. Warren Commission, *Report of the President's Commission on the Assassination of President John F. Kennedy*, 379.
15. Sid Moody, "Science Probes Violence Motive," *Los Angeles Times*, June 7, 1964, 2; George S. Stevenson, "The Mixed-up Child: If a Youngster Is Mentally Disturbed, What Should the School Do About It?," *Baltimore Sun*, November 8, 1964, TW12.
16. Tolchin, "Judges Asked Aid for Oswald at 13."
17. "Interview of Reginald Lourie, by Spafford Ackerly," 4; "Mental Care Bill Framed by Ribicoff," *Washington Post*, January 16, 1965, A5; Robert D. Byrnes, "Committee Approves Ribicoff Amendments," *Hartford Courant*, July 6, 1965, 2; Robert D. Byrnes, "Most Ribicoff Changes Used in Security Bill," *Hartford Courant*, July 16, 1965, 2; Robert D. Byrnes, "Ribicoff Submits Bill to Aid Disturbed Child," *Hartford Courant*, January 16, 1965, 2.
18. John Leo, "12% of Children Found Disturbed: Study in Manhattan Calls 34% of Others 'Impaired,'" *New York Times*, April 3, 1969, 40.
19. *The Negro Family, the Case for National Action* (Washington, DC: Government Printing Office, 1965). On the Moynihan Report and its impact, see Ruth Feldstein, *Motherhood in Black and White: Race and Sex in American Liberalism, 1930–1965* (Ithaca, NY: Cornell University Press, 2000); Alice O'Connor, *Poverty Knowledge: Social Science, Social Policy, and the Poor in Twentieth-Century U.S. History* (Princeton, NJ: Princeton University Press, 2001); James T. Patterson, *Freedom Is Not Enough: The Moynihan Report and America's Struggle over Black Family Life: From LBJ to Obama* (New York: Basic Books, 2010); Daryl Michael Scott, *Contempt and Pity: Social Policy and the Image of the Damaged Black Psyche, 1880–1996* (Chapel Hill: University of North Carolina Press, 1997). Moynihan was by no means the first to point to the so-called matriarchal African American family as a cause of psychological distress; both white and black social scientists had described this pattern in the 1940s, 1950s, and early 1960s (Ellen Herman, *The Romance of American Psychology: Political Culture in the Age of Experts* [Berkeley: University of California Press, 1995], 187). However, the prominent role of the report in directing Johnson's War on Poverty initiative and its popular media coverage made these theories more prominent and more immediately relevant.
20. Mical Raz, *What's Wrong with the Poor? Psychiatry, Race, and the War on Poverty* (Chapel Hill: University of North Carolina Press, 2013).
21. Joint Commission on Mental Health of Children, *Crisis in Child Mental Health*, 215.
22. Ibid., 216.
23. Ibid., 221–29, 228.
24. Ibid., 217–29.

25. Herman, *The Romance of American Psychology*, 193–98. Also see Gerald E. Markowitz and David Rosner, *Children, Race, and Power: Kenneth and Mamie Clark's Northside Center* (Charlottesville: University Press of Virginia, 1996); Gabriel N. Mendes, *Under the Strain of Color: Harlem's Lafargue Clinic and the Promise of an Antiracist Psychiatry* (Ithaca, NY: Cornell University Press, 2015).
26. Joint Commission on Mental Health of Children, *Crisis in Child Mental Health*, 227.
27. Ibid., 272.
28. Ibid., 271. Calculation from U.S. Bureau of Labor Statistics, "CPI Inflation Calculator," at http://www.bls.gov/data/inflation_calculator.htm.
29. Anthony N. Maluccio and Wilma D. Marlow, "Residential Treatment of Emotionally Disturbed Children: A Review of the Literature," *Social Service Review* 46, no. 2 (June 1972): 237.
30. Bowsher, "Disturbed Children."
31. James K. Whittaker, "The Changing Character of Residential Child Care: An Ecological Perspective," *Social Service Review* 52, no. 1 (March 1, 1978): 32; Joint Commission on Mental Health of Children, *Crisis in Child Mental Health*, 271.
32. Bruno Bettelheim, "The Future of Residential Treatment in the Society of the Future," in *Healing through Living: A Symposium on Residential Treatment*, ed. Morris Fritz Mayer and Arthur Blum (Springfield, IL: Thomas, 1971), 195. Although the childhood background of Martin Luther King's assassin, James Earl Ray, received much less press than that of Lee Harvey Oswald, the Associated Press reported that Ray had regularly skipped school as a young boy and quoted his former school principal, who stated that Ray "rebelled against authority and his approach to most of his teachers was very bad." Like most children labeled emotionally disturbed, Ray's home background was "broken": his father was an alcoholic and two of his siblings died young (Associated Press, "King Suspect Described as Perennial Rebel," *Hartford Courant*, April 29, 1968, 29).
33. Mayer and Blum, *Healing through Living*, 196.
34. Ibid., 195–96.
35. Waggoner, "President's Message."
36. Gerald N. Grob, "Origins of DSM-I: A Study in Appearance and Reality," *American Journal of Psychiatry* 148, no. 4 (April 1, 1991): 427, and *From Asylum to Community: Mental Health Policy in Modern America* (Princeton, NJ: Princeton University Press, 1991), 5, 42, 98.
37. Grob, *From Asylum to Community*, 49–60, 168.
38. Ibid., 227, 237.
39. Ibid., 241–42.
40. Several argued that mental illness was categorically nonexistent, making psychiatric hospitalization a tool of social control. For example, psychiatrist Thomas Szasz argued that there was no somatic basis for mental illness. Rather, he believed that when physicians labeled people mentally ill, they were simply medicalizing behavior that deviated from dominant cultural norms (*The Myth of Mental Illness: Foundations of a Theory of Personal Conduct* [New York: Harper & Row, 1968]). British psychiatrist R. D. Laing similarly characterized schizophrenia as a host of behaviors that the dominant culture deemed abnormal. According to Laing, psychiatrists could learn a lot by attempting to understand the patient's individual journey to escape a set of unlivable conditions in the external world (*The Politics of Experience* (New York: Pantheon Books, 1967]). Most notably, sociologist Erving Goffman argued that mental hospitals were a type of total institution that penetrated every

element of an inmate or patient's experience, dehumanizing him and forcing him to assume and enact the roles assigned him by authorities (*Asylums; Essays on the Social Situation of Mental Patients and Other Inmates* [Garden City, NY: Anchor Books, 1961]). Although these scholars shared skepticism toward psychiatry, they did not comprise a unified movement. However, their work flourished in the countercultural milieu of the 1960s, much of it based in critiques of institutions and authority. On these thinkers, see Gerald N. Grob, "The Attack of Psychiatric Legitimacy in the 1960s: Rhetoric and Reality," *Journal of the History of the Behavioral Sciences* 47, no. 4 (2011): 398–416; Michael E. Staub, *Madness Is Civilization: When the Diagnosis Was Social, 1948–1980* (Chicago: University of Chicago Press, 2011); Norman Dain, "Psychiatry and Anti-Psychiatry in the United States," in *Discovering the History of Psychiatry*, ed. Mark S. Micale and Roy Porter (New York: Oxford University Press, 1994).

41. Gerald N. Grob and Howard H. Goldman, *The Dilemma of Federal Mental Health Policy: Radical Reform or Incremental Change?* (New Brunswick, NJ: Rutgers University Press, 2006), 47–59, 140.
42. Steven J. Taylor, *Acts of Conscience: World War II, Mental Institutions, and Religious Objectors* (Syracuse, NY: Syracuse University Press, 2009), 369–72; Burton Blatt, *Christmas in Purgatory: A Photographic Essay on Mental Retardation* (Syracuse, NY: Human Policy Press, 1974).
43. David J. Rothman and Sheila M. Rothman, *The Willowbrook Wars* (New York: Harper & Row, 1984), 23.
44. Ibid., 45. For Rivera's complete footage on WABC, see Albert Primo, prod., *Willowbrook: the Last Great Disgrace* (Sproutflix, 1972).
45. Marshall B. Jones, "Decline of the American Orphanage, 1941–1980," *Social Service Review*, 67, no. 3 (1993): 471; James Whittaker, telephone interview with the author, March 4, 2012.
46. Joint Commission on Mental Health of Children, *Crisis in Child Mental Health*, 42.
47. Sid Ross and William Kilpatrick, "Shame of the Nation: Snakepits for Mentally Ill Children," *Boston Globe*, October 17, 1965, G4; Seth Kantor, "Substandard Child-Care Centers Flourish: Industry Thrives on Disturbed Youngsters from Other States," *Los Angeles Times*, November 27, 1975, A1.
48. James K. Whittaker and Albert E. Trieschman, *Children Away from Home: A Sourcebook of Residential Treatment* (Chicago: Aldine-Atherton, 1972), 5.
49. Martin Leichtman, "Residential Treatment of Children and Adolescents: Past, Present, and Future," *American Journal of Orthopsychiatry* 76, no. 3 (2006): 286; Whittaker and Trieschman, *Children Away from Home*, 5.
50. Rosemary Stevens, *In Sickness and in Wealth: American Hospitals in the Twentieth Century* (New York: Basic Books, 1989), 259.
51. M. Gregg Bloche and Francine Cournos, "Mental Health Policy for the 1990s: Tinkering in the Interstices," in *Health Policy and the Disadvantaged*, ed. Lawrence D. Brown (Durham, NC: Duke University Press, 1991), 148; Grob, *From Asylum to Community*, 265–68.
52. Leichtman, "Residential Treatment of Children and Adolescents," 286.
53. Michelle Dally Johnston, *Out of Sorrow and into Hope: The History of the Emma Pendleton Bradley Hospital* (East Providence, RI: Bradley Hospital, 1991), 35.
54. Ibid., 37–39.
55. "Bradley Hospital Reaches Agreement with Blue Cross of Rhode Island," in *Bradley Scope* 4, no. 1 (Winter 1977): 1, RIHS.

56. Raymond W. Waggoner, "President's Message," in "Annual Report 1979," RIHS.
57. "Annual Report, 1961," RIHS; "Annual Report, 1963," RIHS; "Referrals, Patients Increase at Bradley," *Bradley Scope* 7, no. 2 (October 1980): 1, RIHS; "Bradley Hospital Fiftieth Annual Report, 1980," RIHS, 17.
58. "Bradley Hospital Fiftieth Annual Report, 1980," 18.
59. "Intensive Treatment Unit Opens," *Bradley Scope* 4, no. 1 (Winter 1977): 2, RIHS; "ITU Full; Expansion Sought," *Bradley Scope* 4, no. 2 (Spring 1977): 1, RIHS.
60. Bloche and Cournos, "Mental Health Policy for the 1990s."
61. Frank E. Joseph to Victor Gelb, November 22, 1978, Series 2, Box 1, Folder 2, BA.
62. I. S. Anpff to Frank R. Joseph, November 20, 1978, Series 2, Box 1, Folder 2, BA.
63. Sam Kelman, "Sectarian Issue," 1978, Series 2, Box 1, Folder 2, BA.
64. "Bellefaire Priorities 1980–1981," Series 2, Box 1, Folder 4, BA.
65. Robert Hackey, *Cries of Crisis: Rethinking the Rhetoric of Health Care Reform* (Reno: University of Nevada Press, 2012): 8.
66. Ibid.; Mayes, "The Origins, Development, and Passage of Medicare's Revolutionary Prospective Payment System," 21–29; Paul Starr, *The Social Transformation of American Medicine* (New York: Basic Books, 1982), 381–408; Rosemary Stevens, *In Sickness and in Wealth: American Hospitals in the Twentieth Century* (New York: Basic Books, 1989), 284–94; Frank J. Thompson, *Health Policy and the Bureaucracy: Politics and Implementation* (Cambridge, MA: MIT Press, 1981), chap. 2; Lawrence D. Brown, "Introduction to a Decade of Transition," in *Health Policy in Transition: A Decade of Health Politics, Policy, and Law*, ed. Lawrence D. Brown (Durham, NC: Duke University Press, 1987), 4–5. Hackey demonstrates that in many ways this crisis was more perceived than actual. Health-care costs had been increasing dramatically during the 1950s and 1960s, but this trend was interpreted largely as a worthwhile investment in Americans' health. By the 1970s, the growing conservative movement began to question the value of spending so much money, and the liberal consensus had become too fractured to fight back. Meanwhile, Nixon was contributing millions of dollars to the War on Cancer, creating a stark double standard in which medical research was a priority but basic health care was not (Hackey, *Cries of Crisis*, 33, 61–63).
67. Fawn Brodie, "How Did We Get Here, Anyway?" *Los Angeles Times*, February 4, 1968, B12.
68. Harry Nelson and Daryl Lembke, "Turnback to Custodial Care Seen for Mental Hospitals," *Los Angeles Times*, April 23, 1967, I1.
69. Brodie, "How Did We Get Here, Anyway?"; Nelson and Lembke, "Turnback to Custodial Care Seen for Mental Hospitals."
70. Maluccio and Marlow, "Residential Treatment of Emotionally Disturbed Children," 231–32; Whittaker, "The Changing Character of Residential Child Care," 22–24.
71. "Regaining the Magic Childhood: The Bradley Pre-School," *Bradley Scope* 2, no. 2 (June 1975): 2, RIHS.
72. Johnston, *Out of Sorrow and into Hope*, 36; Donald Scott, "At Home in the Samuel B. Swan House," in *Bulletin of the Emma Pendleton Bradley Hospital* (June 1966), Emma Pendleton Bradley Hospital, Miscellaneous Material, RIHS, 1–2.
73. "More Than Halfway to Making It," *Bradley Scope* 4, no. 3 (Summer 1977): 3, RIHS.
74. "Day Hospital Program," *Bradley Scope* 2, no. 1 (January 1975): 2, RIHS.
75. "Day Hospital Renovated," *Bradley Scope* 2, no. 3 (December 1975): 6, RIHS.
76. "Day Hospital Program, 2.

77. Ibid.; "Day Hospital Census Increases," *Bradley Scope* 5, no. 3 (June 1978): 2, RIHS; Bradley Signs Blue Cross Contract," 1.
78. "Day Hospital Census Increases," 2.
79. "Appendix B: Jewish Board of Guardians Hawthorne Cedar Knolls School," in Joint Commission on Mental Health of Children, *Crisis in Child Mental Health,* 305.
80. Andrew L. Ross and Lawrence J. Schreiber, "Bellefaire's Day Treatment Program: An Interdisciplinary Approach to the Emotionally Disturbed Child," *Child Welfare* 54, no. 3 (1975): 183–84.
81. Ibid., 184.
82. Ibid., 190–93.
83. "A New Avenue for Help," *TPR* 28, no. 6 (October–November 1969), in Box 4.2, A New Avenue for Help, KSHS; Allan Smart, "Editorial," *TPR* 28, no. 6 (October–November 1969), in Box 4.2, A New Avenue for Help, KSHS; "The Carriage House Project," pamphlet, Box 4.2, Publicity, KSHS; "For Youngsters Adrift: A Place to Come Down," *Midway* (March 8, 1970), Box 4.2, A Place to Come Down, March 8, 1970, KSHS.
84. "For Youngsters Adrift: A Place to Come Down."
85. Nicholas Hobbs, "Helping Disturbed Children: Psychological and Ecological Strategies," *American Psychologist* 21, no. 12 (1966): 1107.
86. Nicholas Hobbs, "Appendix D: Project Re-Ed: New Ways of Helping Emotionally Disturbed Children," in Joint Commission on Mental Health of Children, *Crisis in Child Mental Health,* 312.
87. Ibid., 311–12.
88. Hobbs, "Helping Disturbed Children," 1108.
89. Nicholas Hobbs, "Project Re-ED: From Demonstration Project to Nationwide Program," *Peabody Journal of Education* 60, no. 3 (April 1, 1983): 10; Joint Commission on Mental Health of Children, *Crisis in Child Mental Health,* 274.
90. Hobbs, "Project Re-ED," 14.
91. Although RTC professionals were surprisingly open to discussing failures, at least among themselves, they still believed that their work was a valuable enterprise. For example, one 1952–53 study of Bellefaire found that twenty-five of thirty-nine children treated there had made positive or moderate changes in their personality or behavior and that treatment was more effective "with the neurotic child than with the acting-out child." Despite the fourteen children doing no better or even worse, the report concluded that "Bellefaire is dealing with some situations for which no one has found the answer." In short, Bellefaire staff and allies believed that efforts to cure these "cancers of the human personality" were valuable even if they could help some proportion of children get better (Child Welfare League of America and Council of Jewish Federations and Welfare Funds, *Bellefaire Survey: 1952–1953,* Container 19, Folder 4, BA, 53–54).
92. Howard W. Polsky, *Cottage Six: The Social System of Delinquent Boys in Residential Treatment* (New York: Russell Sage Foundation, 1962), 133.
93. Ibid.
94. Whittaker, interview with the author.
95. Maluccio and Marlow, "Residential Treatment of Emotionally Disturbed Children," 240–41; Joint Commission on Mental Health of Children, *Crisis in Child Mental Health,* 273.
96. Whittaker, "The Changing Character of Residential Child Care," 30.

97. Hobbs, "Helping Disturbed Children," 1107.
98. L. Bedford and L. D. Hybertson, "Emotionally Disturbed Children: A Program of Alternatives to Residential Treatment," *Child Welfare* 54, no. 2 (February 1975): 113.
99. Gisela Konopka, foreword to Whittaker and Trieschman, *Children Away from Home*, vi.
100. Trieschman and Whittaker, "Dialogue," in ibid., 5.
101. Ibid.
102. Albert E. Trieschman, James K. Whittaker, and Larry K. Brendtro, *The Other 23 Hours: Child-Care Work with Emotionally Disturbed Children in a Therapeutic Milieu* (Chicago: Aldine Pub. Co, 1969).
103. Whittaker and Trieschman, *Children Away from Home*.
104. Atlee L. Stroup et al., "Residential Treatment Centers for Emotionally Disturbed Children, United States, 1983," *Mental Health Statistical Note*, no. 188 (April 1988), 10.
105. James W. Trent, *Inventing the Feeble Mind: A History of Mental Retardation in the United States*, Medicine and Society, no. 6 (Berkeley: University of California Press, 1994), 236–42; Kathleen Jones, "Education for Children with Mental Retardation: Parent Activism, Public Policy, and Family Ideology in the 1950s," in *Mental Retardation in America: A Historical Reader*, ed. Steven Noll and James W. Trent (New York: New York University Press, 2004).
106. Carl Fenichel, "Appendix C: The League School for Seriously Disturbed Children: Education as Therapy for the Seriously Disturbed," in Joint Commission on Mental Health of Children, *Crisis in Child Mental Health*, 307.
107. Ibid.
108. Ruth L. LaVietes, Wilfred C. Hulse, and Abram Blau, "A Psychiatric Day Treatment Center and School for Young Children and Their Parents," *American Journal of Orthopsychiatry* 30, no. 3 (July 1960): 468–82; LaVietes et al., "Day Treatment Center and School: Seven Years Experience," *American Journal of Orthopsychiatry* 35, no. 1 (January 1965): 160–69. Godmother's League exists today as the West End Day School (http://www.westenddayschool.org/) and the League School is still in operation as well (http://www.leaguecenter.org/).
109. "Emotionally Handicapped Students Will Receive Special Instruction," *Los Angeles Times*, September 26, 1965, SG A3.
110. "For Disturbed Children—an Experiment," *Boston Globe*, May 29, 1966, 29.
111. "New School for Disturbed Children Opens This Week," *Chicago Daily Defender*, October 5, 1966, 4.
112. Arnold L. Scheuer, "Certification, Teacher Preparation, and Special Classes for the Emotionally Disturbed and Socially Maladjusted: Report by States," *Exceptional Children* 33, no. 2 (October 1966): 121. Scheuer's survey included fifty U.S. states, as well as the District of Columbia, Puerto Rico, Guam, and the Canal Zone.
113. Although special education offerings had been growing steadily since the 1930s, the 1960s saw a particularly dramatic growth in the availability of these services, in part due to federal government support from President Kennedy, who initiated the 1961 Panel on Mental Retardation to study existing accommodations for the intellectually disabled, and from President Johnson, who established the Committee on Mental Retardation and under whom the 1965 Elementary and Secondary Education Act and its Title VI amendments provided federally funded grants to states for special education programs. Federal involvement, along with parent advocacy through the National Association of Retarded Children, led to an era of un-

precedented growth in special education. However, by the end of the 1960s only a fraction of the children who needed special education services were receiving them (Robert L. Osgood, *The History of Inclusion in the United States* [Washington, DC: Gallaudet University Press, 2005], 63–66, 74–75). For a more general history of special education in the United States, see Margret A. Winzer, *The History of Special Education: From Isolation to Integration* (Washington, DC: Gallaudet University Press, 1993); Robert L. Osgood, *The History of Special Education: A Struggle for Equality in American Public Schools* (Westport, CT: Praeger, 2008).

114. The act defined "handicapped" children as "mentally retarded, hard of hearing, deaf, speech impaired, visually handicapped, seriously emotionally disturbed, crippled, or other health impaired children who by reason thereof require special education" (Elementary and Secondary Education Act Amendments of 1965, Public Law 89-313, U.S. Statutes at Large 79 [1965]). I use "handicapped" here rather than disabled as it was used as an organizing category by policy makers and parents of disabled children in the 1960s and 1970s.

115. David Milofsky, "Schooling the Kids No One Wants," *New York Times*, January 2, 1977, 145; "Highlights of Chapter 766," *Boston Globe*, June 8, 1975, A4. The law defined handicaps as "arising from intellectual, sensory, emotional or physical factors, cerebral dysfunctions, perceptual factors, or other specific learning disabilities or any combination thereof" (ibid.).

116. Ibid.

117. Osgood, *The History of Inclusion in the United States*, 101–3; Education for All Handicapped Children Act, Public Law 94-142, U.S. Statutes at Large 94 (1975).

118. Education for All Handicapped Children Act, Public Law 94-142; Alan Abeson and Jeffrey Zettel, "The End of This Quiet Revolution: The Education for All Handicapped Children Act of 1975," *Exceptional Children* 44, no. 2 (October 1977): 114–28; Joseph Ballard and Jeffrey Zettel, "Public Law 94-142 and Section 504: What They Say about Rights and Protections," *Exceptional Children* 44, no. 3 (November 1977): 177–85. Although distinct from the special education movement in its primary actors and aims (disabled persons vs. parents; achieving normalization vs. celebrating difference), the disability rights movement flourished in the 1960s and 1970s, employing the rights-based language in use by other minority groups. For reviews of the disability rights movement, see Doris Zames Fleischer, *The Disability Rights Movement: From Charity to Confrontation* (Philadelphia: Temple University Press, 2001); Duane F. Stroman, *The Disability Rights Movement: From Deinstitutionalization to Self-Determination* (Lanham, MD: University Press of America, 2003).

119. Education Amendments of 1974, Public Law 93-380, U.S. Statutes at Large 93 (1974); Education for All Handicapped Children Act, Public Law 94-142; Nicholas A. Vacc and Nancy Kirst, "Emotionally Disturbed Children and Regular Classroom Teachers," *Elementary School Journal* 77, no. 4 (March 1, 1977): 310.

120. Osgood, *The History of Inclusion in the United States*, 43–53.

121. Ibid., 76–81.

122. Ibid., 87–89.

123. Ibid., 106–7.

124. For example, see Larry Molloy, "The Handicapped Child in the Everyday Classroom," *Phi Delta Kappan* 56, no. 5 (January 1, 1975): 337–40; A. J. Pappanikou and James L. Paul, *Mainstreaming Emotionally Disturbed Children* (Syracuse, NY: Syracuse University Press, 1977).

125. Milofsky, "Schooling the Kids No One Wants."

126. Mike Ward, "Special School Opens Doors to Disturbed Youth," *Los Angeles Times*, August 13, 1978, SG1.
127. Milofsky, "Schooling the Kids No One Wants."
128. "The Special Child: from Isolation to Life's Mainstream," *Boston Globe*, June 8, 1975, A1.
129. Leo Kanner, "Autistic Disturbances of Affective Contact," *Nervous Child* 2, no. 1943 (1943): 217–50. For an excellent overview of changing models of autism in the twentieth century, see Chloe Silverman, *Understanding Autism: Parents, Doctors, and the History of a Disorder* (Princeton, NJ: Princeton University Press, 2012), chap. 1. On Bettelheim, see Richard Pollak, *The Creation of Dr. B: A Biography of Bruno Bettelheim* (New York: Simon & Schuster, 1997); Theron Raines, *Rising to the Light: A Portrait of Bruno Bettelheim* (New York: Alfred A. Knopf, 2002); Nina Sutton, *Bettelheim: A Life and a Legacy* (New York: Basic Books, 1996).
130. Gil Eyal et al., *The Autism Matrix: The Social Origins of the Autism Epidemic* (Cambridge: Polity, 2010), 127–32.
131. Kanner, "Autistic Disturbances of Affective Contact"; Charles Bradley, *Schizophrenia in Childhood* (New York: Macmillan, 1941); Lauretta Bender, "Childhood Schizophrenia: Clinical Study on One Hundred Schizophrenic Children," *American Journal of Orthopsychiatry* 17, no. 1 (1947): 40–56, and "Childhood Schizophrenia," *Nervous Child* 1, no. 1 (1941): 138–41.
132. Peter Tanguay, interview with the author, October 26, 2010, New York City.
133. Eyal et al., *The Autism Matrix*, 205; Silverman, *Understanding Autism*, 39–40.
134. Anthony Davids, "Therapeutic Approaches to Children in Residential Treatment. Changes from the Mid-1950s to the Mid-1970s," *American Psychologist* 30, no. 8 (August 1975): 813.
135. Anthony Davids, "Childhood Psychosis: The Problem of Differential Diagnosis," *Journal of Autism and Childhood Schizophrenia* 5, no. 2 (June 1975): 129–38.
136. For example, a 1972 edited collection on residential treatment only mentioned autism with respect to the importance of attracting a wide variety of children and in an example of a father learned patience after visiting his autistic son (George H. Weber and Bernard J. Haberlein, eds., *Residential Treatment of Emotionally Disturbed Children* [New York: Behavioral Publications, 1972], 8, 114).
137. Eyal et al., *The Autism Matrix*. Eyal and his colleagues are largely talking about the perceived autism "epidemic" of the 1990s, but their origin story should theoretically also apply to the growing prevalence of autism among American children in the 1970s.
138. Silverman, *Understanding Autism*, 47–48.
139. Ibid., 106.
140. Ibid., 106–18.
141. Barry C. Feld, *Bad Kids: Race and the Transformation of the Juvenile Court* (New York: Oxford University Press, 1999), chap. 3.
142. William S. Bush, *Who Gets a Childhood? Race and Juvenile Justice in Twentieth-Century Texas* (Athens: University of Georgia Press, 2010), 151–52.
143. On the children's rights movement of the 1960s and 1970s, see Joseph M. Hawes, *The Children's Rights Movement: A History of Advocacy and Protection* (Boston: Twayne Publishers, 1991), chap. 8.
144. C. R. Margolin, "Salvation versus Liberation: The Movement for Children's Rights in a Historical Context," *Social Problems* 25, no. 4 (1978): 441–52.
145. Bush, *Who Gets a Childhood?* See chaps. 6 and 7.

146. Kenneth Wooden, *Weeping in the Playtime of Others: America's Incarcerated Children* (New York: McGraw-Hill, 1976), 27.
147. Howard James, "What about Reform Schools?," *Christian Science Monitor*, May 5, 1969.
148. Wooden, *Weeping in the Playtime of Others*, 98.
149. Milton J. E. Senn, "Interview with Dr. Jerome Miller, November 2, 1978 in Washington, D.C." n.d., Box 3, Folder 13, NLM.
150. Ibid.; C Holden, "Massachusetts Juvenile Justice: De-Institutionalization on Trial," *Science* 192, no. 4238 (April 30, 1976): 447–48.
151. Bush, *Who Gets a Childhood?*, chaps. 6 and 7.
152. Hawes, *The Children's Rights Movement*, 105–9.
153. Feld, *Bad Kids*, 98–103.
154. Ibid., 100–101, 105.
155. Title I, Findings and Declaration of Purpose, Sec. 101, Juvenile Justice and Delinquency Prevention Act of 1974, Public Law 93-415, U.S. Statutes at Large 93 (1974).
156. Title II, Juvenile Justice and Delinquency Prevention, Part B, Sec. 223, Juvenile Justice and Delinquency Prevention Act of 1974; Title V, Miscellaneous and conforming amendments, Part A, Sec. 501, Juvenile Justice and Delinquency Prevention Act of 1974.
157. Joann Stevens, "New Juvenile Code Troubles Officials: Police See Code as Bar to Aiding Youths," *Washington Post*, December 1, 1977, 148.
158. Craig Turner, "Reform of Juvenile Justice Faces Trial: Reactions Vary as Officials Prepare to Enforce New Law," *Los Angeles Times*, December 26, 1976, OC1.
159. Ibid.
160. Holden, "Massachusetts Juvenile Justice," 449.
161. See Feld, *Bad Kids*, chap. 5.

CHAPTER 8

1. "Treatment Program," Box 3, Folder 9, circa 1979, in Camarillo State Hospital Collection, California State University, Channel Islands.
2. Evolution of Camarillo State Hospital's Youth Program (1947–86), Camarillo State Hospital Collection, California State University, Channel Islands, accessed February 19, 2015, http://repository.library.csuci.edu/bitstream/handle/10139/6268/CSH0028%24.pdf?sequence=1.
3. Richard Simon, "Camarillo Upset by Prison Proposal," *Los Angeles Times*, April 25, 1982, sec. Valley, V1. On the War on Crime, see Elizabeth Hinton, "From Social Welfare to Social Control: Federal War in American Cities, 1968–1988," PhD diss., Columbia University, 2013; on the War on Drugs, see Kathleen J. Frydl, *The Drug Wars in America, 1940–1973* (New York: Cambridge University Press, 2013). On the War on Drugs and the mass incarceration of black men, see "Winning the War on Drugs: A 'Second Chance' for Nonviolent Drug Offenders," *Harvard Law Review* 113, no. 6 (April 1, 2000): 1485–1502; Michelle Alexander, *The New Jim Crow: Mass Incarceration in the Age of Colorblindness* (New York: New Press, 2010); Lawrence D. Bobo and Victor Thompson, "Unfair by Design: The War on Drugs, Race, and the Legitimacy of the Criminal Justice System," *Social Research* 73, no. 2 (July 1, 2006): 445–72.
4. James Quinn, "Backers Fear Move Is Afoot to Close Camarillo Hospital: Employees, Parents Fear Reductions," *Los Angeles Times*, June 8, 1985, sec. Valley, V_A8, http://articles.latimes.com/1985-06-08/local/me-7284_1_camarillo-state-hospital.

5. James Quinn, "Mental Hospital Sheds Image of Grim 'Snake Pit,'" *Los Angeles Times*, March 9, 1986, sec. Valley, V_A4, http://articles.latimes.com/1986-03-09/local/me-18040_1_mental-hospital.
6. "Camarillo Hospital Scheduled to Close," *Los Angeles Sentinel*, February 27, 1997, sec. Health, A10.
7. According to a study funded by the National Institute of Mental Health, at the end of 1983 there were 15,791 children in residential treatment (Atlee L. Stroup et al., "Residential Treatment Centers for Emotionally Disturbed Children, United States, 1983," *Mental Health Statistical Note*, no. 188 [April 1988], 10). Although statistics are difficult to interpret because they measure the number of children in "residential treatment" differently, it appears that this number increased during the 1980s. A congressional study of children placed outside the home estimated that the number of children in "residential treatment" was 19,215 in 1983 and 25,334 in 1986. However, the study defined residential treatment as "overnight mental health care in conjunction with supervised living and other supportive services in a setting other than a hospital, e.g. halfway houses, community residences, and group homes," which would have overestimated the number of children in RTCs (*No Place to Call Home: Discarded Children in America: A Report Together with Additional and Dissenting Views of the Select Committee on Children, Youth, and Families, U.S. House of Representatives, One Hundred First Congress, First Session* [Washington, DC: Government Printing Office, 1989], 108). Another study estimated that 66,000 children were living in RCTs in 1997, although how the authors defined residential treatment was unclear ("Nearly 66,000 Youth Live in U.S. Mental Health Programs," *Latest Findings in Children's Mental Health* 2, no. 1 [Summer 2003]: 1, http://www.ihhcpar.rutgers.edu/downloads/summer2003.pdf).
8. Ronald Reagan, "Address Before a Joint Session of the Congress on the State of the Union," February 6, 1985, Washington, DC, transcript by Gerhard Peters and John T. Woolley, *The American Presidency Project*, accessed November 22, 2015, http://www.presidency.ucsb.edu/ws/?pid=38069. Full video posted by the Ronald Reagan Presidential Foundation and Library, May 4, 2009, https://www.youtube.com/watch?v=q2hx19SLNHo. Transcripts of the speech uniformly cite his words as "if [as] the family goes," but Reagan in fact said "as the family goes," as per the video recording.
9. Education for All Handicapped Children Act, Public Law 94-142, U.S. Statutes at Large 94 (1975).
10. "Adoption Assistance and Child Welfare Act of 1980," P.L. 96-272, *United States Statutes at Large*, 94 Stat. 500, H.R. 3434, 96th Congress, June 17, 1980.
11. Robert E. Lieberman, "Future Directions in Residential Treatment," *Child and Adolescent Psychiatric Clinics of North America* 13, no. 2 (April 2004): 281.
12. Marilyn C. McManus and Barbara J. Friesen, eds., *Families as Allies, Conference Proceedings: Parent-Professional Collaboration toward Improving Services for Seriously Emotionally Handicapped Children and Their Families (Portland, Oregon, April 28–29, 1986)* (Portland, OR: Research and Training Center to Improve Services to Emotionally Handicapped Children and Their Families, Portland State University, 1986), at https://eric.ed.gov/?id=ED288328; Robert M. Friedman et al., "Unlicensed Residential Programs: The Next Challenge in Protecting Youth," American Journal of Orthopsychiatry 76, no. 3 (2006): 296; Barbara J. Friesen et al., "Improving Services for Families," *Children Today* 17, no. 4 (August 1988): 19.
13. Beth A. Stroul and Robert M. Friedman, *A System of Care for Severely Emotionally Dis-*

turbed Children & Youth (Washington, DC: CASSP Technical Assistance Center, July 1986), http://eric.ed.gov/?q=system+of+care+for+severely&id=ED330167.

14. Ibid., 13.
15. Ibid., 14.
16. Ibid., 81. For example, the authors cited the status of "Discharged Pending Placement" in New Jersey, a designation that meant a child in residential treatment no longer required it but had nowhere else to go (82).
17. Beth A. Stroul and Robert M. Friedman, "Principles for a System of Care," *Children Today* 17, no. 4 (1988): 12.
18. Ibid., 11. For example, the authors list "institutional" care at "state hospitals, training schools, and other restrictive institutional facilities" in opposition to community-based care" (11).
19. Mareasa R. Isaacs and Sybil K. Goldman, *Profiles of Residential and Day Treatment Programs for Seriously Emotionally Disturbed Youth* (Washington, DC: CASSP Technical Assistance Center, Georgetown University Child Development Center, 1985), 6.
20. *Children of Darkness*, written by Richard Kotuk and Ara Chekmayan, aired May 4, 1983, on PBS, https://www.youtube.com/watch?v=tTCSfx47R1w.
21. Ibid.
22. Martin Leichtman, "Residential Treatment of Children and Adolescents: Past, Present, and Future," *American Journal of Orthopsychiatry* 76, no. 3 (2006): 286; John M. Jemerin and Irving Philips, "Changes in Inpatient Child Psychiatry: Consequences and Recommendations," *Journal of the American Academy of Child and Adolescent Psychiatry* 28, no. 3 (May 1989): 397; Ronald Geraty, "Administrative Issues in Inpatient Child and Adolescent Psychiatry," *Journal of the American Academy of Child and Adolescent Psychiatry* 28, no. 1 (January 1989): 21; Isaacs and Goldman, *Profiles of Residential and Day Treatment Programs*, 6.
23. Jane Knitzer and Lynn Olson, *Unclaimed Children: The Failure of Public Responsibility to Children and Adolescents in Need of Mental Health Services* (Washington, DC: Children's Defense Fund, 1982).
24. Ibid., ix.
25. Ibid., 6–7.
26. Ibid., ix.
27. Ibid., 6.
28. Ibid., ix.
29. Ibid., 4.
30. National Mental Health Association, *Invisible Children Project: Final Report and Recommendations of the Invisible Children Project* (Alexandria, VA: National Mental Health Association, 1989). The National Mental Health Association is now known as Mental Health America.
31. Ibid., 8.
32. "Average undergraduate tuition and fees and room and board rates charged for full-time students in degree-granting institutions, by type and control of institution: 1964–65 through 2006–07," Digest of Education Statistics, National Center for Education Statistics, accessed November 29, 2015, https://nces.ed.gov/programs/digest/d07/tables/dt07_320.asp.
33. National Mental Health Association, *Invisible Children Project*, 3, 7.
34. Ibid., 19.
35. Ibid., 10; Jacqueline Smollar and Larry Condelli, "Residential Placement of Youth: Pathways, Alternatives and Unresolved Issues," *Children Today* 19 (December 1990):

4–8; "NMHA Presents Invisible Children Project," *Update: Improving Services for Emotionally Disturbed Children* 4, no. 1 (Winter 1988–89), 1, 16, http://files.eric.ed.gov/fulltext/ED357525.pdf.

36. Knitzer and Olson, *Unclaimed Children*, 44.
37. Stroul and Friedman, *A System of Care for Severely Emotionally Disturbed Children & Youth*, 41.
38. Ibid.
39. Friesen et al., "Improving Services for Families," 18.
40. Ibid.
41. Ibid., 19.
42. Ibid. On the history of CASSP, see Albert J. Duchnowski and Robert M. Friedman, "Children's Mental Health: Challenges for the Nineties," *Journal of Mental Health Administration* 17, no. 1 (Spring 1990): 3–12.
43. *Proceedings of the Conference on the Care of Dependent Children Held at Washington, D.C., January 25, 26, 1909* (Washington, DC: Government Printing Office, 1909); *White House Conference on Child Health and Protection, The Delinquent Child; Report of the Committee on Socially Handicapped—Delinquency* (New York: Century, 1932), 297.
44. Ethan G. Sribnick, "Rehabilitating Child Welfare: Children and Public Policy, 1945–1980" (PhD diss., University of Virginia, 2007), 126–27.
45. Robert O. Self, *All in the Family: The Realignment of American Democracy since the 1960s* (New York: Hill and Wang, 2012).
46. Jeffrey M. Jenson and Mark W. Fraser, *Social Policy for Children and Families: A Risk and Resilience Perspective* (Los Angeles: Sage, 2015), 138–40. As of 2011, these grants totaled more than $1.6 billion (Beth A. Stroul and Robert M. Friedman, *Effective Strategies for Expanding the System of Care Approach: A Report on the Study of Strategies for Expanding Systems of Care* [Atlanta: ICF Macro, 2001], available at http://gucchdtacenter.georgetown.edu/publications/SOC%20Expansion%20Study%20Report%20Final.pdf).
47. Family Preservation and Support Services, Omnibus Budget Reconciliation Act of 1993, P.L. 103-66, Sec. 13711, 103rd Congress, August 10, 1993. Sixty million dollars was allocated in 1994, increasing yearly to a maximum of $600 million in 1998.
48. Children's Bureau, Administration for Children, Youth and Families, U.S. Department of Health and Human Services, "Implementation of New Legislation: Family Preservation and Support Services, Title IV-B, Subpart 2," January 18, 1994.
49. Ibid.
50. Mary-Lou Weisman, "When Parents Are Not in the Best Interests of the Child," *Atlantic Monthly* 274 (July 1994): 60.
51. Marian Wright Edelman, "Child Watch: Family Preservation at Its Best," *Atlanta Daily World*, November 17, 1992, 4.
52. Weisman, "When Parents Are Not in the Best Interests of the Child," 62.
53. Ibid.
54. Ibid., 46–47, 62.
55. Michael A. Pawel, "Public Policy and the 'Wicked Stepmother': The Ideological War against Institutional Child Care," *Humanist* 55 (February 1995): 16–21.
56. Richard Small, Kevin Kennedy, and Barbara Bender, "Critical Issues for Practice in Residential Treatment: The View from Within," *American Journal of Orthopsychiatry* 61, no. 3 (1991): 335–36.
57. Flynn O'Malley, "Contemporary Issues in the Psychiatric Residential Treatment of

Disturbed Adolescents," *Child and Adolescent Psychiatric Clinics of North America* 13, no. 2 (April 2004): 255–56.

58. Brian C. Jones, *Bradley Hospital: Legacy of Hope* (Warwick, RI: Emma Pendleton Bradley Hospital, 2006), 65.
59. National Mental Health Association, *Invisible Children Project*, 23.
60. John F. Curry, "Outcome Research on Residential Treatment: Implications and Suggested Directions," *American Journal of Orthopsychiatry* 61, no. 3 (1991): 348.
61. U.S. General Accounting Office, *Residential Care: Some High-Risk Youth Benefit, But More Study Needed* (Washington, DC, 1994).
62. Small, Kennedy, and Bender, "Critical Issues for Practice in Residential Treatment," 327.
63. Ibid., 332–33.
64. Isaacs and Goldman, *Profiles of Residential and Day Treatment Programs*, 135.
65. Children's Division, Program/Service/Discipline Review, February 1993, Program: Child and Adolescent Day Treatment Center, Administrative Records, Menninger Foundation Archives, Menninger Foundation Corporate Records, Menninger Clinic, Box 2, Children's Statistics, Children's Prog. Descriptions, PSDTC info [hereafter Box 2, Children's Program Descriptions], KSHS, 1.
66. Isaacs and Goldman, *Profiles of Residential and Day Treatment Programs*, 45–48.
67. Eileen McNamara, "Citing Budget, State Agency Cuts Aid to Disturbed Youth," *Boston Globe*, December 2, 1983, 1. The day after this article was published on the front page of the *Boston Globe*, Governor Michael Dukakis ordered the Department of Social Services "to provide the appropriate services to all eligible children without delay and without interruption" (Eileen McNamara, "Dukakis Orders DSS to Provide Youth Care," *Boston Globe*, December 3, 1983, 1).
68. Isaacs and Goldman, *Profiles of Residential and Day Treatment Programs*, 44; Weisman, "When Parents Are Not in the Best Interests of the Child," 51. Adjustment for inflation obtained using U.S. Bureau of Labor Statistics, "CPI Inflation Calculator," at http://www.bls.gov/data/inflation_calculator.htm.
69. "Bellefaire Priorities 1980–1981," Bellefaire Series 2, Box 1, Folder 4, BA, 1–2. Although without author, this document is stapled to a January 28, 1980, letter from Bellefaire President David I. Warren to Charles Ratner, Chairman of the Budget Committee of the Jewish Community Federation of Cleveland.
70. Isaacs and Goldman, *Profiles of Residential and Day Treatment Programs*, 45, 167, 172.
71. Jones, *Bradley Hospital*, 65–67.
72. Isaacs and Goldman, *Profiles of Residential and Day Treatment*, 33.
73. Weisman, "When Parents Are Not in the Best Interests of the Child," 44.
74. U.S. Bureau of the Census, *1980 Census of Population*, vol. 1, *Characteristics of the Population* (Washington, DC: Government Printing Office, 1983), chap. B, pt. 1, "U.S.Summary," "Table 37: Summary of General Characteristics," 19, accessed November 30, 2015, http://www2.census.gov/prod2/decennial/documents/1980/1980censusofpopu8011u_bw.pdf.
75. Smollar and Condelli, "Residential Placement of Youth: Pathways, Alternatives and Unresolved Issues."
76. Mical Raz, *What's Wrong with the Poor? Psychiatry, Race, and the War on Poverty* (Chapel Hill: University of North Carolina Press, 2013).
77. Isaacs and Goldman, *Profiles of Residential and Day Treatment Programs*, 152. As discussed in chap. 7, "schizophrenic" and "autistic" were descriptive and diagnostic terms used in overlapping ways.

78. Ibid., 159.
79. On Bradley's use of benzedrine in the 1930s for hyperactive children, see Elizabeth Bromley, "Stimulating a Normal Adjustment: Misbehavior, Amphetamines, and the Electroencephalogram at the Bradley Home for Children," *Journal of the History of the Behavioral Sciences* 42, no. 4 (Fall 2006): 379–98; Madeleine P. Strohl, "Bradley's Benzedrine Studies on Children with Behavioral Disorders," *Yale Journal of Biology and Medicine* 84, no. 1 (March 2011): 27–33.
80. Isaacs and Goldman, *Profiles of Residential and Day Treatment Programs*, 38.
81. Ibid., 146–47.
82. Ibid., 212, 362.
83. William M. Bolman, "Pharmacologic Advances in Residential Treatment," *Residential Treatment for Children & Youth* 13, no. 2 (October 10, 1995): 16.
84. Ibid., 17.
85. See David Healy, *The Antidepressant Era* (Cambridge, MA: Harvard University Press, 1997).
86. Bolman, "Pharmacologic Advances in Residential Treatment," 23.
87. On the development of depression as a diagnostic category, see Laura D. Hirshbein, *American Melancholy: Constructions of Depression in the Twentieth Century* (New Brunswick, NJ: Rutgers University Press, 2009).
88. Daniel F. Connor et al., "Combined Pharmacotherapy in Children and Adolescents in a Residential Treatment Center," *Journal of the American Academy of Child and Adolescent Psychiatry* 36, no. 2 (February 1997): 251.
89. Daniel F. Connor et al., "Prevalence and Patterns of Psychotropic and Anticonvulsant Medication Use in Children and Adolescents Referred to Residential Treatment," *Journal of Child and Adolescent Psychopharmacology* 8, no. 1 (1998): 27–38.
90. Martin Leichtman, telephone interview with the author, July 20, 2011.
91. Children's Division, Outpatient Department Program Description, February, 1993, Box 2, Children's Program Descriptions, KSHS, 2, 5; Children's Division Program Description, Outpatient Department Medication Clinics, Box 2, Children's Program Descriptions, KSHS, 1–2.
92. Children's Division Program/Service/Discipline Review, February, 1993, Program: Hillcrest Residential Treatment Unit, Box 2, Children's Program Descriptions, KSHS, 1.
93. Nancy S. Cotton, *Lessons from the Lion's Den: Therapeutic Management of Children in Psychiatric Hospitals and Treatment Centers* (San Francisco: Jossey-Bass, 1993), 226.
94. As Cotton explained, "Socialization on an inpatient unit incorporates 'corrective steps' in the normal socialization process in order to address the consequences of pathological development" (ibid., 3). Although Cotton's book is about an inpatient child psychiatry unit in a larger hospital, she positions the unit within the larger history of residential treatment for children (ibid., 4–5).
95. Ibid.
96. Phyllis Vine, *Families in Pain: Children, Siblings, Spouses, and Parents of the Mentally Ill Speak Out* (New York: Pantheon Books, 1982).
97. Ibid., 48–54, 71–83.
98. Ibid., 81–82.
99. Katharin A. Kelker, *Taking Charge: A Handbook for Parents Whose Children Have Emotional Handicaps* (Portland, OR: Families as Allies Project, Research and Training Center to Improve Services to Emotionally Handicapped Children and Their

Families, Regional Research Institute for Human Services, Portland State University, 1988), 13.

100. Ibid., 15.

101. Friesen et al., "Improving Services for Families," 21; information on Wisconsin Family Ties can be found at https://www.wifamilyties.org/ (accessed August 20, 2018) and on Facebook at https://www.facebook.com/wisconsinfamilyties (accessed October 23, 2017).

102. Katie S. Yoakum and Barbara J. Friesen, *National Directory of Organizations Serving Parents of Seriously Emotionally Handicapped Children and Youth.* (Portland, OR: Families as Allies Project, Research and Training Center to Improve Services to Emotionally Handicapped Children and Their Families, Portland State University, 1986), 1.

103. This definition was first put forth in the Elementary and Secondary Education Act Amendments of 1965 and was described in detail in the Education for All Handicapped Children Act in 1975 (Elementary and Secondary Education Act Amendments of 1965, Public Law 89-313, U.S. Statutes at Large 79 [1965], Education for All Handicapped Children Act, Public Law 94-142, U.S. Statutes at Large 94 [1975]). The latter defined "emotionally disturbed" children as those who had "(a) an inability to learn which cannot be explained by intellectual, sensory, or health factors; (b) an inability to build or maintain satisfactory interpersonal relationships with peers and teachers; (c) inappropriate types of behavior or feelings under normal circumstances; (d) a general pervasive mood of unhappiness or depression or (e) a tendency to develop physical symptoms or fears associated with personal or school problems."

104. Kelker, *Taking Charge*, 64.

105. Ibid., 66.

106. Ibid., 20.

107. Ibid.

108. Diana Cuthbertson, "Parents' Voices Heard on the Hill," *Exceptional Parent* 23, no. 5 (June 1993): 51.

109. Joseph P. Shapiro, "The Mothers of Invention," *U.S. News & World Report*, January 10, 1994, 38.

110. Mark A. Mlawer, "Who Should Fight? Parents and the Advocacy Expectation," *Journal of Disability Policy Studies* 4, no. 1 (1993): 105–16.

111. Allison C. Carey, "Citizenship and the Family: Parents of Children with Disabilities, the Pursuit of Rights, and Paternalism," in *Civil Disabilities: Citizenship, Membership, and Belonging*, ed. Nancy J. Hirschmann and Beth Linker (Philadelphia: University of Pennsylvania Press, 2015), 165–85.

112. Kelker, *Taking Charge*, 21.

113. On the language of "crisis" in health care since the 1970s, see Robert B. Hackey, *Cries of Crisis: Rethinking the Health Care Debate* (Reno: University of Nevada Press, 2012).

114. Michael S. Jellinek, "Changes in the Practice of Child and Adolescent Psychiatry: Are Our Patients Better Served?," *Journal of the American Academy of Child and Adolescent Psychiatry* 38, no. 2 (February 1999): 16.

115. Carey Goldberg, "Children Trapped by Mental Illness," *New York Times*, July 9, 2001, A1.

116. Abigail Trafford, "War Stories from the Battle for Boarder Children," *Washington Post*, September 12, 2000, WH5.

117. On this process, see Stuart A. Kirk and Herb Kutchins, *The Selling of DSM: The Rhetoric of Science in Psychiatry*, Social Problems and Social Issues (New York: A. de Gruyter, 1992).
118. Carl Ginsburg and Helen Demeranville, "Sticks and Stones: The Jailing of Mentally Ill Kids," *Nation* 269, no. 21 (December 20, 1999): 17–20.
119. Anne-Marie Cusac, "Arrest My Kid: He Needs Mental Health Care," *Progressive* 65, no. 7 (July 2001): 22–26.
120. National Alliance for the Mentally Ill, *Families on the Brink: The Impact of Ignoring Children with Serious Mental Illness*, a national survey conducted by Commonwealth Institute for Child and Family Studies, Department of Psychiatry, Virginia Commonwealth University, July 1999, available at http://citeseerx.ist.psu.edu/viewdoc/download?doi=10.1.1.554.4268&rep=rep1&type=pdf. See table 4 for specific responses to the Likert scale.
121. Cusac, "Arrest My Kid."
122. Maia Szalavitz, *Help at Any Cost: How the Troubled-Teen Industry Cons Parents and Hurts Kids* (New York: Riverhead, 2006).
123. Friedman et al., "Unlicensed Residential Programs," 296–97.
124. Szalavitz, *Help at Any Cost.*
125. Friedman et al., "Unlicensed Residential Programs," 296–97.
126. Ibid., 298.
127. Ibid.
128. Kathryn Whitehead et al., "Definition and Accountability: A Youth Perspective," *American Journal of Orthopsychiatry* 77, no. 3 (2007): 348.
129. Gregory D. Kutz and Andy O'Connell, *Residential Treatment Programs: Concerns regarding Abuse and Death in Certain Programs for Troubled Youth: Testimony before the Committee on Education and Labor, House of Representatives* ([Washington, DC]: U.S. Govt. Accountability Office, 2007), http://www.gao.gov/products/GAO-08-146T; U.S. House of Representatives, *Cases of Child Neglect and Abuse at Private Residential Treatment Facilities: Hearing before the Committee on Education and Labor, U.S. House of Representatives, One Hundred Tenth Congress, First Session* (Washington, DC: Government Printing Office, 2008), 2.
130. U.S. House of Representatives, *Cases of Child Neglect and Abuse at Private Residential Treatment Facilities*, 8, 30.
131. Ibid., 31.
132. Ibid., 36–38.
133. Ibid., 42. For a detailed account of Aaron Bacon's death, see Szalavitz, *Help at Any Cost.*
134. U.S. House of Representatives, *Cases of Child Neglect and Abuse at Private Residential Treatment Facilities*, 32.
135. Maia Szalavitz, "New Efforts to Crack Down on Residential Programs for Troubled Teens," *Time*, October 7, 2011, http://healthland.time.com/2011/10/07/new-efforts-to-crack-down-on-residential-programs-for-troubled-teens/.
136. Stop Child Abuse in Residential Programs for Teens Act. H.R. 5876, 110th Cong. (2008); H.R. 6358, 110th Cong. (2008); H.R. 911, 111th Cong. (2009); H.R. 3126, 112th Cong. (2011); S. 1667, 112th Cong. (2011); S. 2054, 113th Cong. (2014); H.R. 3060, 114th Cong. (2015); S. 3031, 114th Cong. (2016); H.R. 3024 (115th Cong.), 2017.
137. Alliance for the Safe, Therapeutic, and Appropriate Use of Residential Treatment, accessed October 24, 2017, http://www.astartforteens.org/.

138. For more on the Teen Revitalization program, see www.teenrevitalization.com, accessed October 24, 2017.
139. For example, see Diana Schemo, "Report Recounts Horrors of Youth Boot Camps," *New York Times*, October 11, 2007, A26.
140. Andres J. Pumariega, "Residential Treatment for Children and Youth: Time for Reconsideration and Reform," *American Journal of Orthopsychiatry* 77, no. 3 (2007): 344.
141. Joint Commission on Mental Health of Children., *Crisis in Child Mental Health: Challenge for the 1970's: Report* (New York: Harper & Row, 1970), 38.
142. American Academy of Child and Adolescent Psychiatry, *Child and Adolescent Psychiatry Workforce Crisis: Solutions to Improve Early Intervention and Access to Care*, brochure (Washington, DC: American Academy of Child and Adolescent Psychiatry, 2013).

EPILOGUE

1. Jerome G. Miller, *Last One over the Wall: The Massachusetts Experiment in Closing Reform Schools* (Columbus: Ohio State University Press, 1991).
2. State of Connecticut Office of Governmental Accountability, "Investigation into the Death of Tabatha B.," conducted by the Child Fatality Review Panel, November 30, 1998, available at http://www.ct.gov/oca/cwp/view.asp?a=1301&q=254870, 2. Although it had replaced a coeducational institution, the training school was limited to male offenders.
3. Colin Poitras, "Juvenile Center Comes under Fire; State Report Says Staff, Inmates Don't Feel Safe," *Hartford Courant*, June 25, 2002; State of Connecticut Office of Governmental Accountability, "Report of the Child Advocate and Attorney General Regarding Connecticut Juvenile Training School," September 19, 2002, http://www.ct.gov/oca/cwp/view.asp?a=1301&q=254858.
4. Ibid., 18.
5. Ibid.
6. Ibid., 46–47.
7. *CJT$: At What Cost? A Film about Youth Incarceration in Connecticut* (New Haven, CT: Youth Rights Media, 2004), DVD; Alison Leigh Cowan, "Juvenile Center Is Star in State Scandal, and a Film," *New York Times*, June 26, 2004, B1.
8. "About Us," State of Connecticut Office of Governmental Accountability, Office of the Child Advocate, http://www.ct.gov/oca/cwp/view.asp?a=1300&q=254830.
9. Stacey Stowe, "Tape Shows Boys' Abuse at Correctional Center," *New York Times*, June 29, 2004, B5.
10. Stacey Stowe, "Juvenile Center Improves, but Officials Remain Wary," *New York Times*, August 31, 2004, B5.
11. Colin Poitras, "Rell OKs $1.2 Million for Juvenile Center," *Hartford Courant*, October 27, 2004, B3; Christopher Keating and Colin Poitras, "Rell Proposes Closing Training School," *Hartford Courant*, April 2, 2005, B1; William Yardley, "Rell Announces Closing of Center for Juveniles," *New York Times*, August 2, 2005, B7. The term "prisonlike" is quoted in Yardley.
12. Shawn R. Beals, "Secure Lockup Aimed at Girls," *Hartford Courant*, August 7, 2013, A1.
13. Josh Kovner, "Debate Rises over Locked Unit for Girls," *Hartford Courant*, August 7, 2014, A1.
14. State of Connecticut, Office of the Child Advocate, *Investigative Facility Report: Connecticut Juvenile Training School and Pueblo Unit* (Hartford, CT: Office of the Child Ad-

vocate, 2015), http://www.ct.gov/oca/lib/oca/oca_investigative_cjts_pueblo_report_july_22_2015.pdf, 6.

15. Ibid., 7.
16. Ibid., 7, 19, 36–37, 45.
17. Josh Kovner, "Connecticut Juvenile Training School Closes," *Hartford Courant*, April 12, 2018, http://www.courant.com/news/connecticut/hc-cjts-closes-20180412-story.html.
18. Ibid.; Julie Miller, "Fight to Close Youth Prisons Doesn't End There, Advocates Say," *Juvenile Justice Information Exchange*, August 7, 2018, https://jjie.org/2018/08/07/fight-to-close-youth-prisons-doesnt-end-there-advocates-say/; Jacqueline Rabe Thomas, "Controversy Surrounds Closure of Juvenile Prison," *CT Mirror*, January 2, 2018, https://ctmirror.org/2018/01/02/state-ceases-admissions-to-locked-facility-for-boys-who-break-the-law/.
19. *Connecticut Juvenile Training School Advisory Board Report to the Commissioner of the Department of Children and Families* (Middletown: Connecticut Juvenile Training School, 2015), https://assets.documentcloud.org/documents/2434412/2015-legislative-report-on-cjts.pdf, 7–8.
20. Ibid., 4.
21. U.S. Census Bureau, "QuickFacts: Connecticut," accessed August 14, 2018, https://www.census.gov/quickfacts/table/RHI225215/09.
22. Gail A. Wasserman et al., "The Voice DISC-IV with Incarcerated Male Youths: Prevalence of Disorder," *Journal of the American Academy of Child and Adolescent Psychiatry* 41, no. 3 (March 2002): 317; Linda A. Teplin et al., "Psychiatric Disorders in Youth in Juvenile Detention," *Archives of General Psychiatry* 59, no. 12 (December 2002):1133–43; Kevin Whitley and John S. Rozel, "Mental Health Care of Detained Youth and Solitary Confinement and Restraint within Juvenile Detention Facilities," *Child and Adolescent Psychiatric Clinics of North America* 25, no. 1 (January 2016): 71–80. On the racial distribution of psychiatric diagnoses among detained youth, see Katherine S. L. Lau et al., "The Effects of Racial Heterogeneity on Mental Health: A Study of Detained Youth across Multiple Counties," *American Journal of Orthopsychiatry* 85, no. 5 (September 2015): 421–30.
23. Teplin et al, "Psychiatric Disorders in Youth in Juvenile Detention," 1140.
24. U.S. President's New Freedom Commission on Mental Health, ed., *Achieving the Promise: Transforming Mental Health Care in America: Final Report*, DHHS Publication, no. SMA-03-3832 (Rockville, MD: President's New Freedom Commission on Mental Health, 2003), 43. Despite national reports such as this, efforts to decrease incarceration of mentally ill youth have been focused almost entirely at the state level.
25. Committee on Adolescence, "Health Care for Youth in the Juvenile Justice System," *Pediatrics* 128, no. 6 (December 1, 2011): 1219–35; Joseph V. Penn and Christopher Thomas, "Practice Parameter for the Assessment and Treatment of Youth in Juvenile Detention and Correctional Facilities," *Journal of the American Academy of Child and Adolescent Psychiatry* 44, no. 10 (October 1, 2005): 1085–98.
26. "Serious mental illness" in the juvenile justice context was defined by the Senate Appropriations Committee in 1993 as "schizophrenia, schizoaffective disorder, manic depressive disorder, autism, as well as severe forms of other disorders such as major depression, panic disorder, and obsessive compulsive disorder" (Chris D. Erickson, "Using Systems of Care to Reduce Incarceration of Youth with Serious Mental Illness," *American Journal of Community Psychology* 49, nos. 3–4 [June 1, 2012]: 404–5).

27. Alison Evans Cuellar, Larkin S. McReynolds, and Gail A. Wasserman, "A Cure for Crime: Can Mental Health Treatment Diversion Reduce Crime among Youth?," *Journal of Policy Analysis and Management* 25, no. 1 (2006): 197–214.
28. Erickson, "Using Systems of Care to Reduce Incarceration of Youth with Serious Mental Illness," 413.

INDEX

Page numbers in italics refer to illustrations.